Endurance Sports Nutrition

Suzanne Girard Eberle, MS, RD

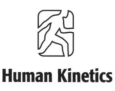

jjohnson@triathlete.com

Human Kinetics

Library of Congress Cataloging-in-Publication Data

Eberle, Suzanne Girard, 1962-
   Endurance sports nutrition / Suzanne Girard Eberle.
     p. cm
   Includes bibliographical references and index.
   ISBN 0-7360-0143-3
    1. Athletes--Nutrition. I. Title.
   TX361.A8 E39 2000
   613.2'024'796--dc21

                                           00-025081

ISBN: 0-7360-0143-3
Copyright © 2000 by Suzanne Girard Eberle

Acquisitions Editor: Martin Barnard; **Developmental Editor:** Cassandra Mitchell; **Assistant Editor:** Wendy McLaughlin; **Copyeditor:** Robert Replinger; **Proofreader:** Jim Burns; **Indexer:** Marie Rizzo; **Permission Manager:** Cheri Banks; **Graphic Designer:** Nancy Rasmus; **Graphic Artist:** Tara Welsch; **Photo Editor:** Clark Brooks; **Cover Designer:** Jack W. Davis; **Photographer (cover):** © Greg Crisp/Sports Chrome USA; **Photographers (interior):** ©Al Bello/ALLSPORT 27; ©Bob Allen 253; ©C. Yarbrough 259; ©David Sanders 35, 78, 172, 261; ©Jon Gnass/Gnass Photo Images 127; ©International Stock 30, 123, 130, 214, 232; ©iPhotoNews.com 207, 217, 241; ©J. A. Photographics 39, 111; ©Ken Lee 237; ©Rich Pomerantz Photography 135; ©SportsChrome USA 48, 59, 149, 156, 179, 185, 255; ©Terry Wild 149; ©Todd Patrick Photography 225; ©Victah Sailer 203; **Illustrator:** Craig Newsom and Kim Maxey; **Printer:** United Graphics

Human Kinetics books are available at special discounts for bulk purchase. Special editions or book excerpts can also be created to specification. For details, contact the Special Sales Manager at Human Kinetics.

Printed in the United States of America   10 9 8 7 6 5 4 3 2

Human Kinetics
Web site: www.humankinetics.com

United States: Human Kinetics
P.O. Box 5076
Champaign, IL 61825-5076
800-747-4457
e-mail: humank@hkusa.com

Canada: Human Kinetics
475 Devonshire Road, Unit 100
Windsor, ON N8Y 2L5
800-465-7301 (in Canada only)
e-mail: orders@hkcanada.com

Europe: Human Kinetics
Units C2/C3 Wira Business Park
West Park Ring Road
Leeds LS16 6EB, United Kingdom
+44 (0)113 278 1708
e-mail: hk@hkeurope.com

Australia: Human Kinetics
57A Price Avenue
Lower Mitcham, South Australia 5062
08 8277 1555
e-mail: liahka@senet.com.au

New Zealand: Human Kinetics
P.O. Box 105-231, Auckland Central
09-523-3462
e-mail: hkp@ihug.co.nz

To Flip,
forever following in my footsteps

Contents

Preface

A properly hydrated and fueled body is an amazing machine. Give it enough water and the proper mix of fuels, and it can go on forever. Or at least long enough to swim 2.4 miles, bike 112 miles, and run 26.2 miles (in an Ironman triathlon); bike 2,900 miles across America in less than a week (in the Race Across America); or run 100 miles in less than a day (in an ultrarun). It would be impossible to accomplish these and other difficult endurance feats without eating and drinking while on the move.

Equally important is how you meet your fluid and fuel needs on a daily basis. Even if you're just starting out, running your first 10K road race or hiking along local trails, frequent colds and illnesses, injuries, and poor training days can stop you in your tracks. Paying attention to your nutritional needs will help you stay on course. Unfortunately, athletes often spend more time, effort, and money picking out a pair of shoes or researching the latest technical gadget than they do cultivating healthy eating habits. Sure, it requires some discipline, motivation, and commitment to read labels on food packages, fit nutritious meals into a crammed schedule, and keep a ready supply of healthy snacks on hand. Yet who is better qualified to tackle and master the challenge than an endurance athlete? Besides, soon enough you'll be dreaming of running your first marathon or ascending one of the world's tallest mountains. You will definitely need to have a sound nutritional program in place for that.

Most athletes, luckily, don't need a complete dietary overhaul (although I've met a few who did)—just a tweak here and there, like tinkering to find just the right seat height on a bike or trying on several pairs of running shoes until you hit upon the right fit. Establishing a balanced eating style based on foods that taste good and are good for you means one less thing to worry about on the big or, in this case, long day.

This sport nutrition book is unique in two aspects. First, it's geared to the endurance athlete. The person who understands the saying "No guts, no story." (Who does these crazy things for the glory anyway?) Second, I've tried to draw on my background as both a registered dietitian and an endurance athlete to sort through what health and science professionals recommend versus what really works in real life. Besides my own experience, I had a lot of help from some of the best endurance athletes in the country.

Some themes ring loud and clear when speaking with top-notch runners, cyclists, triathletes, adventure racers, long-distance swimmers, mountaineers, and winter athletes involved in Nordic and backcountry skiing. They know their bodies extremely well. They always go into an endurance event or race with a well-thought-out nutritional game plan. Most important, they are always thinking about their food and fluid needs while on the move.

Part I of this book offers eight chapters geared to deliver practical nutrition information that you can apply the next time you open the refrigerator door, hear about the latest supplement, worry about your weight, or wonder, now that you've signed up, how you're ever going to go that far or last that long. Part II looks at how some elite endurance athletes get the job done as they share their experience through real-life situations and offer tried-and-true advice. All of it is offered to you, the endurance athlete, as food for thought.

Acknowledgments

My greatest appreciation goes to acquisitions editor Martin Barnard for believing in my ability to write this book and to developmental editor Cassandra Mitchell for her extraordinary patience through the process.

Many thanks to the athletes who brought this book to life by willingly sharing their time and wisdom and to all the others who believe I have something to say. Thanks also to my colleagues Sandy, Jenny, Shannon, Patti, and Levi for their advice, Kate for her guiding hand, and Cousin Denise for home-cooked meals and true friendship. Lastly, this book never could have been written without the support of two special people: my husband, John, who has run through life with me for the past 18 years, and my brother, Michael, who made the time to read and comment on every word.

part I

Performance Eating

Endurance Nutrition Checkup

"I try to eat a semibalanced diet—some protein, mostly carbohydrates, and I certainly don't restrict my fat intake. It backfires if you try to be too spartan in your diet. Just eat everything in moderation. Sure, I snack on fruit, pretzels, and fig newtons, but I love Oreo cookies too, and I'm addicted to Starbucks coffee ice cream."

—Karen Smyers, 1995 winner of the International Triathlon Union World Championship and the Hawaii Ironman

Three factors figure predominantly in the success of any athlete: genetics, training, and nutrition. Because you can't do anything about your genetic makeup, it's wise to concentrate on the other two. Indeed, these two factors are inextricably linked: the intense and exhaustive efforts endurance athletes often undertake wouldn't be possible unless they eat the right foods in optimal amounts. How else do you think you can tackle an early morning swim workout, a full day at the office, and a long bike ride or run in the evening? More important, how do you think you can get up the next day and do it all over again? It goes without saying that runners, cyclists, swimmers, rowers, triathletes, hikers, mountaineers, backcountry and Nordic skiers, and adventure racers would enjoy little success if they didn't pay attention to their food and fluid needs while attempting to race or complete endurance events.

Eating a well-balanced, healthy diet doesn't guarantee success, but poor eating habits can literally stop you in your tracks or, at the very least, keep you from reaching your true potential. The foods and fluids you consume before, during, and after exercise provide the fuel and nutrients your body needs to perform at its best. Frequent colds and illnesses, nagging injuries, and poor training days may signal that your nutrition program is out of sync with your training program. The most successful endurance athletes have learned that getting the most out of their bodies requires paying attention to their nutrition needs as they put in the miles.

Besides being good for you, the foods you choose to eat must taste good; otherwise, you won't eat them! The key is to follow an eating style that satisfies both these needs—quality nutrition and good taste. On top of that, unless you like to spend time in the kitchen or can afford to hire a personal chef, you probably want to figure out how to eat a healthy, well-balanced diet without expending too much time and energy.

How Healthy Is Your Daily Diet?

You may already know a great deal, or think you do, about what constitutes a healthy diet for an endurance athlete. It never hurts to look at what you're actually eating though. Being knowledgeable about a topic doesn't always translate into putting that knowledge into practice. Knowing what you are currently eating will help you answer for yourself the question I hear most often from athletes of all abilities, "What should I be eating?"

A Personal Pyramid

Before you read any further, grab a pencil and get ready to analyze your current eating habits. First, familiarize yourself with the Food Guide Pyramid (see figure 1.1), which serves as a guideline for making healthful food choices. The Food Guide Pyramid organizes foods by the nutrients they contain into five major food groups. In addition it's topped by a catch-all category containing foods high in fat and/or sugar, and foods that contain

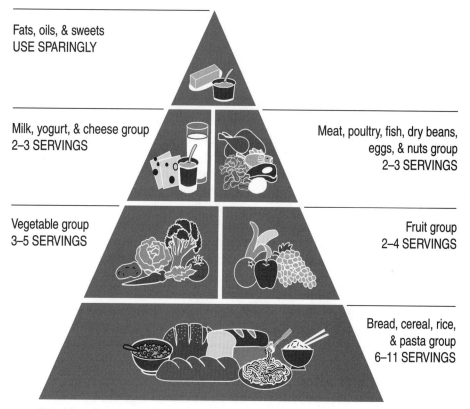

Fats, oils, & sweets
USE SPARINGLY

Milk, yogurt, & cheese group
2–3 SERVINGS

Meat, poultry, fish, dry beans,
eggs, & nuts group
2–3 SERVINGS

Vegetable group
3–5 SERVINGS

Fruit group
2–4 SERVINGS

Bread, cereal, rice,
& pasta group
6–11 SERVINGS

United States Departments of Agriculture and Health and Human Services.

Figure 1.1   Food guide pyramid.

few or no nutrients, such as coffee, tea, and alcohol. As the pyramid depicts, eating generous amounts of plant-based foods, such as breads, cereals, and whole grains, and fruits and vegetables forms the foundation of a healthful diet. Consuming adequate amounts of meat and other protein foods and dairy products ensures that you are eating a well-balanced sports diet. Capping off your daily diet with a limited amount of "empty calorie" foods, such as fats and sweets that are high in calories but low in most nutrients, makes eating an enjoyable experience. These foods also help endurance athletes meet their high-energy needs by supplying extra calories.

As you take a closer look at the pyramid, you may wonder where some foods belong. The bread and cereals group, the fruit and vegetable group, and the dairy group contain foods that you most likely would expect. Note that the meat group, however, includes a variety of protein-rich foods, including meat, fish, and poultry, as well as dried beans and peas, eggs, tofu, nuts and seeds, and peanut butter and other nut butters. The tip of the pyramid (fats, oils, and sweets) is home to such foods as coffee and tea, soda, fruit-flavored drinks, alcohol, cream cheese, butter and margarine, salad dressing, jam and jelly, mayonnaise, nondairy creamer, condiments, sour cream, sugar, honey, maple syrup, pickles, olives, sauces, gravy, vegetable oils, bacon, French fries, onion rings, chips and snack foods, oil-popped popcorn, candy, gelatin desserts, sherbet, high-fat ice cream and frozen yogurt, cookies, doughnuts, pastries, cakes, and pies.

Take a few minutes to recall what you had to eat (and drink) yesterday from the time you arose until you went to bed. If yesterday was unusual, for example, if you were ill or traveling, choose another day that you can recall. Turn to the blank Your Personal Pyramid worksheet (see figure 1.2 on page 7) and write down in the margin of the pyramid a list of all the foods and beverages you consumed in one day. You may want to photocopy and enlarge this to use for several days. Once you've completed that list, transfer each item into the appropriate food group on the lines provided. You may prefer simply to write each item down directly in the appropriate box as you recall it. For example, if you ate a bagel with cream cheese and orange juice for breakfast, you would write bagel in the base of the pyramid (bread and cereals group), orange juice in the fruit group box, and cream cheese in the tip of the pyramid (fats, oils, and sweets).

Don't forget to include snacks, beverages, and foods eaten on the run, such as the energy bar you downed in the car on the way home following a workout or the cheese and crackers you grabbed on the way through the kitchen. Be sure to record condiments or additions to food, such as the parmesan cheese (dairy group) you covered your plate of spaghetti with or the olive oil (fats, oils, and sweets) in which you soaked your bread. Obviously, many of the foods you eat will fit into more than one food group. A slice of pizza with green peppers, for example, would count in the bread and cereals group (crust), the vegetable group (tomato sauce, green peppers) and the dairy group (cheese). Count only the major ingredients in mixed foods.

Next, take a stab at estimating the amount you ate by comparing it with what counts as one serving in each group (see table 1.1, p. 8). For example, count the bagel as two servings (a half bagel is a serving) and the tomato sauce and green peppers on the pizza as one serving (it takes a half cup of cooked vegetables or sauce to equal a full serving). Legumes, such as kidney, garbanzo, and black beans, provide hefty doses of carbohydrates and other key nutrients, as well as protein, and thus can be counted in either the base of the pyramid (bread and cereals group) or the meat group. Tally up the number of servings you ate in each food group and put a circle around the number.

Keeping the particular needs of athletes in mind, I've modified the base of the personal food guide pyramid to emphasize the importance of drinking a minimum of eight to ten glasses of fluid a day. Estimate your fluid intake by checking off one water glass (as depicted at the base of the pyramid) for every cup (eight ounces) of fluid you consumed. Count water, fruit juice, milk, sports drinks, and other non caffeinated beverages, but not alcoholic drinks (including beer). For more accurate tracking, pencil in the actual source of fluid under each water glass that you mark.

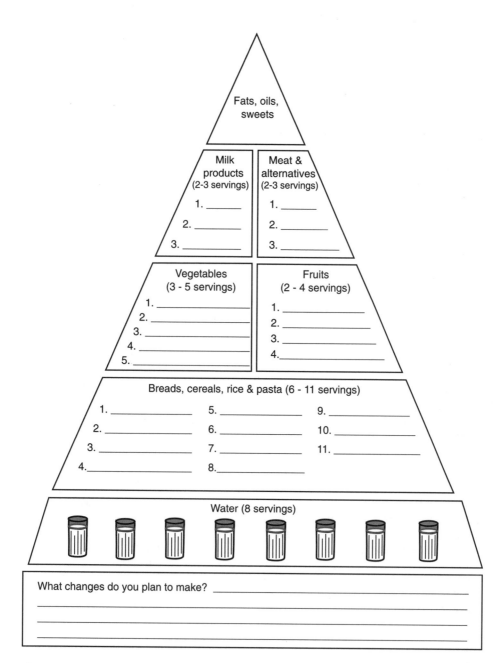

Figure 1.2 Your personal pyramid.

Adapted from SMART CHOICES for Health™ by Sandy S. Miller, MS, RD, LD. Copyright 1999. Providence Health System.

Table 1.1   What Counts as One Serving?

Bread and cereals group (6-11 servings)

bread	1 slice
tortilla, pita bread	1 six-inch
roll, biscuit, muffin	1 small (2 oz or less)
small bagel, hamburger bun, English muffin	1/2
large croissant	1/2
dry cereal	1 oz
cooked cereal, pasta, rice	1/2 c.
small crackers	4-6
pancake	1 four-inch
pretzels	1 oz
rice cakes	2
air-popped popcorn	3 c.

Vegetable group (3-5 servings)

raw, leafy vegetables	1 c.
cooked or chopped raw vegetables	1/2 c.
vegetable juice	3/4 c.
spaghetti sauce	1/2 c.
scalloped potatoes or potato salad	1/2 c.
potato	1 medium

Fruit group (2-4 servings)

fruit	1 medium piece
chopped, cooked, canned fruit	1/2 c.
melon	1/4
grapefruit, banana	1/2
fruit juice	3/4 c.
dried fruit	1/4 c.

Meat group (2-3 servings)

cooked, lean meat, poultry, fish	2 1/2 - 3 oz
These foods count as one ounce of meat:	
cooked beans/peas	1/2 c.
tofu	3 oz
egg	1
egg whites	2
peanut butter	2 tbsp.
nuts	1/3 c.

Dairy group (2-3 servings)

milk	1 c.
yogurt	1 c.
natural cheese	1 1/2 oz
processed cheese	2 oz
cottage cheese	1 c.
fat-free or low-fat frozen yogurt or ice cream	1 c.

Fats, oils, and sweets

No specific serving sizes recommended for this category

Granted, one day of tracking your eating habits doesn't give you a complete picture of your diet, but it can be a useful reality check. You may be pleasantly surprised at how well you're doing at meeting your nutrition needs, or you may be prompted to rethink some of your current choices.

The recommended servings listed on the Food Guide Pyramid provide a range of calories (about 1,600 to 2,800) depending not only on the number of servings you eat from each group, but on the specific foods you choose. Some endurance athletes will require far more than 2,800 calories a day to fuel their needs. Before you analyze your personal pyramid, assess your calorie needs and the corresponding number of servings you need from the Food Guide Pyramid by completing the following sections.

Part One: Estimating Your Daily Calorie Needs

Determining how many calories you require on a daily basis is as much an art as it is a science. You don't need to begin counting calories, but estimating your calorie requirement can help you better understand your energy needs as an endurance athlete. Use the simple method listed below to estimate the range of calories you need daily. (For those athletes desiring further information, a more sophisticated method can be found in chapter two.)

Less active: little or no purposeful exercise, such as when you're taking a break from training or recuperating from an injury or illness.

Body weight (in pounds) × 14 to 15 calories per pound = _____ calories

Moderately active: approximately 45 to 60 minutes a day of purposeful exercise (moderate intensity), most days of the week.

Body weight (in pounds) × 16 to 20 calories per pound = _____ calories

Very active: approximately 60 to 120 minutes a day of purposeful exercise (moderate intensity), most days of the week.

Body weight (in pounds) × 21 to 25 calories per pound = _____ calories

Extremely active: training for an ultraendurance event, such as an Ironman triathlon or 100-mile ultrarun

Body weight (in pounds) × 25 to 30 calories (or more) per pound = _____ calories

Table 1.2 Translating Calories Into Pyramid Servings

	Estimated Calories*						
	About 1,600-1,800	About 2,200	About 2,500	About 2,800	About 3,300	About 3,800	About 4,200
	Recommended Number of Daily Servings Based on the Food Pyramid						
Bread and cereal group	6-8	9	11	14	18	22	24
Vegetable group	3	4	4	5	6	6	7
Fruit group	2-3	3	3	4	5	5	6
Dairy group**	2-3	3	4	4	4	5	5
Meat group	2	3	3	3-4	4-5	5	6
Fats, oils, and sweets	No recommendation. Enjoy foods from this category if you can afford the calories after eating the recommended servings from the five food groups.						

Notes:

*Obtain additional calories by choosing higher-calorie items, eating more servings from the five food groups and enjoying foods from the fats, oils, and sweets category. Athletes who have trouble meeting their energy needs can add high-carbohydrate drinks to meals and snacks. Meal replacement beverages and energy bars can also be used to supplement a balanced diet.

**Teenagers, young athletes up to age 24, and women who are pregnant or breast-feeding need 3 or more servings a day from the dairy group.

Adapted from the U.S. Department of Agriculture and the U.S. Department of Health and Human Services.

Part Two: Translating Calories Into Pyramid Servings

Once you've estimated the number of calories you need daily, use table 1.2 as a guideline to translate your calories into pyramid servings. Eating at least the minimum recommended number of servings from each food group daily will help you get the nutrients, as well as the calories, you need. Compare your circled values with the recommendations in table 1.2.

Analyzing Your Diet

Here are some points to consider as you look at your current eating style.

A well-balanced sports diet takes the shape of the Food Guide Pyramid. Does the personal pyramid you just filled out look like a pyramid or is it top heavy or missing sections altogether? Did you build a strong base by eating at least 6 to 11 servings or more of wholesome foods, such as rice and other grains, pasta, whole-grain breads and cereals? These foods provide complex carbohydrates, B vitamins, fiber, and numerous other nutrients without contributing much unnecessary fat.

Carbohydrates provide the most readily available form of energy to fuel endurance exercise. Glycogen (stored carbohydrate) is the primary fuel your body uses as you exercise more intensely. Your glycogen reserves also play a vital role in determining how long you can exercise. You need to consume a daily dose of carbohydrate-rich foods to replace the muscle glycogen you use during exercise. Failing to do so can leave you feeling sluggish and tired, and unable to maintain your normal training intensity. Eating foods such as bread, cereal, rice, and pasta, as well as ample amounts of fruits and vegetables, legumes, and dairy foods will ensure that approximately 60 percent of your total calories come from carbohydrates—the foundation of any serious endurance athlete's diet. Eating a high-carbohydrate diet every day, not just the night before an endurance endeavor, is the best way to maximize your glycogen stores and increase your endurance capacity.

Moving up the pyramid, did your fruit and vegetable servings total up to at least five each day? Consuming nine or more servings a day is an even better goal. Chock full of vitamins A and C, fiber, phytochemicals, and other nutrients, fruits and vegetables are nature's vitamin pills. They're certainly a lot more tasty and fun to eat than a bunch of supplements. Several national health organizations, including the American Heart Association and the American Cancer Society, have recently petitioned the government to revise the Food Guide Pyramid and consider fruits and vegetables the core of a healthy diet. To date, hundreds of studies have shown the health benefits of eating a diet rich in fruit and vegetables.

As important as carbohydrates are, endurance athletes cannot perform their best by ignoring their protein requirements. Protein is needed daily to fulfill numerous jobs in the body: building, maintaining, and repairing muscles and other body tissues, making hemoglobin, which carries oxygen to exercising muscles, forming antibodies to fight off infection and disease, producing enzymes and hormones that help regulate processes in the body, and, for endurance athletes, supplying energy in the latter stages of endurance events. Up to 20 percent of your total daily calories should come from protein.

Lean meats, dried beans, soy foods such as tofu and tempeh, eggs, and other protein-rich foods supply protein and varying amounts of two crucial nutrients—iron and zinc. Low-fat dairy foods also supply high-quality protein, as well as large doses of calcium, a nutrient needed for healthy nerves, muscles, and bones. How did you do at consuming two to three servings of foods from the meat and beans group and at least two servings (three for women and younger athletes up to age 24) from the dairy group? Athletes often go to one extreme or another when it comes to eating foods from these two groups. Some have little trouble exceeding their requirements, thanks to supersize burgers and pints of ice cream. Others, concerned about eating a meat-free diet or reducing their fat intake, skimp on or eliminate animal products with little regard to finding alternatives. In either case, the athlete is no longer eating a well-balanced diet.

Fat, by the way, is an appropriate part of a healthy sports diet. Besides providing a concentrated dose of energy, the fat you eat allows the body to absorb and use fat-soluble vitamins (A, D, E, and K) and consume an adequate amount of linoleic acid, an essential fatty acid needed for growth and healthy skin and hair. A well-balanced sports diet obtains at least 20 percent of its total calories from fat. If you're an elite swimmer, distance runner, triathlete, or cyclist who requires upwards of 4,000 calories a day, you may need to consume a greater percentage of your calories as fat to help meet your high energy needs.

The tip of the pyramid houses fats, oils, and sweets, as well as other foods that offer little in the way of nutrients, such as coffee and soda. These foods can round out a healthy diet and help you meet your energy requirements. Go ahead and enjoy the taste, pleasure, and psychological boost these foods provide. The question to ask yourself, however, is whether the foods in the tip of your pyramid routinely throw your diet off balance by squeezing out healthier options from the five food groups. How do you tell? Your diet no longer resembles the triangular shape of the Food Guide Pyramid.

A healthy sports diet is full of variety. No single food or food group can supply all the nutrients you need (see appendix A for vitamins and minerals needed for performance). Each food group contains foods that are particularly rich in a package of nutrients. Fruits and vegetables, for example, mainly serve up vitamins A, C, and fiber, and dairy group foods supply protein, calcium, and riboflavin. Eliminating entire groups of food puts you at risk for being low in certain essential nutrients needed for good health and optimal athletic performances. How well do you do at eating from all five food groups on a daily basis?

Eating a varied diet also refers to eating many different foods from each of the five major food groups of the pyramid. If you always drink apple juice for breakfast and grab a banana for a snack, you've missed opportunities to boost your vitamin C intake, as well as experiment with other great-tasting foods rich in vitamin C, such as cantaloupe and tangerine juice. (Apple juice provides no vitamin C unless it's been fortified, and bananas, although rich in potassium, carbohydrates, and fiber, provide minimal amounts of vitamin C.)

Keep in mind that some foods are nutritional powerhouses compared to others. Although you can certainly meet your carbohydrate needs by eating bagels, plates of spaghetti, and an energy bar or two, your health and performance (never mind your taste buds) would undoubtedly benefit from including more whole grains, such as kashi or oatmeal for breakfast, brown rice or couscous for dinner, and whole-wheat fig newtons as a snack.

Taking a multivitamin can help ensure you get an adequate intake of most nutrients, but it's no guarantee that the nutrients will be as well absorbed as those from food. Supplements also don't supply all the health benefits, such

Do Energy Bars Fit Into a Healthy Sports Diet?

Run this diet by your taste buds: carrot cake for breakfast, an almond brownie for lunch or an afternoon snack, and a chocolate praline following your evening workout. It's possible—thanks to the newest crop of energy bars now available to athletes. You may even believe that energy bars (also called sports or endurance bars) are, well, real food.

Beyond simple and complex carbohydrates, energy bars now include varying amounts of protein, fat, vitamins, and minerals, as well as antioxidants, herbs, and other potentially performance-enhancing substances (although little evidence exists that these "enhancers" have any effect on athletic performance). You may also be consuming items you don't want, such as caffeine, palm kernel oil (a saturated fat common in coated bars), or high-fructose corn syrup (a refined sweetener).

The Food Guide Pyramid was designed with real foods in mind. From that perspective energy bars don't fit neatly into any food group. Despite being fortified with vitamins and minerals, most carbohydrate-rich bars are high in sugar and contain little or no fiber. "Balanced" bars may provide protein but without the accompanying iron and zinc found in protein-rich foods. Some bars really aren't much different than a candy bar or a bunch of fat-free cookies combined with a vitamin pill.

Think about energy bars as being in the tip of the pyramid, as a sports or fuel supplement to an otherwise healthy diet based on real food. Consider that this food is more than just the sum of its parts. The nutrients in food work together to produce a desired effect greater than a single nutrient could produce. It's not exactly clear what quantity or combination of nutrients the body requires. On top of that, some potential health boosters, like the phytochemicals ("plant chemicals" that may help the body ward off aging and disease) found in fruits and vegetables, haven't yet been fully identified, so they can't possibly be in your favorite bar. That's why routinely replacing meals or snacks with manufactured foods doesn't make sense for your health or your performance.

Fill in or round out your diet with energy bars, but don't make them the main part of it. At their best, energy bars supply a convenient dose of energy. They work well as an easily digestible preworkout or prerace meal, as fuel during exercise (as tolerated), and following exercise to help replenish muscle glycogen stores. You might also rely on energy bars (meal-replacement products, too) as a backup, perhaps on busy days or while traveling when you would otherwise miss or skip a meal or snack. To be sure of what you're getting and what you're missing out on, check the nutrition label and ingredients list of whatever bar you choose. Many bars lack substantial amounts of some key nutrients that athletes are often low in, such as vitamins A and C, calcium, iron, and fiber.

as fiber, phytochemicals, and other yet undiscovered nutritional boosters, contained in food. What efforts do you typically make to eat a variety of foods from each of the five food groups?

Moderation is the key to a healthy sports diet. Endurance athletes are good at doing things in extreme, and often struggle with eating in moderation. Many shun nutrient-rich foods because such foods also contain fat, or they continually rely on sugar and caffeine for a pickup instead of obtaining the energy they need from real foods. No foods are good or bad for you; your overall diet is what counts. Eating a single food, a specific type of energy bar, for example, won't save an otherwise poor diet, nor will eating a bowl of premium high-fat ice cream or a fast-food meal erase all your healthier choices.

Look at your personal eating habits. Instead of eliminating foods or entire food groups, do you select healthier versions (less fat, sodium, calories, and so on) or work at incorporating alternatives into your diet? For example, if you choose not to eat dairy foods, do you replace milk with fortified soy or rice milk and eat plenty of dark green leafy vegetables to obtain calcium? If you're watching your weight or just trying to eat more healthfully, do you eat high-fat foods in smaller amounts or less frequently? Keep in mind that you need to consider the fat and added sugars in your choices from all the food groups, not just fats, oils, and sweets from the pyramid tip.

For many athletes, performing a diet makeover or losing weight without skimping on good nutrition hinges on cutting out excess fat. A gram of fat supplies nine calories compared with the four calories in a gram of protein or carbohydrate. But this doesn't mean you should bypass a sandwich and a glass of milk to eat an entire box of fat-free cookies! Eating in moderation means you strive to fit all foods into a healthy sports diet.

Quick Fixes for Six Common Dietary Downfalls

You're not alone if your personal pyramid doesn't quite measure up to the standard. Athletes of all abilities, beginners to world-class, shortchange their health and performance by not paying enough attention to their daily diet. This section provides quick fixes for the six most common dietary downfalls that can trip up even the fittest endurance athlete.

1. Filling in Missing Food Groups

Eliminating entire food groups or shortchanging yourself by barely squeezing in the required servings every now and then can cause you, in the end, to run low on some essential nutrients. Athletes often struggle with eating enough fruits and vegetables and meeting their requirements from the meat and dairy group.

Fulfilling the Fruits and Vegetables Requirement

Here are some tips for adding more vegetables to your diet. As a rule, choose colorful fruits and vegetables to obtain the most nutrients.

- Drink tomato or vegetable juice.
- Include a cup of vegetable soup with lunch.
- Order vegetable-based soup as an appetizer instead of another pale green nutrition-poor salad.
- Buy fresh, ready-to-eat varieties, such as bags of baby carrots and salad-in-a-bag, or stop by the salad bar and pick up your precut favorites. It's no more expensive then throwing away heads of slimy lettuce, wilted carrots, and mushy tomatoes. Keep your favorite low-fat salad dressing on hand for dipping and dressing salads.

> ## Best Bets: Fruits and Vegetables
>
> **High in Vitamin A:** apricots, cantaloupe, carrots, kale, collards, romaine lettuce, spinach, sweet potatoes, winter squash
>
> **High in Vitamin C:** broccoli, cabbage, bell peppers, cantaloupe, grapefruit, kiwi, mangoes, oranges, spinach, strawberries, tomatoes
>
> **High in Fiber:** apples, bananas, berries, carrots, cherries, dates, figs, pears, spinach, sweet potatoes

- Keep frozen or canned vegetables on hand and toss them into whatever else you're heating up during the last few minutes—soup, spaghetti sauce, stew, casseroles, or mashed potatoes.
- Buy a vegetable steamer, available for $25 or less, or microwave your veggies. Either way it takes only minutes.
- Bake a potato or sweet potato in the microwave. Add your favorite low-fat topping.
- Eat more of the ones you like, especially if you eat vegetables at one only meal. Serving sizes are small (a half cup cooked or one cup of raw leafy greens) and add up quickly.
- Choose fast food with veggies—vegetarian pizza, Chinese stir-fry, vegetable curries, and so on.
- Learn to like vegetables you hated as a kid, such as Brussels sprouts, cauliflower, and squash. When you find yourself smiling and having a good time, simply take one bite (no more) of the veggie you dislike. Do this at least a half dozen times, a few days to a week or more apart, and make sure your brain is always dialed into a happy mode. After several times of no misery or adverse reactions (like being sent to your room), your brain may decide this isn't so bad after all.

The following are some tips for adding more fruit to your diet.

- Get a leg up by starting out the day right. Drink 100 percent fruit juice or add a piece of fruit to your morning meal. Try a banana, peach, or berries on cereal, pancakes, or waffles, or stir extra fruit into yogurt.

- Keep dried fruit such as raisins, dates, apples, cherries or dried apricots stashed in your briefcase or desk drawer.
- Keep bananas in the refrigerator (only skins turn black) so they ripen more slowly.
- Purchase ready-to-eat fruit from the salad bar. You will be more likely to eat it if you don't have to prepare it first.
- Make or choose desserts that emphasize the fruit, such as fruit tarts or crustless pies.
- Keep frozen berries in the freezer and use them as a topping for ice cream, frozen yogurt, plain cakes, or make fruit parfaits.

Fulfilling the Meat and Beans Requirement

Endurance athletes need ample amounts of protein, iron, and zinc to train and perform consistently at a high level. Iron is needed to form hemoglobin and myoglobin, the oxygen-carrying compounds in blood and muscles. Without enough iron to produce new red blood cells, iron-deficiency anemia results, leaving you feeling fatigued and unable to perform at your best. Zinc is required to fight off infections and help wounds and injuries heal properly, including the cellular microdamage caused by logging an ambitious number of daily training miles.

Animal foods, such as red meat and seafood, provide the most readily absorbable form of iron (heme iron) and zinc. Boost your absorption of non-heme iron from plant foods by eating a food rich in vitamin C at the same time, for example, a glass of orange juice with your morning bowl of oatmeal. If you're eating enough protein, you are most likely getting enough zinc. Coffee and the tannins in tea (regular and decaffeinated) block the absorption of iron and zinc from foods, so drink these beverages between meals, not with them.

The following are some tips for meeting the servings for meats and beans.

- To limit the fat that often accompanies meat, choose lean cuts (rounds and loins, such as tenderloin, sirloin, and round steak) and trim all visible fat. Choose the leanest ground beef you can afford or substitute ground turkey breast instead. Buy boneless, skinless poultry or remove the skin.

Best Bets: Iron

Animal sources

Beef, pork, lamb, liver, and other organ meats
Poultry (especially dark meat)
Fish/shellfish

Plant sources

Dark leafy greens: spinach, beet, collard and turnip greens, Swiss chard
Tomato and prune juice
Dried fruit: apricots, raisins
Legumes: chickpeas, black, kidney, lima, navy, and pinto beans
Lentils
Soy foods: tofu, tempeh, textured vegetable protein, soy milk
Whole-grain and enriched breads and cereals (including hot cereals, such as oatmeal and Cream of Wheat)
Wheat germ

- Use low-fat cooking methods, such as baking, broiling, and grilling. Remember, a three-ounce serving for any type of meat, poultry, or fish is only the size of a deck of cards.

- Eat more fish. It takes only minutes to prepare. Order fish when you dine away from home. Buy ready-to-eat shellfish, such as precooked shrimp.

- Eat more beans. Keep several canned varieties on hand, buy from a salad bar to add to salads, or serve as a side dish instead of potatoes or rice. Choose soups made from beans or peas (minestrone, split pea, black bean, or lentil) and try meatless meals such as tacos or burritos stuffed with beans, vegetarian chili, or black beans with rice.

- Don't shy away from eggs. Inexpensive and easy to prepare, eggs provide high-quality protein. Most endurance athletes can afford to follow the American Heart Association guidelines and eat up to four eggs a week. Beyond that, use egg whites (toss the yolks) to get protein without the fat and cholesterol. Egg substitutes (such as Egg Beaters) provide another easy option.

Best Bets: Zinc
Animal Sources
Shellfish: oysters, crab, shrimp, clams
Red meat: beef, pork, lamb, liver and other organ meats
Poultry
Fish
Dairy foods: milk, yogurt, and cheese
Plant Sources
Legumes: chickpeas, kidney, lima, navy, and pinto beans, split peas
Lentils
Spinach
Soy foods: Tofu, tempeh, textured vegetable protein
Peanut butter
Peanuts, cashews, Brazil nuts
Sunflower seeds
Whole-grain and enriched breakfast cereals, including oatmeal
Wheat germ

- Toss tofu (rich in high-quality protein and a good source of iron, magnesium, and zinc) into soups, stews, and lasagna, mash it with cottage cheese and seasonings to make a sandwich spread or dip, or blend it with lemon juice and salt for a baked-potato topping.

- Other time-savers include canned tuna (packed in water) or chicken, cubed meat for kebabs and stir-fries, precooked rotisserie chickens, and frozen veggie-burgers or gardenburgers.

- Aim to include some protein at each meal. Don't eat your grains plain. Smear your bagel with peanut butter, toss baked beans over noodles, or throw seafood into your favorite sauce and pour it over pasta, rice, or couscous.

Fulfilling the Dairy Requirement

Don't shortchange yourself when it comes to getting enough calcium. If your diet doesn't supply the calcium you need, your body will steal from the only source it has—your bones! To reduce the risk of osteoporosis, build for the future by optimizing your bone mass before you reach age 25. You can still build some bone up to age 35; after that, your goal becomes holding on to

Best Bets: Calcium*

1 cup of milk (nonfat, low-fat, or whole)

1 cup of yogurt

1 1/2 oz of cheese

2 cups of cottage cheese

1 1/2 cups of ice cream or frozen yogurt

1 cup of fortified soy or rice milk

1 cup of fortified orange juice

1 1/2 cups of cooked collards, turnip greens, or kale

3 cups of cooked broccoli

1 1/2 cup of baked beans

1 cup (8 oz) of tofu (prepared with calcium sulfate)

1/2 cup of soy nuts

4 oz of canned salmon (with bones)

2 1/2 oz of canned sardines (with bones)

*Contains at least 300 milligrams per serving.

what you have. Because many endurance athletes hit their stride later in life, every day counts in consuming enough calcium.

If you choose not to drink milk or consume dairy foods, incorporate other calcium-rich foods into your daily diet. Aim for 1,000 milligrams a day (1,300 milligrams for younger athletes age 9 to 18 and 1,200 milligrams for adults over age 50). It's easy to determine how much calcium a food provides. Check the nutrition facts section of the food label and add a zero to the percent daily value for calcium. For example, a food supplying 35 percent of the daily value provides 350 milligrams of calcium.

Here are some tips to help boost your intake of dairy and dairy alternatives.

- Sneak in milk—any variety will do. Drink milk shakes, fruit smoothies, latte, and flavored milks (check the dairy case for chocolate and other varieties or stir in flavored syrups). Enjoy pudding or custard for dessert.

- Prepare foods such as hot chocolate, oatmeal, or tomato soup with milk rather than water. Snack on yogurt or use it to make a salad dressing or vegetable dip.

- Add a slice or two of low-fat cheese to a sandwich or burger, snack on low-fat string cheese or a slice of cheese pizza, and sprinkle low-fat parmesan or mozzarella cheese on foods.

- Don't let other less nutritious beverages, such as soda (diet and regular), coffee, tea, iced tea, lemonade, and fruit drinks, squeeze milk out of your diet.

- If you suffer from lactose intolerance, try drinking milk or eating ice cream with a meal, not on an empty stomach. Experiment with lactose-reduced and lactose-free milk and milk products or take lactase tablets before you consume dairy foods. You can also substitute soy or rice milk (choose a brand fortified with calcium and vitamin D) for regular milk. Yogurt and natural aged cheeses, such as cheddar and Swiss, tend to produce fewer symptoms.

- To boost your calcium intake beyond that contained in dairy foods, make sure the tofu you consume is prepared with calcium sulfate (check the label) and add or substitute other calcium-fortified foods to your

Performance-Enhancing Snacks

Peanut butter and jelly or banana sandwich (half or whole)

Trail gorp (nuts, raisins, dried fruit, etc.)

Instant oatmeal with dried apricots

Cereal or low-fat granola with fruit and yogurt

Banana, pumpkin, or date bread and a carton of milk

Cookies (oatmeal raisin, fig bars, vanilla wafers, gingersnaps, animal crackers, or graham crackers) and milk

Low-fat cheese and crackers or rice cakes

Tuna fish and crackers

Pita bread with low-fat cheese

An English muffin or bagel topped with peanut or another nut butter

Low-fat muffin with milk, yogurt, or juice

Rice cakes or crackers and humus

Slice of pizza (thick crust and vegetable toppings)

Baked potato topped with salsa, cottage cheese, or low-fat cheese

Cup or bowl of soup and crackers

Three-bean, pasta or potato salad (low-fat dressing) and a roll

Raw veggies dipped in low-fat salad dressing or salsa

Nonfat refried beans or salsa and baked chips or crackers

Piece of fresh fruit and pretzels or low-fat popcorn

Fresh fruit dipped in yogurt or chocolate-flavored syrup

Frozen fruit juice bar or low-fat frozen yogurt

Angel food cake with fresh berries or dipped in yogurt

Half a papaya or cantaloupe filled with yogurt or cottage cheese

Breakfast drink or shake made with low-fat milk, ice cream, or yogurt

Fruit smoothie (fruit, yogurt, and milk or juice)

Meal-replacement drink

diet, such as calcium-fortified cereals, soy or rice milk, and orange juice. Eat plenty of dark green leafy vegetables such as kale, collard, and turnip greens, bok choy, and broccoli. (Don't count on the calcium in spinach as it's poorly absorbed.)

2. Righting a Top-Heavy Pyramid

Who deserves to enjoy sweets, treats, and some extra fat more than endurance athletes putting in the miles? Occasional indulgences are good for the body and the spirit. Keep in mind the 80-20 rule. If you're eating nutritious foods most of the time (80 percent or more), then go easy on yourself the rest of the time (20 percent or less).

Eating foods high in fat or sugar and otherwise low in nutrients becomes a problem, though, when you squeeze out healthy foods and fill up on these empty calories. The fact that you're physically active doesn't mean you don't have to pay attention to your health. Consuming excess fat, saturated fat, cholesterol, sodium, and calories can increase your risk for heart disease, diabetes, and some cancers. It's also unlikely to do much for your performance.

The following are some quick fixes for righting a top-heavy pyramid.

- Snack on "real food" from the five food groups. Aim to include at least one food group (two is even better) in your snack choices. Instead of plowing through a box of cookies, for example, enjoy a reasonable amount with a glass of milk. Better yet, on some occasions pour a bowl of your favorite cereal and add milk. Think of your snacks as minimeals or opportunities to get the nutrients you need. Selecting foods that are more nutritious is particularly important if you tend to graze throughout the day instead of eating defined meals.

- Don't let yourself get too hungry. Plan to eat every three to five hours while you're awake to keep your blood sugar (fuel for your brain) from dipping too low. If you allow yourself to get too hungry, you're apt to toss your good intentions out the window and simply eat whatever food is in sight, which may not be the healthiest fare. You'll also consume more calories and have more energy when you need it most during the day, not the few hours between dinner and bedtime. Of course, this means you'll have to plan and keep healthy "fast food" on hand.

- Savor your favorites. When you treat yourself, treat yourself! Slow down and savor whatever it is you crave or desire. Sit down, serve it on a plate, and consciously enjoy every bite. Rushing can leave you feeling unsatisfied and cause you to overeat. Feeling guilty afterward dilutes the pleasure and can also lead you to overeat. Guilt can also have the opposite effect, causing you to skimp on healthier foods to make up for the foods you indulge in.

- Cut down on soda and other caffeinated beverages. Drinking too much coffee, tea, and soda fills you up and may temporarily perk you up, but that's it. Ask yourself if what you really need is something to eat. Sustainable energy comes from the calories provided by foods and nutritious beverages. On top of that, you can only consume so much fluid, and water, low-fat milk, juice, and sports drinks make far healthier choices. Make your own healthy soda by mixing fruit juice and seltzer half and half.

3. Strengthening a Weak Base by Eating More Whole Grains

Most athletes have little trouble racking up enough servings from the bread and cereals group, especially because serving sizes are small and add up quickly. Consuming a few of these servings, if any, as whole grains can be another matter. The complex carbohydrates provided by these foods (as well as starchy vegetables and legumes) replenish the glycogen used by working muscles and are superior to the carbohydrates in simple sugars found in candy bars and soda. Whole grains supply more fiber, vitamin E, vitamin B_6, zinc, copper, manganese, and potassium than refined grains.

The following are some quick fixes for increasing your intake of whole grains.

• Choose whole-wheat bread more often, instead of white, wheat, multigrain, rye, or pumpernickel. Check the ingredients list and look for *whole* wheat (the key word is whole) as the first ingredient or at least listed before any other flour. Try whole-wheat tortillas, bagels, pitas, and rice cakes, too.

• Experiment with whole-wheat pasta or other whole grains, such as couscous, bulgur, kasha, quinoa, or brown rice. Look for prepackaged, quick-cooking (15 minutes or less) whole-grain mixes.

• Eat a whole-grain breakfast cereal (hot or cold) like oatmeal, Wheatena, Ralston, Roman Meal, shredded wheat, Grape-Nuts, Cheerios, Wheaties, or Total. Bran cereals like raisin bran, All-Bran, or 100% Bran count, too.

• Eat more whole-grain crackers like Triscuits, Ry Krisp, and whole-grain crispbreads.

4. Controlling Your Calories by Eating Regular Meals

Whether you need to reduce or expand your food selections to meet your daily needs (including calories), eating regular meals and snacks will help you be more conscious of what you eat. You'll boost your metabolism and have more energy during the day when you need it most. Besides, ignoring your hunger and skipping meals often leads to making poor choices and overeating at the next meal.

When planning meals, even as you wait in line at your favorite eatery or stand in front of the refrigerator with the door open, remember this guideline: try to eat from at least three food groups at every meal. (Aim for one to two food groups when you snack.) Some athletes take this concept a step further by creating their own meal plan. To do this, take the recommended servings you need from the Food Guide Pyramid and divvy them up among three meals and however many snacks you typically have (two to three for most endurance athletes). Having a written plan may help you stay on track.

Eating breakfast improves your ability to perform at school and work and helps with weight control. Making time to eat lunch can reduce stress, enhance productivity, and recharge you for the afternoon, especially if you train at the end of the day. Preparing a gourmet meal for dinner isn't necessary or required, but sitting down is. You deserve a break at the end of a long day and need to refuel for the next one. Besides, sitting down for dinner is an enjoyable way to reconnect with family and friends. Remember, many poor training days can be linked to poor eating days.

Here are some quick fixes to help you eat regular meals.

• Choose to eat breakfast. If you've gotten out of the habit (and that's what it is) or conditioned your body not to be hungry, rethink the importance of this meal. If you're not hungry, check out your current eating habits. You're most likely eating too much or too late at night. Stop eating an hour earlier at night. Keep cutting down the time until you are hungry enough to eat breakfast. Anything goes for this meal from traditional breakfast foods to leftovers. The ultimate quick breakfast is a glass of juice and a glass of milk.

• Make lunch a priority. Again, anything goes. Brown bagging has the advantage of always being available, especially if you can't get away from your desk or other commitments. Pack your lunch the night before and keep stashes of nonperishable items (instant oatmeal, peanut butter, crackers, dried soup, dried fruit, energy bars, and so forth) in your briefcase, locker, or desk drawer for the days you forget. Drink liquid lunches, such as meal-replacement supplements or instant breakfast drinks, when you're really pressed for time or need more calories. If you eat out or at a cafeteria, do your best to make wise choices. Concentrate on eating carbohydrate-rich lunches, not fat-laden meals. Compensate for what you don't eat or can't get at lunch at other meals or snacks.

• Sit down for dinner. To help meet the challenge of what to eat for dinner, save time and mental energy by planning ahead.

TIPS FOR QUICK MEAL PLANNING

1. Work out a system beforehand. Plan five simple meals for the upcoming week concentrating on what the main entrée will be. (Between leftovers and eating out you should be covered.) At dinnertime, simply select one. Some athletes do well with even more of a routine, for instance, chicken every Monday, pasta on Tuesday, fish or seafood on Wednesday, and so on. To add variety, prepare the entrée a different way or vary the side dishes you serve it with (for example, couscous or instant stuffing instead of rice).

2. Keep staples on hand to throw together quick, nutritious meals: milk and cereal, scrambled eggs and toast or toaster waffles, baked potato (use the microwave) topped with beans or cottage cheese, pasta and sauce, soup and sandwich, canned chili and crackers, and so on. Round out your meal with some fresh, frozen, or canned fruit, juice, or vegetables (raw or cooked).

3. Keep a running list of items you need to restock your staples or prepare special meals. Take it with you when you shop. A well-stocked kitchen is the key to preparing tasty, timesaving meals. Shop at a familiar store so you can locate items quickly.

4. Buy part of dinner and prepare the rest. For example, buy a rotisserie chicken or meatloaf and add your own healthy sides, such as instant mashed potatoes and microwaved or steamed vegetables without sauces

or butter. Alternatively, take advantage of preprepared foods, such as boneless, skinless chicken breasts, cubed or sliced cooked turkey, skinned fish filets, prepeeled shrimp, canned beans, instant-cooking grains, salad-bar produce or salad-in-bag, and grated cheese.

5. Cook for more than one meal. Cook meals in bulk on the weekends and then date and freeze them in family-size or individual-size containers or prepare at least enough at dinnertime so you have leftovers to eat at another meal the following day.

6. Stock your kitchen with all or some of these timesaving devices: a sharp knife, freezer-to-microwave-friendly cookware, small electric or hand-operated food chopper, blender, vegetable steamer (no pots to watch), rice cooker, toaster oven (toasts, bakes, or broils small amounts of food), microwave, and a Crock-Pot or slow cooker (requires more preparation time in the morning but dinner is ready when you arrive home).

5. Energizing Your Eating Style by Adding Variety

Eating the same few foods or too much of any single food can be boring and get you into trouble. You can miss vital nutrients that you require and rack up too much of what you don't need, such as excess fat, sugar, or cholesterol. Just as important, eating should be an enjoyable experience that you look forward to. A healthy diet doesn't need to be bland or boring. Reading food labels can help you choose nutritious and good-tasting foods. (See chapter 2 for tips on how to read a food label.)

Here are some tips for adding variety to your diet.

• Experiment with new foods. Have fun with food; buy one new food from the grocery store each week or try a new recipe once a month. Don't get bogged down by thinking you have to create an entire new meal; just make one new item and serve it with some familiar standbys. Keep the best and toss the rest.

• Order something unusual or different when you dine away from home (but don't try this the night before an important endurance event or race.) Not everything you experiment with will be a hit, but you'll never know unless you try.

• Just because you didn't like a food the first time, try it again prepared or seasoned a different way.

• Plan ahead so you can be more creative when it comes time to select or prepare meals and snacks. If you get too hungry or don't have the right ingredients on hand, you'll end up doing what you always do, grabbing whatever is the easiest.

• Forget about observing your forbidden foods list. Depriving yourself of what you really want usually backfires in the end. All foods can fit in a healthy diet; just eat sweets, treats, and other indulgences less frequently or in smaller amounts.

6. Drinking Enough Water

Before the advent of fruity juice concoctions, caffeinated beverages that take longer to make than to drink, and sports drinks full of ingredients athletes don't need while exercising, there was water. Pure, clear, calorie-free, fat-free water. Humble and unpretentious, water does yeoman's service in an athlete's body with barely a hint of recognition. Sure, you may crave it when you feel thirsty or curse the lack of it when you become dehydrated, but how much credit do you give water on a daily basis? (Take another look at your personal pyramid and see how many cups of *water* you actually drank.)

Water is the ultimate nutrient, especially for athletes. Roughly three-quarters of your body weight is water. Muscles are 70 to 75 percent water. Water is the medium in which the body conducts almost all of its activities. Go a month without food and you can survive. Go a few days without water and you may not make it.

Working quietly behind the scenes, water has many functions.

- It helps digest food through saliva and stomach secretions.
- Water helps lubricate joints and cushion organs.
- It transports nutrients, hormones, and oxygen through the blood (of which water is the main ingredient) to working muscles and removes waste products such as carbon dioxide and lactic acid.
- In urine, water carries waste products out of the body.
- In sweat, it helps regulate body temperature during exercise by absorbing the heat generated by muscles and transporting it to the skin where it can evaporate.

Under normal conditions, you lose a minimum of eight cups of water a day through your skin, lungs, feces, and urine. You can easily sweat off several more cups every hour during exercise. Sweat losses of as little as 2 percent of your body weight (3 pounds for a 150-pound athlete) can impair your ability to perform athletic feats. How? Sweating reduces your blood volume, especially if you don't drink while exercising. This drop in blood volume will reduce your ability to take in and use oxygen, which decreases your endurance as well as your ability to handle the heat. Classic early signs of inadequate hydration (even when you're not exercising) include dizziness, light-headedness, headaches, loss of appetite, darkly colored urine, lack of energy, and fatigue.

Don't wait until your tongue sticks to the roof of your mouth to think about your fluid needs. In fact, waiting until you're thirsty means you've waited too long. Stay on top of your fluid needs by drinking a *minimum* of 8 to 10 cups of fluid a day, emphasizing water, fruit juice, milk, sports drinks,

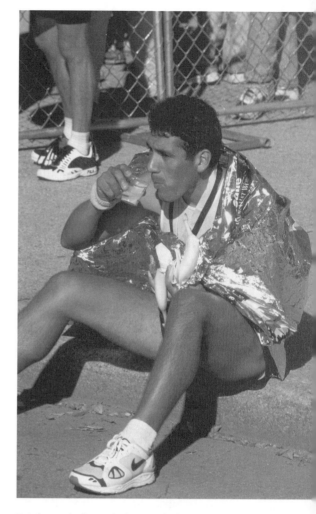

Drink up—before, during, and after exercise.

and other decaffeinated beverages. To prevent kidney stones and reduce your risk of colon and bladder cancer, aim to drink at least four cups as water. Alcohol, soda, and caffeinated beverages like coffee aren't the best hydrating choices. Besides being nutrition "zeros", alcohol and caffeine are diuretics (cause you to urinate), and the carbonation in fizzy beverages may cause you to drink less.

The following are some tips for increasing your fluid intake.

• Begin the day conscious of the need to stay hydrated. Drink an eight-ounce glass of water when you get up in the morning.

• If you take vitamins or other supplements, take them with a full glass of water, not just a few sips.

• Drink beverages with all your meals.

• Drink an extra half-cup of a caffeine-free beverage for every cup of coffee you consume. (It's true that coffee is primarily water, but you don't retain as much fluid from a cup of coffee as you do a glass of water due to caffeine's diuretic effect.)

• For easy access, keep a jug of water on your desk or carry a water bottle with you when traveling or running errands.

• Hydrate and fuel up before you head out to exercise by drinking a sports drink—aim for two cups during the two hours before exercise.

• Have a large glass of water along with your beer, wine, or other alcoholic drink. An added bonus is that you'll handle the alcohol better.

• Make your own healthy soda by mixing fruit juice and seltzer half and half.

Keeping a Food Journal

To get an even better handle on your eating habits, keep track of your food intake for three days (two weekdays and one weekend day) or, if you're really committed, for a full week. Be sure to compile an overall picture of your food intake by recording it on a personal pyramid form (like that on page 7). You'll be able to see patterns develop, such as how you might starve yourself during the week only to feast on weekends, or how you may be missing some nutrients if you routinely skimp on certain food groups.

One of my clients, a health-conscious 20-year-old soccer player, came for a nutrition checkup before heading back to college. A vegetarian, she was worried that she wasn't getting enough protein to perform at her best and help her team return to the NCAA soccer tournament. After transcribing her food records for three days onto the pyramid, she saw for herself that she needed to boost her protein intake slightly by consuming more protein-rich foods such as eggs, beans, and tofu. She was most shocked, though, to see that she hadn't eaten any vegetables in three days!

The value of using the Food Guide Pyramid to guide your eating habits is that you don't need to worry about tracking individual nutrients. Who has time to worry about the more than 40 nutrients the body needs each day? Remember, each food group contains foods that are rich in a package of nutrients. Eating a variety of foods in the recommended amounts from all five food groups helps ensure that you get all the nutrients you need. Besides, you don't need to worry about throwing your system off balance by taking supplements that can contain too much of certain nutrients and not enough of others.

Sometimes a quick nutrition checkup using the pyramid is particularly useful. Whenever you gear up your training another notch, you'll want to gear up your diet too. Keeping nutrition records can be as useful as keeping a training log to determine what works and what doesn't. If you fall into a period of poor training days, take a look at both your diet and your training log. Poor nutrition habits, such as skimping on carbohydrates or eating too few calories can leave you feeling unusually tired and stale in a matter of days. On the other hand, failing to consume enough iron may take a few weeks to a few months to slow you down, but eventually it will as your body's iron reserves become depleted. Your constant battle with one injury after another may also be linked with poor nutrition habits. Athletes who routinely exercise with low muscle glycogen stores incur more injuries. Finally, if you're trimming calories to lose weight make sure you don't trim nutrients by eliminating food groups. Keeping food records will help you be more aware of what you're eating and will help those trying to lose weight stick to a plan.

Energy for Hardcore Training

"When I was racing, everyone was so keen on my diet. It gave me a great psychological edge. In reality, I worked at eating a sound diet that complemented my training and recovery. For example, I shifted my eating habits so I was consuming more calories during the day including a big breakfast (25 to 30 percent of my total daily calories), and I made sure to consume 400 to 800 calories within 30 to 90 minutes following exercise. Every single meal I ate included protein. My diet played a huge role in my success because it allowed me to train more consistently."

—Dave Scott, six-time winner of Hawaii Ironman Championship

Consuming enough calories is key to a performance-enhancing diet. The more arduous the activity, the more important becomes the proper mix of nutrients that supply energy thru carbohydrates, fats, and proteins. As you read in chapter 1, eating a well-balanced, healthy diet will supply the nutrients and calories you need to perform prolonged bouts of exercise. This chapter will provide more detailed information about obtaining the correct mix of fuel based on your training and competitive needs as an endurance athlete.

This chapter is for the athlete who wants to look "under the hood" to understand how to prepare his or her body for future endurance endeavors. The fuel you provide your body affects daily training, your performances, and your overall health. Your training program also influences the fuel the body uses. All of us have heard conflicting advice about eating for endurance activities. What you'll come to understand as the formula for athletic success is this: carbohydrates make up the backbone of a sound sports diet, but protein and fat play crucial roles, too.

Sources of Fuel

The foods you eat provide the potential energy, or fuel, your body needs in three forms: carbohydrate, fat, and protein. Your body can store some of these fuels in a form that offers your muscles an immediate source of energy. Carbohydrates, such as sugar and starch, for example, are readily broken down into glucose, the body's principal energy source. Glucose can be used immediately or it can be stored in the liver and muscles as glycogen. During exercise, muscle glycogen is converted back into glucose and used as fuel by muscle fibers. The liver also converts its glycogen back into glucose and releases it directly into the bloodstream to maintain your blood-sugar or blood-glucose level. During exercise, your muscles pick up this glucose and use it in addition to their own private glycogen stores. Blood glucose also serves as the brain's sole source of energy at rest and during exercise. Your body constantly uses and replenishes its glycogen stores. The carbohydrate content of your diet and the type and amount of training you undertake influence the size of your glycogen stores.

Your body's capacity to store muscle and liver glycogen is limited, though, providing approximately 1,800 to 2,000 calories worth of energy, or enough fuel for approximately 90 to 120 minutes of vigorous activity. If you've ever "hit the wall" while exercising you know what it feels like to deplete your muscle glycogen stores. As your muscle glycogen stores run low, blood glucose plays a larger role in meeting the body's energy demands. To keep up with the high demand for glucose, the body can rapidly deplete its liver glycogen stores. As blood glucose levels fall, hypoglycemia or low blood sugar results. As an athlete, you may be more familiar with the term "bonking." Foods that you eat or drink during exercise that supply carbohydrate can help delay the depletion of muscle glycogen and prevent hypoglycemia.

Fat is the body's most concentrated source of energy, providing more than twice as much potential energy as carbohydrate or protein (nine calories per gram versus four calories per gram). During exercise, the body's stored fat (in the form of triglycerides in adipose tissue) is broken down into fatty acids. These fatty acids are transported through the blood to muscles for fuel. This process occurs relatively slowly as compared to the mobilization of carbohydrate for fuel. Fat is also stored within muscle fibers where it can be more easily accessed during exercise. Unlike your glycogen stores, which are limited, body fat is a virtually unlimited source of energy for athletes. Even if you are lean and mean, the fat stored in muscle fibers and fat cells can supply up to 100,000 calories—enough for over a hundred hours of marathon running!

Fat is a more efficient fuel per unit of weight than carbohydrate. Carbohydrate must be stored along with water. Our weight would double if we stored the same amount of energy as glycogen (plus the water glycogen holds) that we do as body fat! Most of us have sufficient stores of fat, and the body readily converts and stores excess calories from any source (for example, carbohydrates and protein) as body fat. In order for fat to fuel exercise, though, sufficient oxygen must be simultaneously consumed. The second part of this chapter explains how the intensity and the length of time you exercise affect fat use.

When it comes to protein, the body doesn't maintain any official stores for use as energy. It would rather use protein to build, maintain, and repair body tissues, as well as to synthesize important enzymes and hormones. Under ordinary circumstances, protein supplies only 5 percent of the body's need for energy. In drastic cases, such as crash diets, starvation, or the latter stages of endurance exercise when your glycogen stores become depleted, some amino acids (the building blocks of protein) within skeletal muscle can be converted into glucose to provide fuel for working muscles. The brain also needs a constant supply of glucose to keep functioning.

Energy Release From Food

Our ability to run, bicycle, ski, swim, and row hinges on the body's capacity to extract energy from ingested food. As potential fuel sources, the carbohydrates, fat, and protein in the foods you eat follow different metabolic paths in the body, but they all ultimately yield water, carbon dioxide, and a chemical energy called adenosine triphosphate (ATP). Think of ATP molecules as high-energy compounds or batteries that store energy. Anytime you need energy—to breathe, to tie your shoes, or to cycle 100 miles—your body uses ATP molecules.

The body stores a small reserve of ATP and another high-energy compound called phosphocreatine within muscles to power activity instantly. This reserve is enough to fuel several seconds of explosive, all-out exercise, such as when you sprint into the shop to grab the last pair of your soon-to-be-discontinued running shoes. When you perform exercise lasting beyond 10 seconds, though, your body requires an additional energy source for the continual resynthesis of ATP. Fat and glycogen represent the major energy sources the body uses.

The second energy system the body relies on is glycolysis, which is a series of biochemical reactions that don't require oxygen to convert glycogen stored in muscles into useable energy. Carbohydrates are the only nutrient whose stored energy can be used to generate ATP anaerobically (without oxygen). This factor becomes important during high-intensity exercise of short duration. The anaerobic breakdown of muscle glycogen generates ATP (as well as lactic acid) rapidly for a short amount of time and it serves as the primary fuel for all-out exercise lasting one to two minutes, such as running

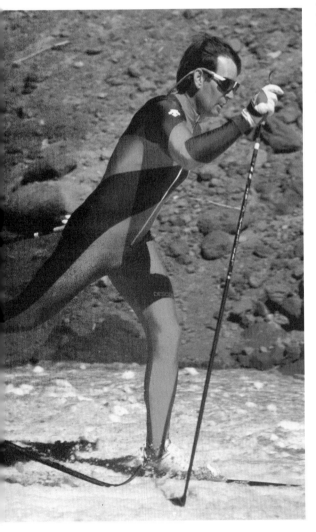

800 meters. During anaerobic metabolism, every molecule of glucose burned yields two molecules of ATP.

As an endurance athlete interested in completing longer bouts of exercise, you predominately rely on aerobic metabolism or oxygen-requiring reactions to generate a fairly constant supply of ATP. Endurance and ultraendurance activities require the body to take in more oxygen (hence your slower pace) so that carbohydrates and fats will be oxidized more completely and yield a more substantial amount of ATP. During aerobic metabolism, every molecule of glucose oxidized yields 36 ATP. For example, during the first 20 minutes of moderately paced, submaximal exercise, liver and muscle glycogen are broken down to glucose and the ATP generated supplies about half the energy the body requires.

The remainder of energy is supplied by the breakdown of fat stores. The complete oxidation of a triglyceride molecule yields 460 ATP. During light to moderate exercise, fat supplies about

Fill up on carbohydrates, not fat, to avoid running out of energy while training or racing.

50 percent of the energy required. The oxidation of fat gradually increases as exercise continues past an hour or two and muscle glycogen stores become depleted. During prolonged exercise, the oxidation of fatty acid molecules can provide nearly 80 percent of the energy the body needs. The complete breakdown of fatty acids, however, depends in part on the breakdown of carbohydrate. When carbohydrate levels (that is, glycogen and blood glucose) in the body fall, the body's ability to break down fat for fuel also falls. So, think of the well-known phrase "fats burn in a carbohydrate flame."

If not enough carbohydrate and fat are present to meet energy needs, the body will turn to using protein for energy. It must first be converted into a form that can enter various metabolic pathways to produce ATP aerobically. In some cases, amino acids can be broken down directly in muscles and the by-products converted into glucose and used for energy. In other cases, amino acids are converted into intermediate products in the liver, and then broken down through the same pathways as glucose to yield energy.

Demand: Intensity and Duration of Exercise

Don't think in terms of burning only carbohydrates or only fat during exercise. Your body uses a mixture of fuels during every activity you do, including resting on the couch. How hard you work (the intensity) and how long you go (the duration) ultimately determine what proportion of fuels the body uses. At rest, you use more fat than carbohydrate (blood glucose) to meet your energy needs. During low-intensity exercise (25 percent of your maximal aerobic capacity), such as walking, fat continues to supply almost all the energy you need. As long as you eat enough calories and carbohydrates, your body won't have to resort to using protein to fuel everyday activities or exercise.

If the intensity of the exercise you perform remains low to moderate (up to 65 percent of your maximal aerobic capacity), your body relies on a mixture of fat and carbohydrate (glycogen and blood glucose) as fuel. As you pick up the pace (increase the intensity above 70 percent of $\dot{V}O_2$max), you have trouble consuming enough oxygen to meet your needs. Your body responds by relying less on fat for energy, shifting instead to burning more glycogen (see figure 2.1). First, fat cannot be mobilized (broken down into free fatty acids and brought to the muscle from adipose tissue) or burned quickly enough to meet the energy demands of intense muscle contractions. Second, the burning, or oxidation, of carbohydrate for energy requires less oxygen than does the oxidation of fat, so carbohydrates become the preferred fuel whenever oxygen is a limiting factor. On top of that, as lactic acid accumulates (as a by-product of the breakdown of glycogen when enough oxygen isn't available), it further hinders the ability of muscles to burn fat. At times of very high-intensity exercise (90 to 95 percent of aerobic capacity), your body relies essentially on glucose.

You've probably figured out by now that how long you go (duration) is inversely related to how fast you go (intensity). For example, no matter how talented you may be, your average speed in a marathon won't be as fast as it is during a 10K race. Fat becomes more important as a fuel source as the intensity of exercise decreases, which occurs as the distance or time you exercise increases. The oxidation of fat, for example, contributes up to 70 percent of the energy needed during moderate-intensity exercise lasting four to six hours. As exercise continues and glycogen stores run low, the break-down of fat supplies most of the energy needed (see figure 2.2). Because the burning or oxidation of fat supplies ATP at a significantly slower rate, however, you cannot maintain the same intensity or pace. Intensity becomes limited to approximately 60 percent or less of aerobic capacity, and only if some carbohydrate is still available.

The limiting factor on performance, therefore, even during low- to moderate-intensity exercise, remains the body's limited carbohydrate stores. No matter how ample your fat stores, once you deplete your muscle glycogen stores, you will experience fatigue to some degree and be unable to sustain your current pace. On top of that, your brain needs a constant supply of glucose. As previously mentioned, if you exhaust your liver glycogen stores and thus cannot maintain an adequate blood sugar level, your body simply shuts down. Remember, too, that a certain amount of carbohydrate breakdown is required for the complete burning of fat as fuel. The longer you exercise past an hour, the more important an outside source of glucose (for example, sports drinks or carbohydrate-rich foods) becomes to compensate for the body's depleted glycogen reserves.

Endurance events, such as marathons and short-course triathlons, and ultraendurance events, such as the Race Across America (a 3,000 mile coast-to-coast cycling event) or 50- and 100-mile foot races, provide particularly challenging situations. Elite marathoners typically race at paces equivalent to 86 percent of $\dot{V}O_2$max, with runners finishing over three hours running at 65 percent of $\dot{V}O_2$max—exercise intense enough to require a substantial amount of glycogen for fuel. Glycogen depletion can also be a concern in ultraendurance cycling, such as the Race Across America and other multistage events, because these athletes generally cycle at an intensity greater than 70 percent of $\dot{V}O_2$max. Riders must constantly ingest carbohydrate-rich foods and beverages on a daily basis (before, during, and after their rides) to replenish their glycogen stores.

Hypoglycemia, or bonking, on the other hand, is often more likely than glycogen depletion at the exercise intensities of most ultraendurance running events (less than 60 percent of $\dot{V}O_2$max), such as 50- and 100-mile races. Well-prepared ultraendurance runners may be very efficient at burning fat as fuel, but nevertheless, the brain needs a constant supply of carbohydrates to function well. As a protective mechanism when muscle and liver glycogen levels run low, the brain shuts down the body until another source of carbohydrate comes along.

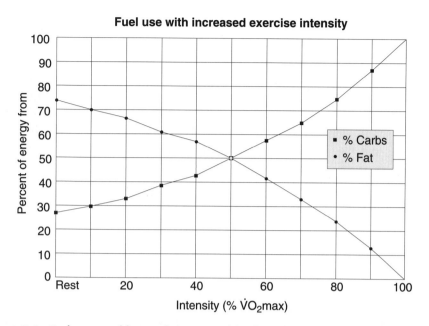

Figure 2.1 Endurance athletes rely on a combination of fat and carbohydrates for fuel, depending on the intensity and duration of exercise.

Reprinted, by permission, from P. Pfitzinger, 1999, "Fat facts," *Running Times*.

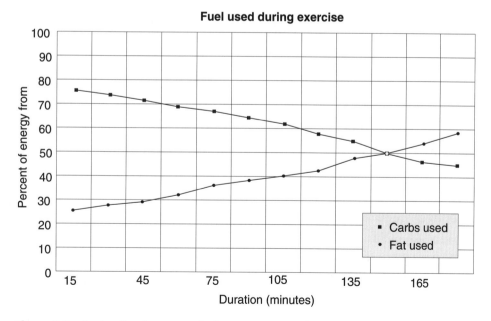

Figure 2.2 As duration increases, fat becomes a more important source of fuel.

Reprinted, by permission, from P. Pfitzinger, 1999, "Fat facts," *Running Times*.

What is $\dot{V}O_2$max?

$\dot{V}O_2$max is a measurement of your aerobic capacity—the ability of your body to take in, transport, and use oxygen. As you exercise more intensely, the rate at which you consume oxygen increases. At some point, however, your body reaches a limit on the amount of oxygen it can consume, even if the intensity of the exercise continues to increase. This point is known as your maximal oxygen uptake, or $\dot{V}O_2$max. As an indicator of aerobic fitness, $\dot{V}O_2$max can predict which athletes will perform well in endurance activities, but it can't determine who will win the race!

Two other factors influence your performance in endurance activities: your ability to perform at a higher percentage of your $\dot{V}O_2$max for a prolonged period (referred to as your lactate threshold) and your efficiency or skill at performing an exercise. Your lactate threshold is the exercise pace above which lactic acid begins to accumulate significantly in the blood. This occurs when glycogen and glucose are broken done rapidly because insufficient oxygen is unavailable (during anaerobic metabolism). Developing a higher lactate threshold means you can exercise more intensely without accumulating lactate—a distinct advantage because the buildup of lactate contributes to fatigue. Becoming more skilled or economical at performing an exercise means your body needs less oxygen to perform the same rate of work (that is, you work at a lower percentage of your maximal $\dot{V}O_2$max), which helps you conserve energy over the long run.

Supply: Diet and Training

Endurance athletes vary tremendously in their energy needs depending on their size, gender, and the sport they engage in. Some athletes have been reported to need over 10,000 calories per day! Endurance athletes, in particular, can have trouble consuming enough calories to balance the energy demands of a rigorous training schedule. No magic foods or formulas exist per se, but all athletes can benefit from taking a closer look at the quantity and blend of carbohydrate, fat, and protein in their daily diet.

Carbohydrate Intake

Carbohydrates are critical for an endurance athlete. You can tap into the power of carbohydrates in four main ways

- by eating a carbohydrate-rich training diet,
- taking advantage of the "carbohydrate window" immediately following exercise,
- loading up on carbohydrate-rich foods for three days before long events and races, and

- consuming sports drinks and other carbohydrate-rich foods (if applicable) during exercise.

Athletes who consistently eat a carbohydrate-rich diet have greater muscle glycogen stores to draw on during training and racing efforts. Remember, adequate muscle glycogen stores help delay the onset of fatigue as you pick up the pace or exercise more intensely (such as in a 10K running race or a sprint triathlon) or when you exercise longer than 90 to 120 minutes (such as a marathon or an olympic or ironman distance triathlon.) Another bonus is that workouts (and races) will seem easier to complete when you have enough glycogen on board to fuel the entire session.

Eating a daily training diet based on three to four grams of carbohydrate per pound of body weight (six to eight grams per kilogram) will speed your recovery from daily training bouts so you can get out the door the next day. You'll also reduce your chance of being sidelined, as athletes who exercise with low muscle glycogen stores tend to incur more injuries. As discussed in chapter 1, breads, cereals, pasta, rice and other grains, fruit and vegetables, dried beans and lentils, as well as milk and yogurt, are the best options for meeting your carbohydrate needs. Foods that contain a great deal of sugar, such as cookies and other desserts, ice cream, frozen yogurt, candy, and soft drinks, supply carbohydrates, but few nutrients. Eat these foods in moderation to round out your carbohydrate intake.

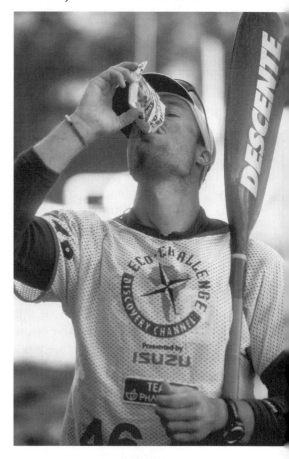

Poor training days or feeling unusually sluggish or stale is often caused by poor eating habits. Why? The effects of glycogen depletion are cumulative. If you don't replenish your stores on a daily basis, you run the risk of digging yourself into a hole. You'll be forced either to back off or to take time off to recover completely. By the way, planning rest days into your training schedule is a good idea. It gives your body time to fully replenish its glycogen stores, which takes about 20 hours.

Refueling after a workout is the last crucial step to getting the most out of your training. A 15- to 30-minute window exists following exercise when muscles are most receptive to replacing glycogen. Unfortunately, many athletes spend this time

Refuel as soon as possible after exercise when muscles are most receptive to replacing glycogen.

stretching, showering, and racing back to their desk, or in the car traveling home after running or riding their favorite trail.

Furthermore, since exercise elevates your body temperature, which in turn depresses your appetite, you can't rely on feeling hungry to prompt proper refueling.

Get in the habit of immediately consuming a recovery drink that supplies both fluid and carbohydrates, such as a sports drink, fruit juice, or a meal replacement beverage (even a soft drink in a pinch). Aim to consume approximately half a gram of carbohydrate per pound of body weight within the first 30 minutes following exercise, which equates to 50 to 100 grams for most athletes. Ease in carbohydrate-rich foods as soon as you can tolerate them. Popular choices include yogurt, fruit, a low-fat milk shake or "smoothie," cereal, bagels, baked potatoes, and energy bars. (To determine the carbohydrate content of sports drinks and foods, check the nutrition facts panel on food labels.)

TIPS FOR READING FOOD LABELS

1. Always check the *serving size* first and compare it to the amount you actually eat. Adjust the rest of the nutrition information contained on the label accordingly. For example, if you eat twice as much as the listed serving size, double all the values given. Use labels to compare food products. Similar foods generally have the same serving size.

2. Don't confuse *calories from fat* with *total fat* or percent of calories from fat. *Calories from fat* tells you the total calories you'll get from fat (in this example, a one cup serving provides 150 calories from fat). *Total fat* gives you the grams of fat in a serving (in this example, one cup provides four grams). To determine percent of calories from fat, use the formula listed in the box titled Calories from Fat [in this example, (150 calories from fat / 330 total calories) x 100 = 45 percent of calories from fat].

   Remember, a healthy sports diet obtains at least 20 percent of calories from fat. This goal applies to your total diet over a day or more, not to a single food or meal. Some foods, such as a slice of bread, will contain little or no fat (12 percent of calories from fat), but others, such as the butter or margarine you spread on, will supply a great deal of fat (100 percent of calories from fat).

3. Use *percent daily value* (% Daily Value or % DV) to quickly tell if a serving of food is high or low in nutrients. A low % Daily Value means the food provides a small amount and a high % Daily Value means it contributes a large amount (based on a 2,000-calorie diet). Check to see if the nutrients most athletes need more of, such as fiber, vitamins A and C, calcium, and iron, have high % Daily Values (20 percent or more indicates the food is a significant source). Your daily goal is to select foods that together provide 100 percent or more of each nutrient (or

average close to 100 percent over a few days). For nutrients that athletes need to eat in moderation, such as fat, saturated fat, cholesterol, and sodium, choose foods that together provide 100 percent or less of the daily value.

4. Check the *ingredients list* (required on most foods) for information on ingredients you may be trying to eat more of (whole wheat, for instance) and others you want to avoid for health, religious, or other reasons. Labels list ingredients by weight from most to least.

Serving Size
Always check the serving size. You may eat more or less than one serving; adjust the numbers accordingly. Keep in mind that the labeled serving size is not a recommended portion size.

Calories
Shows total calories (from fats, carbohydrates and proteins) in one serving.

Total Fat
Lists the total fat contained in one serving (includes monounsaturated, polyunsaturated and saturated fats). All fats listed are rounded off to the nearest .5 gram.

Saturated Fat
This is one of several fats that constitute Total Fat. It's most responsible for raising blood cholesterol levels. Less than 10% of total calories should come from saturated fat.

Cholesterol
Not as significant as saturated fat, dietary cholesterol can also raise blood cholesterol levels. Eat less than 300 mg per day (less than 200 mg if you have high blood cholesterol levels).

Vitamins & Minerals
Your goal is 100% of each for the day, provided by a combination of healthy foods. One food can't do it all!

Calories from Fat
This helps you see how fatty a food is. You can calculate % fat as follows:
(Calories from fat ÷ Total Calories) X 100
Example:
(150 Calories from Fat ÷ 330 Total Calories) X 100 = 45% Calories from Fat.

% Daily Value
This value shows how a food fits into the overall daily diet. Labels use a 2,000 calorie diet as a standard.
Note: If a food has 20% or more of the Daily Value, it's considered a "significant" source of the nutrient. A "low" source would be less than 5%.

Sodium
No more than 2,400 mg a day is recommended for healthy adults. Endurance athletes may need more.

Total Carbohydrate
This total includes several carbohydrate sources: complex carbohydrates (e.g. grains), sugars and dietary fiber.
Fiber: Foods containing 2.5 grams or more are good sources of fiber.
Sugars: This number isn't very precise; it includes naturally occurring fruit and milk sugars.
Tip: 1 teaspoon sugar = 4 grams of carbohydrate.

Nutrition Facts

Serving Size 1 cup (225g)
Servings Per Container 2 1/2

Amount Per Serving

Calories 330   Calories from Fat 150

	% Daily Value*
Total Fat 17g	26%
Saturated Fat 6g	30%
Cholesterol 30mg	10%
Sodium 940mg	39%
Total Carbohydrate 31g	10%
Dietary Fiber 2g	8%
Sugars 6g	
Protein 14g	

Vitamin A	2%	Vitamin C	0%
Calcium	30%	Iron	2%

* Percent Daily Values are based on a 2,000 calorie diet. Your daily values may be higher or lower depending on your calorie needs:

	Calories	2,000	2,500
Total Fat	Less than	65g	80g
Sat Fat	Less than	20g	25g
Cholesterol	Less than	300mg	300mg
Sodium	Less than	2,400mg	2,400mg
Total Carbohydrate		300g	375g
Fiber		25g	30g

Calories per gram:
Fat 9   •   Carbohydrate 4   •   Protein 4

Figure 2.3 Nutrition facts label.

In addition, numerous studies have shown that endurance athletes can enhance their performance during continuous exercise lasting longer than two hours by carbohydrate loading, or "topping off," their glycogen stores. Do this by boosting your carbohydrate intake to four to five grams per pound (8 to 10 grams per kilogram) for three days prior to the event or race. Athletes who have trouble eating enough carbohydrates can supplement their food intake with high-carbohydrate beverages or meal-replacement products.

Last but not least, numerous studies have shown that consuming beverages that contain carbohydrate (such as sports drinks) during exercise lasting longer than 60 to 90 minutes provides muscles with a ready supply of blood glucose for immediate energy, which further spares glycogen stores. Drinking a sports drink may also be valuable during intense anaerobic workouts lasting less than 60 minutes, such as hill repeats or interval sessions, when your body burns glycogen at a rapid rate.

Besides ensuring that you will perform better, consuming carbohydrates during exercise appears to boost the immune system by preventing precipitous dips in blood sugar. A low blood-sugar level signals the body to release large quantities of stress hormones, particularly cortisol. Typically elevated after prolonged exercise, cortisol profoundly suppresses immune function. Take in plenty of carbohydrates and keep your blood-sugar level up during exercise and your cortisol levels will be significantly lower. This may provide just the edge you need to keep a cold, sore throat, or the flu at bay.

The optimal concentration of carbohydrate-containing drinks intended for use during exercise appears to be 6 to 8 percent, the amount found in most commercially available sports drinks, such as Gatorade and PowerAde. (To determine the carbohydrate concentration of your favorite sports drink, divide the number of grams of carbohydrate in an eight-ounce serving by 240 and multiply by 100.) Fruit juice and soft drinks fall outside the established guidelines because they are more concentrated in carbohydrate (as well as low in sodium), which can delay their absorption from the stomach. Above 9 to 10 percent, water may actually be drawn into your gastrointestinal tract to dilute the excess carbohydrates, thereby robbing the blood and muscles of valuable water. Drinking carbonated drinks during exercise may also upset your stomach. Many athletes, however, consume juice and soda with no ill effects.

You may have noticed that sports drinks contain sodium and that some brands taste salty if you drink them when you're not exercising. Sports drinks include sodium for many reasons. It helps speed the rate at which fluid and carbohydrates empty the stomach and are absorbed out of the intestinal tract—good news for working muscles and your brain, which needs a steady supply of glucose to keep functioning. The presence of sodium also makes you feel thirsty (stimulating you to drink), helps replace sodium lost in sweat, and helps you retain the fluids you ingest.

Does Coke Make the Grade as a Sports Drink?

You've seen it happen. An athlete at the top of his or her game drinks Coke during a long race. Is it a smart idea or just something the good guys (and gals) can get away with? To see just how many athletes rely on Coke as a sports drink, researchers at the Australian Institute of Sport surveyed 11 of the 19 men's cycling teams in the 1997 U.S. Professional Championships. How popular was the use of Coke? Every athlete on 6 of the 11 teams and almost two-thirds of the riders on 4 other teams drank Coke. Only one team went for the gold without the beverage in the red and white can. Most of the athletes drank the Coke defizzed in the last half of the two- to six-hour-long competitions.

When it comes to being a winning sports drink, Coke barely qualifies to enter the contest: excessive carbohydrate content (11 percent), limited electrolytes, carbonation, acidity, and artificial colors. Why then does the stuff seem to be the drink of choice for so many athletes? No doubt, the caffeine (30 to 45 milligrams in a 12-ounce can) has something to do with it. Caffeine has been shown to reduce fatigue and enhance muscle strength at the end of exhaustive exercise by working on the nervous system or perhaps by stimulating muscles. And that's not the only good news for athletes who drink Coke during exercise. Research has shown that carbonation doesn't substantially interfere with the rate at which fluids empty the stomach to be absorbed, nor does caffeine taken during exercise act as a diuretic and increase urine output (as it does before or after exercise).

Hundreds of studies have looked at the effects of caffeine on exercise and athletic performance, although the mechanisms responsible for any improvements in endurance still aren't clearly established. Caffeine may help endurance athletes perform better by promoting the release of free fatty acids from muscle and fat stores (thereby conserving muscle glycogen), by helping the body maintain better blood glucose

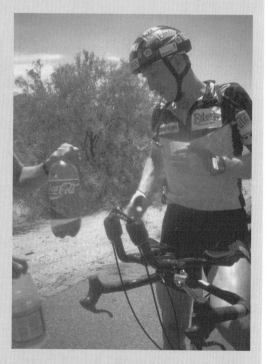

Experiment with soft drinks in training before relying on them in a race.

levels (energy for muscles and the brain), and by stimulating the release of two key hormones—epinephrine and norepinephrine (which also helps increase blood sugar levels as well as enhance the strength of muscular contractions).

Coke certainly isn't the ideal sports beverage for everyone, but keep the following points in mind if you like the taste of it and want to try it during exercise. Diluting Coke with a sports drink (which many athletes do) or water will lower the carbohydrate concentration into the desired range. Drinking it defizzed is the safest (and most comfortable) way to go, especially if you're running. When it comes to the amount needed to boost performance, it's anyone's guess. In order for Coke to supply enough caffeine (most studies use 300 milligrams, or the amount in two cups of strong coffee), you may need to drink quite a bit of it. On top of that, regular caffeine users may not get the same jolt as caffeine neophytes. On the other hand, if you strongly believe that swigging the stuff helps you perform better, you may get the lift you've been looking for. (For more information on the performance-enhancing effects of caffeine, see chapter 4.)

Fat Intake

Since endurance athletes rely increasingly on fat as an energy source during prolonged bouts of exercise, you may be tempted to eat a high-fat diet to improve your performance. Before you begin "fat-loading"(most studies use 50 to 80 percent of total calories), take a look at the research. To date, studies reveal that endurance (also referred to as time-to-exhaustion) doesn't seem to be affected in any consistent manner by following an adaptation period of up to four weeks, a fat-rich diet. In other words, time-to-exhaustion in laboratory trials has been shown to increase (in only one study), remain unchanged, or decrease, when subjects were on a prolonged fat-rich diet as compared with a carbohydrate-rich diet. Consuming a fat-rich diet beyond four weeks has been shown definitively to have a detrimental impact on endurance.

The one study that showed a positive benefit revealed that fat loading did improve trained cyclists' ability to adapt to and use fat as a fuel; however, it did not significantly improve their performance. After four weeks on a diet obtaining 85 percent of calories from fat, the cyclists rode 152 minutes compared to 147 minutes following an average or moderate-carbohydrate diet (50 percent calories from fat). The cyclists rode to exhaustion at an intensity low enough (63 percent of $\dot{V}O_2max$), however, to be fueled primarily by fat oxidation and not limited by glycogen depletion. In fact, most athletes train and compete at an intensity of 70 percent of their $\dot{V}O_2max$ or above, levels at which glycogen depletion is a limiting factor.

Fat loading, or following a high-fat diet that weighs in much above the recommended 30 percent of total calories, doesn't make sense for most athletes. It squeezes carbohydrates out of the diet and lowers muscle glycogen stores, which reduces endurance. In the long term, eating a fat-rich diet could also increase your risk for heart disease and certain cancers. (Despite training heavily, the above mentioned competitive road cyclists saw their cholesterol levels rise while on the high-fat diet.) Don't forget that even very lean athletes have more than enough body fat stored to fuel their endurance endeavors. If you want to improve your performance, manipulate your training program, not the fat content of your diet. Aerobic or endurance exercise stimulates the body to use fat as an energy source. Highly trained endurance athletes are able to use more fat and less glycogen at the same absolute level of exercise compared with less fit athletes.

The news that merely eating more fat won't improve your performance in endurance events doesn't mean you should shun all high-fat foods such as salad dressing, cheese, or an occasional bowl of ice cream. To perform at your best, you need muscles that have adapted to using both fat and carbohydrate as fuel. The metabolism of fats and carbohydrates requires different sets of enzymes. By training hard and long, you train your muscles to burn fat and spare glycogen during exercise. By eating a diet that contains adequate fat (approximately $1/2$ gram per pound of body weight), you also stimulate your muscles to make more of the enzymes necessary for fat metabolism. In other words, you support the efforts of your muscles to build extra cellular machinery for metabolizing fat.

Fat also provides more energy per pound of food. Eating an adequate amount of fat helps athletes obtain enough calories to fuel high-volume training, such as running 10 or more miles per day or participating in multiple training sessions throughout the day. Athletes eating the majority of their calories from carbohydrate-rich foods (about 60 percent) still have plenty of leeway for some fat and, of course, protein too. Besides, how much fun is a diet without some fat in it? Keep in mind though, that even athletes need to watch their intake of unhealthy fats, such as saturated fat and trans fats. Choose lean meats, poultry and fish, and low-fat dairy products, avoid fried foods and don't indulge in fast food and high-fat snacks on a daily basis.

Athletes with high calorie needs often train quite successfully consuming an adequate amount of carbohydrate (for example, 450 to 600 grams a day) and a relatively higher percentage of fat calories (up to 35 percent of total calories). For example, an athlete who consumes 4,000 calories a day (50 percent derived from carbohydrate, 15 percent from protein, and 35 percent from fat) still receives a substantial amount of carbohydrate (500 grams). The calories provided by fat add up quickly and allow the athlete to do something other than train and eat all day. For instance, downing a stack of five pancakes with margarine and syrup is easier, and provides the same amount of calories, as eating 10 plain pancakes.

As for trying to improve your performance by supplementing with fat before or doing exercise, little evidence exists for doing so. The fat in the foods you eat (long-chain triglycerides) takes too long to be digested and absorbed to provide readily available energy during exercise, unless you're planning to be on the move all day. Dietary fat empties slowly from the stomach and the fatty acids it provides typically don't appear in the blood stream (as available energy for active muscles) until three to fours after ingestion.

Medium-chain triglycerides (MCTs) represent another type of fat that could possibly enhance performance during endurance exercise. Unlike long-chain triglycerides, MCTs are rapidly broken down to fatty acids and directly absorbed into the bloodstream and liver. Theoretically, they could be delivered to muscles quickly enough to provide energy, thereby sparing muscle glycogen. MCTs are available as MCT oil, and some energy bars, sports drinks, and meal replacement beverages now contain MCTs.

When it comes to supplementing with MCTs during exercise, the research is inconclusive. Of studies looking at the effect of using a carbohydrate-MCT mixture (delivered by a sports drink) on a time-trial performance, one has shown a positive benefit. After a long low-intensity warm-up (two hours at 60% of $\dot{V}O_2$max), six endurance-trained cyclists immediately rode a simulated 25-mile (40-kilometer) cycling time trial. During the rides, the athletes consumed a carbohydrate drink, an MCT solution, or a combined MCT-carbohydrate drink. The times recorded in the MCT-carbohydrate time trials were significantly faster (by 2.5 percent) than the trials using carbohydrate alone. The riders turned in their worst performances when they drank the MCT (no carbohydrate) beverage.

Other studies, however, have not been able to duplicate the positive effect of ingesting MCTs in conjunction with carbohydrate. Plus, you may not be able to tolerate a large enough amount (the riders in the above study ingested 86 grams) to see a benefit. MCTs can cause cramping and diarrhea when consumed in amounts greater than 30 grams. (To learn more about MCTs, see chapter 4.)

Protein Intake

As much as you might like bagels and pasta, athletes involved in endurance activities can't live on carbohydrates alone. Endurance exercise increases your need for protein. In fact, your daily protein requirement may register higher than that of strength and power athletes.

Endurance athletes need protein to shore up the loss of amino acids oxidized during exercise and to repair exercise-induced muscle damage, especially the trauma that occurs during eccentric muscle work, such as downhill running. Protein typically supplies less than 5 percent of daily energy needs. During prolonged bouts of exercise when glycogen stores run low, however, protein is used as fuel and may contribute as much as 15 percent of the energy needed. Dieting or failing to eat enough calories to match those burned during exercise, which may happen during periods of hard training, also raises daily protein needs.

Endurance athletes require 0.55 to 0.75 grams of protein per pound (1.2 to 1.7 grams of protein per kilogram). For example, a 120-pound athlete needs around 75 grams a day. A 150-pound athlete should get about 95 grams, and a 180-pounder, about 115 grams. Competitive athletes involved in very intense training, such as Ironman triathletes, and growing teenage athletes, may need as much as 0.8 to 0.9 grams of protein per pound.

This may sound like a lot, but most well-nourished athletes easily meet their protein needs. Consider this: eat two eggs and cereal with milk for breakfast, a tuna sandwich and yogurt for lunch, and grilled chicken with baked beans for dinner and you've devoured almost 100 grams of protein. Between-meal snacks can also provide protein, and vegetables, whole grains, nuts, and tofu and other soy products, supply varying amounts as well. Another bonus of including some protein at every meal (and snacks, too) is that it helps stabilize your blood-sugar level so you feel full longer.

Branched-chain amino acids (BCAAs) are of particular interest to endurance athletes due to their potential role in enhancing mental strength and delaying fatigue during prolonged exercise. BCAAs, stored in muscle, can be converted into glucose and utilized as fuel during prolonged exercise. Normally, high levels of BCAAs help block the entry of tryptophan (another amino acid) into the brain, but during the latter stages of prolonged endurance exercise BCAAs levels may fall if they are used as energy to compensate for depleted glycogen stores. Consequently, tryptophan may have an easier time gaining entry to the brain, where it's converted into serotonin, a brain chemical that can induce sleepiness and fatigue.

Although supplementing with BCAAs during exercise to improve performance is sound in theory, the studies to date are limited. Adding BCAAs to sports drinks and other products doesn't appear to provide any additional benefits, nor does it appear to be detrimental, although large doses (most studies use seven to 20 grams) can impair the absorption of water and contribute to gastrointestinal distress. Eating protein-rich foods, such as milk, yogurt, meat, poultry, and fish easily supplies the recommended daily dose (about three grams a day) of BCAAs. (To learn more about BCAAs, see chapter 4.)

Keep in mind that the goal is to maintain lean muscle tissue, not break it down during exercise for fuel! Beginning exercise with adequate glycogen stores and supplementing with carbohydrate (sports drinks, energy gels and so forth) during prolonged exercise remains the best defense against delaying fatigue and preventing the breakdown of muscle tissue. Consuming protein-rich foods shortly after exercise (at your next meal, for example) promotes the rebuilding of muscle proteins and it may help the body replenish its glycogen stores more quickly.

Sources of Fuel During Endurance Exercise

The key functions of carbohydrates, proteins, and fats are summarized below.

Carbohydrates

- Provide an efficient source of energy—Because they require less oxygen to burn than protein or fat, carbohydrates are the body's most efficient fuel. Carbohydrates are vital during high-intensity exercise when the body cannot process enough oxygen to meet its needs.

- Fuel the brain and nervous system—When your carbohydrate stores run low, you become irritable, disoriented, lethargic, and may be incapable of concentrating or performing even simple tasks.

- Aid the metabolism of fat—To burn fat effectively, your body must break down a certain amount of carbohydrate. Because carbohydrate stores are limited compared to the body's fat reserves, consuming a diet inadequate in carbohydrate essentially limits fat metabolism.

- Preserve proteins—Consuming adequate amounts of carbohydrate spares your body from using protein (from your muscles or your diet) as a source of energy. Using protein as a fuel is undesirable because you need adequate protein to grow, maintain, and repair body tissues, as well as synthesize hormones and enzymes.

Fats

- Provide a concentrated source of energy—Fat provides more than twice the potential energy that protein and carbohydrates do—nine calories per gram of fat versus four calories per gram of carbohydrate or protein.

- Help fuel low- to moderate-intensity activity—At rest and during exercise, at or below 65 percent of your aerobic capacity, fat contributes 50 percent or more of the fuel your muscles need.

- Aid endurance by sparing glycogen reserves—Generally, as the distance or time you spend exercising increases and the intensity decreases, fat becomes more important as a fuel source. As the body uses more fat during exercise, limited muscle and liver glycogen reserves are used at a slower rate, thereby delaying the onset of fatigue and prolonging the activity.

Proteins

- Provide energy in late stages of prolonged exercise—When muscle glycogen stores fall, as may occur in the latter stages of endurance activities, the body breaks down amino acids found in skeletal muscle protein into glucose to supply up to 15 percent of the energy needed.

- Provide energy when diet is inadequateæConsuming too few calories or a low-carbohydrate diet causes the body to resort to using protein for fuel, leading to a loss of lean muscle tissue.

High-Protein, Reduced-Carbohydrate Diets

Diets touting higher protein and, consequently, less carbohydrate, are popular among athletes seeking to lose body fat and heighten athletic performance. For instance, proponents of the 40-30-30 plan (40 percent carbohydrate, 30 percent protein, and 30 percent fat) shove carbohydrates aside and claim protein to be the most coveted nutrient for athletes. Carbohydrates are blamed for everything from unwanted pounds to low energy levels. How can this be if glycogen (stored carbohydrate) is the body's preferred fuel during exercise, especially as you pick up the pace?

Take a closer look at this popular, but not necessarily beneficial diet. The 40-30-30 balance of nutrients supposedly keeps the correct balance between two hormones the body produces, insulin and glucagon. Advocates reason that limiting the intake of carbohydrate keeps the body from producing too much insulin, while consuming protein boosts glucagon (a hormone that counteracts the effects of insulin) levels. This optimal insulin-glucagon balance supposedly maintains blood-sugar levels better, improves endurance by increasing the use of fatty acids for fuel, and reduces body fat by increasing the use of stored fat. Incidentally, all the scientific mumbo jumbo referred to in these diets about good and bad eicosanoids (hormone-like substances that regulate a variety of body functions) as being the key to all health and disease is unfounded and unproven by any published scientific research.

High-protein diets hinge on the theory that carbohydrates, not excess calories, do the damage. Eating high-carbohydrate foods, such as rice and potatoes, raises insulin levels. High insulin levels cause the body to store excess carbohydrates as fat instead of burning them for energy. The result is you feel lethargic and fatigue easily as your blood-sugar level dips (insulin moves glucose out of the bloodstream) and you gain weight as high insulin levels inhibit the body's ability to access its fat stores. Eating protein, on the other hand, supposedly increases the level of glucagon, which directs the liver to release glucose, thereby replenishing the body's blood-sugar supply. Lower insulin levels also promote the release of fatty acids from the body's fat cells for use as energy.

Here's a look at the flip side of high-protein, low-carbohydrate diets. First, go too low in carbohyrate and you'll pay the price. It's been known since the 1930s that a high-carbohydrate diet enhances endurance during strenuous athletic events. As you've read in this chapter, consuming carbohydrate before, and especially during, exercise is crucial for endurance athletes. Eating carbohydrate-rich foods (for instance, an hour before exercise) does raise insulin levels and lower blood-sugar levels, but this response is temporary. Most healthy, active people experience no negative effects on performance. Refilling glycogen stores following exercise is also critical. Failing to do so definitely hinders your ability to train and recover effectively.

Second, fat is an important source of energy, particularly at rest and during low-intensity exercise, and training promotes its use as a fuel. The body's limited glycogen (stored carbohydrate) reserves, however, remain the limiting fuel in endurance exercise, even in marathons and ultraendurance events. Plus, the body shifts to burning carbohydrates, not fatty acids, as you increase your pace or exercise more intensely. Your brain needs lots of carbohydrate, too. Who likes having a headache and feeling grumpy and irritable?

Third, losing weight is about expending more calories than you consume. The calories you burn exercising are what counts – not whether you burn fat or carbohydrate. Your body can pull from its fat stores at any time of day or night to compensate for the calories burned during exercise. Besides, eat too much of anything albiet carbohydrate, protein, or fat, and the body stores the excess calories as body fat. As for high insulin levels making people overweight, the reverse is more likely to be true. Being overweight drives insulin levels up. People have trouble regulating their blood-sugar level and consequently, feel hungrier, which makes it easier to overeat. Losing weight through a sound exercise program almost always brings insulin levels back down within the normal range.

By the way, it's not surprising to lose weight quickly on high-protein, low-carbohydrate diets because most provide too few calories for active people. Besides, ketosis (when the body turns to burning fat when insufficient carbohydrates are eaten) promotes water loss and curbs appetite. (Every gram of glycogen is stored with almost three grams of water, so as you deplete your glycogen stores, you lose a great deal of water.) Besides dehydration, ketosis also causes bad breath, lightheadedness, dizziness, and fainting and can be very dangerous in the long run.

Why do some athletes claim to feel, and perform, better on a higher protein, lower carbohydrate diet? Obviously we don't all have the same nutritional needs, and not everyone is an elite athlete training for hours every day. Some active people, especially those who have been on carbohydrate overload (for example, fruit, salad, bagels, pasta, and more bagels), may lose weight or perform better on high-protein diets simply because they're eating a more balanced diet. You'd be amazed at how getting enough high-quality protein, iron, zinc, calcium, and a little more fat can make you feel. Perhaps you've been "fat-phobic"; that is, eliminating protein-rich foods, such as meat and dairy products, because they also contain fat. Adding some protein and fat back to a very low-fat diet means you may eat less because you feel more satisfied and can resist those urges to plow through a box of fat-free cookies in one sitting.

Keep in mind that deciphering complicated formulas and eating specific percentages of nutrients at every meal and snack most likely have little to do with your feeling healthier and performing better. The key lies in eating a balanced diet that tastes good, mixes carbohydrates, protein, and fat at every meal, and meets your energy needs. Eating plenty of carbohydrates, without

Energy Nutrients Needed for Peak Performance

Relying on the Food Guide Pyramid (chapter 1) and your common sense may be all you need most of the time to keep your eating habits on track. At times, however, you may wonder if you're getting the right mix of energy-supplying nutrients (carbohydrate, fat, and protein) to perform up to your true potential. For this approach, keep in mind that the food you eat serves three basic needs; it supplies energy (measured in calories), supports the growth, maintenance, and repair of tissues, and helps regulate the body's metabolism.

Carbohydrate (about 60 percent of total calories):

Training one hour a day—3 grams of carbohydrate per pound of body weight (6-7 grams per kilogram)

Training two hours a day—4 grams of carbohydrate per pound of body weight (8-9 grams per kilogram)

Training three hours a day—5 grams of carbohydrate per pound of body weight (10-11 grams per kilogram)

Protein (about 15 to 20 percent of total calories):

0.55 to 0.75 grams of protein per pound of body weight (1.2 to 1.7 grams per kilogram)

Fat (at least 20 percent of total calories):

Approximately 0.5 grams of fat per pound of body weight (1 gram per kilogram)

- Use the numbers you just derived to estimate your daily calorie needs: (grams of carbohydrate × 4 calories/gram) + (grams of protein × 4 calories/gram) + (grams of fat × 9 calories/gram) = estimated total daily calories

going overboard, makes sense. Otherwise, someone should tell some of the world's fastest runners, the Kenyans, that they're doing it all wrong by eating a diet high in ugali, a starchy corn-based mash that's rich in carbohydrates.

The Body's Response to Training

Athletes often get caught up in manipulating their diet in hopes of performing better, rather than eating to support their training efforts. When you boil it down, the connection between your diet and your training program is simple. Food is fuel. To succeed you must train. To have enough energy to train, you must consume enough energy.

Sure, it's important to be knowledgeable about the recommended nutrition guidelines, however, these recommendations are just that—guidelines. We all know that simply eating properly doesn't guarantee a PR or put you on the winner's podium. You have to do the work. Take Lance Armstrong, winner of the 1999 Tour de France following successful treatment for testicular cancer. When questioned about what substance he was on that led to his success, he replied: I'm on my bike! Your diet plays a key role in your success by enabling you to train consistently and recover quickly. Healthy eating habits also help you avoid days lost to injuries and upper respiratory infections, such as colds.

There are many benefits to endurance training. Keep the following in mind when you're having a hard time riding one more mile, completing one more set of swimming intervals, or running along one more trail in the rain. Endurance training helps you

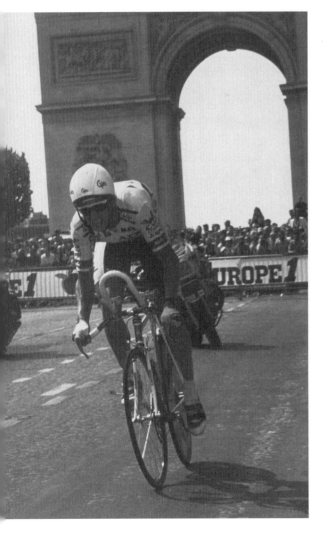

- increase your cardiac output (the maximum amount of blood that can be pumped by the heart every minute), which means you supply your exercising muscles with more oxygen;

- increase the capacity of your muscles to store more glycogen—the fuel the body relies heavily on during prolonged exercise of moderate to high intensity (50 to 90 percent of $\dot{V}O_2max$);

- increase the capacity of your muscles to store fat (triglycerides) and increase the rate at which it's released (as free fatty acids), thereby making free fatty acids more readily available for your muscles to use as fuel during exercise;

- improve your muscles' aerobic energy system by increasing the size and number of mitochondria (site of ATP production) in skeletal muscles, as well as the activity of oxidative enzymes needed to break down carbohydrates and fat to produce ATP. Consequently, a trained athlete has a

The best athletes, like 1999 Tour de France champion Lance Armstrong, eat well to train well, leading to peak performance during races.

greater capacity to burn carbohydrate for fuel during intense endurance exercise and relies less on muscle glycogen and blood glucose as fuel during prolonged sub-maximal exercise; and

• raise your lactate threshold (the pace you can maintain above which lactic acid begins to accumulate significantly in the blood and contribute to fatigue) though, certain types of training, such as fartlek, intervals, circuit training, and sustained tempo exercise, thereby helping to minimize anaerobic metabolism. A unit of glycogen burned aerobically generates nearly 20 times the ATP it could through anaerobic metabolism.

In practical terms, a higher lactate threshold means your oxygen-dependent energy systems have improved and your muscles are better able to clear lactic acid from the blood. You can exercise more intensely without accumulating lactic acid—an obvious benefit because the presence of lactic acid contributes to fatigue and it increases the rate at which glycogen is broken down because it inhibits the body's ability to burn fat as fuel.

All these adaptations help you become more efficient at using fat as a fuel source during exercise. Fats are mobilized and made available to working muscles more rapidly. Training also stimulates your muscles to store more carbohydrate in the form of muscle glycogen. The benefits are twofold: muscles start out with larger glycogen reserves and you use it at a slower rate. This allows you to exercise at a higher absolute level (for example, maintain your pace for longer) before experiencing the fatiguing effects of glycogen depletion.

Remember, a daily diet that supplies key nutrients and adequate calories sets you up to train consistently at a high level. Athletes who accomplish their training goals arrive at the starting line better prepared to handle the rigors associated with endurance sports. Couple the benefits of endurance training with the nutrition strategies for peak racing that follow in chapter 3, and you'll be capable of succeeding at whatever endurance endeavor you choose.

3

Timing Fuel for Peak Racing

"The number one mistake people make is not eating enough. The best nutritionally advanced food is worthless if you start to gag on it after 12 hours. You can't go anywhere without calories, so any food you can swallow is better than nothing. When I'm riding well, I feel like all I have to do is eat enough and I could ride forever. But I can never eat enough."

—John Stamstad, ultramarathon cyclist, world record holder in the Great Divide Mountain Bike Route (2,469 miles)—18 days, 5 hours (self supported)

You've logged many miles and set your sights on completing some personal challenge. It may be scaling a fourteen-thousand-foot peak, finishing your first century ride, or surviving an open-water swim. Or, if the competitive bug has bitten you, the possibilities are endless. Choose your weapon—racing flats, a bike helmet, swim goggles, oars, snowshoes, skis, or trekking poles.

Of course, before you pack all that gear, you want to make certain that your most important piece of equipment is in prime working order. Without a well-hydrated and well-fueled body, you won't be going anywhere very far or very fast. Dehydration and glycogen depletion are two foes you will constantly battle the longer you push your body to perform. Fancy and expensive equipment can get you to the starting line, but adequate fluid and fuel is what gets you to the finish line.

To illustrate the crucial role nutrition plays, especially on race day, read the following accounts from two world-class athletes who were both at the top of their games.

Colleen Cannon, winner of the 1984 World Triathlon Championship in Nice, France, shares her experiences:

> "I really had a hard time eating during long races. When it's hot and you are breathing hard and you try to eat anything at all, it's very unpleasant. During the 1986 Hawaii Ironman, I ate umoboshi plums, which are salty, as well as avocado sandwiches. I totally fell apart even though I had won all the half-Ironmans leading up to that race. I later learned to drink my calories and did much better. Another crazy year I took my juicer to France so I could have fresh carrot juice. I took that during the bike and it made me sick. Then one year I had my husband bring me over a box of Twinkies from the States. That is what I rode on for 100 miles during training and I did great. The Twinkies really made me sick during the race. I did not do well on any of the bars either. In fact, after a PowerBar melted on my bike frame once during a long, hot race, I cannot even look at those things. Everyone is so different, but eating during a long race is an art."

Karen Smyers, winner of the 1995 Hawaii Ironman and the 1995 International Triathlon Union World Championship has had some problems, too.

> "After 1995, I thought I had it all figured out, but I blew it in 1996. I normally go with three bottles on my bike, one with water, two with a sports drink. In the 1996 Hawaii Ironman, I decided to bring more of my own sports drink—two bottles double strength (equivalent to carrying four bottles), which I planned to dilute half and half with water that I would get along the course and one bottle of water. Unfortunately I missed two or three aid stations in a row (either going too fast or dropping the bottle), so for about 15 miles I had no extra water. I was taking my energy gels with the water I did have, but I began to drink my sports drink straight up since I knew I needed

fluid. It was too concentrated and I wasn't absorbing it. I felt like I was bonking, but really, I was behind in water. I totally misread my symptoms. I had my best bike ride ever even though I had a harder time than normal the last 25 to 30 miles. I had enough calories; the problem was that I was dehydrated.

I started the run not feeling good and knew I was in trouble at two to three miles. It was like running in an oven. It was unbearable compared to other years. I was so depressed. I was walking by mile four, whereas the year before I didn't have to walk at all. The next five miles I spent trying different things. I knew I must be bonking now and needed carbohydrates. I would walk and chug Coke, just waiting for the sugar to kick in. My stomach was huge and eventually I threw up at mile 10. I realized I wasn't absorbing anything because I was completely dehydrated. It was almost easier to start from scratch. I knew I needed both water and carbohydrates at that point, but I started to push the water and backed off on the Coke a bit. Finally, two hours into the run I rebounded, pulled myself together, and managed a run of three hours and 23 minutes to hold on to third place overall. In 1996, I was in even better shape than 1995, but I made one error in my drinking regimen and the damage had been done."

These experiences illustrate two very important points about hydrating and refueling for peak performance. First, there's more than one way to get the job done. Second, not even the best athletes always get it right. Paying attention to your need for fluid and fuel is of ongoing importance. After all, success on the big day hinges on your ability to train consistently day after day. This chapter focuses on nutrition strategies for three particularly critical time periods: the week and days before competition, during the race, and immediately following the race.

Timing of Meals

Many athletes I meet would rather not eat than risk being stuck in the bathroom before training sessions or important competitions. Obviously, no athlete wants to start out with a stomachache, cramps, or diarrhea from eating the wrong thing or eating too much of the right thing too close to starting time. On the other hand, studies repeatedly show that athletes who consume carbohydrates up to one hour before exercise improve their performance in endurance events. This extra dose of carbohydrate helps maintain blood-sugar levels and tops off glycogen stores.

Eating carbohydrate-rich foods, such as cereal, yogurt, or a glass of juice, before exercise raises blood-glucose levels. In response, the body releases insulin (a hormone produced by the pancreas). Insulin's job is to move glucose out of the bloodstream and into cells, where it's typically used right away for energy. In the case of the liver and muscle cells, excess glucose can be stowed away as glycogen for later use. In the old days (the 1970s) it was thought that athletes should avoid eating before exercise because high insulin levels were responsible for lowering blood-glucose levels and suppressing the body's ability to access its fat stores. This was bad news for endurance athletes, who need to use fatty acids for fuel to spare limited glycogen stores. Numerous studies since then have revealed that this isn't the case. Although blood-glucose levels may be lowered and insulin levels may be high following a preexercise meal, it's only temporary. Within 15 minutes after the start of exercise, insulin levels fall and glucose levels rise to normal. In most cases, the person exercising doesn't feel a thing, nor is there any detrimental effect on performance.

Eating at least an hour before exercise should allow the body's glucose and insulin levels to normalize before you head out the door. If you don't have that much time, say before an early morning training ride, run, or swim workout, try to eat or drink something containing mostly carbohydrate (a glass of juice, piece of toast with jam, or half of an energy bar) close to the start of exercise. These preexercise carbohydrates may be just the fuel you need in the end, because an overnight fast can cut liver glycogen stores in half. Remember, the body breaks down liver glycogen to keep your blood-sugar level constant during exercise, as well as providing extra fuel to working muscles. A steady blood-sugar level keeps your brain happy and means the pool won't feel quite so cold or the wind quite so strong.

The Glycemic Index

Some athletes are very sensitive to the initial lowering of blood glucose produced by eating within a half hour to even a few hours before exercise, complaining of sugar lows (hypoglycemic reactions) such as sweating and feeling light-headed, dizzy, or shaky. Besides experimenting with the timing of preexercise meals, the type of carbohydrate eaten at preexercise meals may also play a role. The glycemic index (GI), a system that ranks carbohydrate foods on their ability to affect blood-glucose levels, may help athletes enhance their endurance without suffering any negative consequences.

Carbohydrate-rich foods and drinks that enter the bloodstream rapidly after ingestion earn a high glycemic index rating, whereas foods that enter the bloodstream slowly have a low glycemic index. Don't be fooled into thinking that this system neatly divides carbohydrate-containing foods into simple and complex categories or that less healthy simple carbohydrates (candy bar) raise and rapidly lower blood sugar, and wholesome complex carbohydrates (potatoes) produce the desired slow release of glucose and insulin. On the contrary, potatoes produce a rapid blood-glucose response (high GI) and chocolate induces a slow rise in blood glucose (low GI). For a list of low-, moderate-, and high-glycemic foods, see table 3.1.

Table 3.1 Glycemic Indexes of Common Foods

Breads and grains

rice, instant	91	whole wheat bread	69	bulgur	48
waffle	76	cornmeal	68	spaghetti, white	41
doughnut	76	bran muffin	60	whole-wheat	37
bagel	72	rice, white	56	wheat kernels	41
white/wheat bread	70	rice, brown	55	barley	25

Cereals

Rice Krispies	82	Cheerios	74	Life	66
Grape-Nuts Flakes	80	Shredded Wheat	69	oatmeal	61
Corn Flakes	77	Grape-Nuts	67	All-Bran	42

Fruits

watermelon	72	banana	53	pear	36
pineapple	66	grapes	52	apple	36
raisins	64	orange	43		

Starchy vegetables

potatoes, baked	83	potatoes, mashed	73	sweet potatoes	54
potatoes, instant	83	carrots	71	green peas	48

Legumes

baked beans	48	butter beans	31	kidney beans	27
chick peas	33	lentils	29	soybeans	18

Dairy

ice cream	61	milk, skim	32
yogurt, sweetened	33	milk, full fat	27

Snacks

rice cakes	82	angel food cake	67	chocolate	49
jelly beans	80	wheat crackers	67	banana cake	47
graham crackers	74	popcorn	55	peanuts	14
corn chips	73	oatmeal cookies	55		
Lifesavers	70	potato chips	54		

Sugars

honey	73	lactose	46
sucrose	65	fructose	23

Beverages

soft drinks	68	orange juice	57	apple juice	41

Note:
Foods with higher glycemic values produce a faster rise in blood sugar (glucose) than foods with lower values. Nothing produces a faster rise in blood glucose than pure glucose, with a glycemic index of 100. It is generally considered better to have a slow and steady rise in blood glucose rather than a sudden rise in blood glucose. Therefore, foods with a glycemic index below 75 are preferable for usual consumption.

If you're "sugar sensitive," try experimenting with preexercise meals based on low-GI foods. Choosing low-GI carbohydrate foods before exercise, particularly before prolonged efforts, may benefit your performance because of the sustained release of glucose these foods promote (see table 3.2). Conversely, carbohydrate-rich drinks or foods with a moderate to high GI that make glucose readily available work best during exercise. Eating high-GI carbohydrate foods after exercise may also help you more quickly replenish the glycogen you used during exercise. As easy as this sounds, it may not work for all athletes in all cases. Combining foods at meals, including the presence of other nutrients such as fat, protein, and fiber, and even the way carbohydrate-rich foods are prepared, can affect the GI. Other

Table 3.2   Example of Daily Diets With High or Low Glycemic Index

Higher glycemic index	GI	Lower glycemic index	GI
Breakfast			
2 c. corn flakes	77	2 c. All-Bran	42
1 c. 1% milk	33	1 c. 1% milk	33
2 waffles	76	1 apple muffin	44
2 tbsp. syrup	?		
1 c. pineapple chunks	66	1 c. orange juice	57
Lunch			
2 slices white bread	70	1 c. chili with beans	27
3 oz turkey	—		
1 c. watermelon	72	2 bananas	53
3 oz corn chips	73	2 oz potato chips	54
1/2 c. carrots	71	1/2 c. broccoli	?
8 oz cola drink	71		
Dinner			
baked potato	83	2 c. whole wheat spaghetti	37
topping: 2 oz cheese		3/4 c. tomato sauce	?
and 1 oz ham	—		
2 slices cheese pizza	60	1 oatmeal cookie	55
1 green salad	—	1 green salad	—
Snacks			
1 c. ice cream	61	1 c. fruit yogurt	33
1 slice angel food cake	67	1 slice banana cake	47
4 graham crackers	74	1/4 c. peanuts	14

Note:

Each of these diets contains about 2,600-2,700 calories, and 61-63% of this energy is derived from carbohydrate. Those foods listed that have very little carbohydrate do not have a glycemic index (GI) listed. Those foods with a significant carbohydrate content but without published GI are listed with a "?".

practical concerns, such as taste, how easily the food can be prepared and toted around, and how well you tolerate the food, also play an important role in choosing what to eat before, during, and after exercise. Experimenting in training is the best way to find out what works and what doesn't.

Glycogen Depletion and the Bonk

Of course, you don't need to worry about the effect of consuming carbohydrates *during* exercise. Other hormones released during exercise suppress insulin production and single out muscles as the main recipient of glucose. This way, the sports drinks and any carbohydrate-rich foods you consume during exercise help stabilize your blood sugar and provide additional fuel to working muscles, extending the body's limited glycogen stores. In fact, be worried if you weren't planning to consume carbohydrates during continuous exercise lasting 90 minutes or longer, especially if you'll be pushing the pace or really exerting yourself.

Remember, if you eat a normal athlete's diet with about 60 percent of your calories from carbohydrate, you probably store 1,400 to 1,800 calories of glycogen in your muscles a day. An athlete can burn through that in one to three hours of moderate-to high-intensity continuous exercise. When muscle glycogen stores become depleted during exercise, often referred to as "hitting the wall," muscle fibers lack the fuel needed for contraction and fatigue results. Depleted muscle glycogen stores force you to reduce your pace drastically and may even prevent you from finishing the event. Sure, your body continues to burn fat, but it can't turn it into energy quickly enough. If you've ever watched or run a marathon, you may have witnessed even some of the top athletes shutting down and basically shuffling to the finish, running on almost-empty glycogen reserves.

Your blood-sugar level during exercise depends on a balance between the release of glucose by the liver and the uptake of glucose by the muscles. Keep in mind that glucose is the sole source of energy for the brain and nervous system. If exercise continues to the point that the liver can no longer release glucose fast enough to fuel the brain and working muscles, you're in real trouble. Your body needs some carbohydrate to burn as a pilot light while burning fat as the main fuel. What happens if no carbs exist to prime the engine? Your nervous system shuts down, making exercise difficult, if not impossible. Welcome to the bonk.

Because your brain isn't functioning properly due to low energy, bonking means you feel irritable, lose focus, and find it difficult to concentrate. You may become dizzy, disoriented, and even hallucinate. Your vision begins to close in and your balance becomes more difficult to maintain. Molehills turn into insurmountable mountains. Feeling miserable, you can easily make a costly error, such as taking a wrong turn or riding your bike right off the road, or find yourself forced to drop out of the race altogether.

Fluid and Fuel Before the Long Event

After months of deliberation, you finally registered for that killer century ride or mountain run or you're ready to tackle your first triathlon. The check's in the mail. Now what? Better start eating smart. Here's a prerace nutritional countdown that will get you to the starting line a step ahead of the competition.

Weeks in Advance

The best way to prepare for a long race is to do some backward planning. You can't get the job done by stuffing in some pasta the night before or waiting until during the race to experiment with a new food or sports drink. Make the most of your training diet and your training sessions. Just as you experiment with and develop new mental and motor skills in training, you need to experiment with sports foods, including sports drinks, bars, and gels, to establish the types and amounts that you will tolerate in competition or under stressful conditions. Do you really want to lug a fanny pack full of your favorite sports bars only to find that they're hard as rocks and inedible because of the cold or that after being on the road for three hours you can no longer tolerate your favorite candy?

Check out what you can before you arrive at the starting line or head out for your long-anticipated adventure. Talk to other participants and read race applications closely. Look to see what will be provided at aid stations and what you will be expected or allowed to provide for yourself. Adventure races, for example, provide no outside assistance, whereas standard road-running races and cycling events supply fluids and foods along the way. If you don't currently use the sports drink that will be provided by organizers, get used to it by trying it in training. Familiarize yourself with various options for toting fluid and food, such as bladder systems and fanny packs. Rehearse drinking out of a bottle or grabbing cups and swallowing liquid on the move without choking. Test in training what you plan to do during the race.

Travel, particularly to another time zone or country, can interfere with your preparations and routines. Plan ahead by gathering information on restaurants, food stores, and other resources near your lodging and by talking to athletes and coaches who have previously been to the area. If you're traveling into the backcountry, be sure your water filtration device is in working order or have a supply of iodine and neutralizing tablets on hand. Scan outdoor and adventure travel magazines and cookbooks or visit your favorite camping store to research the latest options for lightweight, portable meals.

In some cases, you may find it advantageous to gain a few pounds of padding before you participate in an endurance activity. An extended stay at high altitude or a prolonged backcountry trekking or skiing trip can lead to extensive weight loss when you burn extreme amounts of calories with limited or inadequate options for proper refueling. An experienced mountaineering friend often reminisces about eating a stick of butter every couple of days during his final preparations for expeditions to Everest and other Himalayan adventures.

To put on weight before you depart, you need to increase the amount of calories you consume or reduce the amount you burn through physical activity. If you desire to gain lean weight (muscle mass), you will need to increase your calorie intake and engage in a strength-training or weight-training program. Otherwise, most people can expect to gain a few pounds by eating larger portions of foods they currently consume, adding more snacks or mini-meals throughout the day and before bedtime, and supplementing with high-calorie foods such as commercial or homemade liquid meals or shakes. Tapering your training will also help you create and store excess calories.

One Week to Go

The goal the week before the event is to load your muscles with the glycogen you'll need for the activity. The greater your preexercise muscle glycogen stores, the greater your potential to perform well during endur-

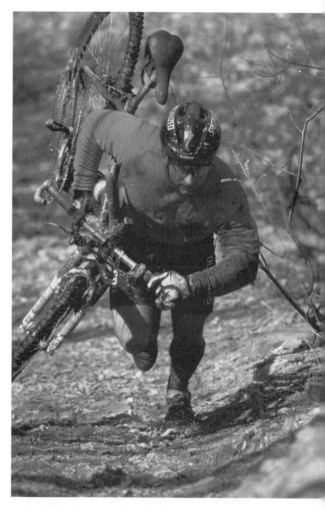

Taper your training and stockpile muscle glycogen by carbo loading for at least three days before long races.

ance events lasting longer than 90 to 120 minutes. Traditionally, endurance athletes prepared for long races by doing a long, hard effort seven days before their event. The rationale behind this exhaustive exercise was to reduce muscle glycogen stores because endurance training itself provides the primary stimulus for the resynthesis and storage of glycogen. After following a high-protein, high-fat, low-carbohydrate diet for the next few days (the depletion phase), you then fed your hungry muscles a high-carbohydrate diet for the three days before the race (loading phase). Although this approach worked well for some athletes, others didn't like feeling poorly so close to their race (during the low-carbohydrate depletion phase) or the stiffness and muscular discomfort associated with superpacked glycogen stores.

You can still maximize your muscle glycogen stores by following a modified carbohydrate-loading regimen. Skip the last strenuous exercise bout (unless it's part of your typical training program) and depletion phase. With a week to go, gradually taper your training while eating your normal diet. For the last few days of the week, further reduce your training, perhaps even resting completely for one to three days, while consuming a high-carbohydrate diet of up to five grams per pound of body weight. If you don't reduce your training, you run the risk of simply using for exercise fuel the dietary carbohydrate you hope to stockpile for the long event. This approach will help superload your muscles with glycogen and it can increase endurance by about 20 percent. If your competitive season involves several races longer than 90 to 120 minutes and you cannot reduce your training each time for the full week, try to back off at least three days before and eat more carbs than usual. It takes about three days of eating a high-carbohydrate diet to achieve maximum glycogen stores.

Many athletes I meet hesitate to cut back their training or eat more carbohydrate-rich foods because they fear gaining weight or feeling heavy the week before a competitive event. You need to realize that gaining weight means you're carbohydrate-loading properly. Every gram of glycogen is stored with almost three grams of water, which can result in a gain of up to five pounds. Remind yourself of the benefits of carbohydrate-loading. You'll arrive at the starting line well fueled and the extra fluid will help delay dehydration during the event. The stiffness and heavy legs you may feel with glycogen loading will dissipate as you exercise. If this is worrisome to you, try resting two days before the event (rather than the day before) and exercise lightly the day before.

You don't need to sit around and eat bonbons for three days either. Use your common sense. Decrease your calorie intake slightly as you taper your training. What needs to increase, however, is the proportion of calories from carbohydrates. Although bonbons and other chocolate-covered treats provide carbohydrates in the form of sugar, they also contain a lot of fat and little else in the way of good nutrition. You don't have to stop eating these familiar foods but save the extra helpings of high-fat candies, cookies, muffins, pastries, doughnuts, chips, and ice cream for after your event or race.

For example, if you typically consume 3,000 calories a day, with 60 percent of your calories coming from carbohydrate, you eat about 450 grams of carbohydrates a day. For example, 60 x 3,000 calories = 1,800 carbohydrate calories. 1,800 carbohydrate calories/4 calories per gram = 450 grams of carbohydrate. To boost your carbohydrate intake to 70 percent of your total calories, you would need to eat about 525 grams of carbohydrates per day. Concentrate on consuming ample servings of complex carbohydrates. Starchy foods, such as bread, cereal, rice, pasta, beans, potatoes, and fruit provide the most carbohydrates (15 grams) per serving. Servings add up quickly at one slice of bread or a small tortilla, half a bagel or bun, three-quarters cup of

Carbohydrate Loading—The Old Days and Now

It's a good idea to get advice from an endurance athlete who really knows what they're doing. Pete Pfitzinger fills the bill. A two-time Olympian, Pfitzinger was the top American finisher in the 1984 and 1988 Olympic Marathons (2:13:53, 11th place in Los Angeles and 2:14:44, 14th place in Seoul, South Korea). Today, Pfitzinger is an exercise physiologist, coach, and the director of the UniSports Centre for Sport Performance in Auckland, New Zealand.

The Old Days: "I did the full carbohydrate depletion and loading diet (three to four days of depletion, three to four days of loading) for 12 of my 18 marathons. The pattern for a Sunday-morning marathon would be as follows: following a long depleting run (17 to 20 miles) the previous Sunday, I would start the depletion phase. For example, a big omelet for breakfast, tuna salad with mayonnaise for lunch, cashews and diet soda (a relative luxury) for a snack, most of a chicken and a salad with diet dressing for dinner. The carbohydrates were low, the calories pretty low, the protein content was high, and the fat content was fairly high also. I would taper my training back during the week and do most of my runs in the morning as I would be too tired to run in the afternoon or evening.

"Wednesday I would run eight to nine miles, with the last three miles at close to race pace to burn off the last bits of glycogen, and I would start to load at either Wednesday dinner or following Thursday morning's run. Loading would consist of a lot of bread, pasta, rice, sweet potatoes, crackers, and cookies. It took a while to realize what was carbohydrate and what was fat. I gradually learned that lasagna was not a good option. I never experienced any particularly negative effects commonly associated with depleting and loading—maybe I was just lucky. The benefit of the depletion phase had a strong psychological component. I thought it worked and, perhaps more importantly, it made me think that if I adhered to it religiously that I deserved to run well in the marathon."

Now: "What I recommend today is a one-day depletion phase. The last week of training before a Sunday marathon looks like this: 13- to 14-mile run on Sunday, 6 miles on Monday and Tuesday, a minidepletion run on Wednesday of 8 miles with 3 miles close to marathon pace, followed by a 5-mile run before breakfast on Thursday morning. Then you start to carbohydrate load. [Lightly jog or rest completely on Friday and Saturday.] There is evidence this one-day depletion provides most of the stimulus of the longer depletion with little or no side effects such as the danger of becoming overtired during depletion or compromising your immune function from the extreme swing in nutrient composition. It also provides the mental reinforcement that the runner has done everything in preparation."

ready-to-eat cereal, a half cup of cooked cereal or pasta, a third cup of cooked beans or rice, one small potato, or one-half cup of corn, peas, or winter squash. A serving of fruit includes a half cup of canned or chopped raw fruit, one cup of berries or melon, a quarter cup of dried fruit, three-quarters of a cup of fruit juice, or one medium-size piece of fruit. Milk and yogurt weigh in next at 12 grams of carbohydrate per cup, with vegetables providing five grams per serving (one cup of raw vegetables, including leafy greens, or a half cup of cooked vegetables, or three-quarters of a cup of tomato or vegetable juice).

Be certain to load up on carbohydrates, not fat (see table 3.3, High-Carbohydrate, Low-Fat Meals). For instance, opt for low-fat frozen yogurt over premium high-fat ice cream, pasta with marinara sauce rather than Alfredo sauce, and thick-crust pizza topped with vegetables instead of meat. If you're having trouble consuming enough carbohydrates from food, supplement your diet with liquid carbohydrates, such as fruit juices, high-carbohydrate energy drinks, or a liquid food supplement.

Check the nutrition facts label of your favorite snack foods, too. As a general rule, snacks that supply at least four grams of carbohydrates for every gram of fat can be considered low-fat, high-carbohydrate foods. A chocolate-covered doughnut, for example, doesn't fill the bill. It supplies only 21 grams of carbohydrate (40 percent carbohydrate) for 13 grams of fat (59 percent fat). A cup of instant pudding made with low-fat milk is a better choice: 56 grams of carbohydrate (75 percent carbohydrate) and five grams of fat (15 percent fat).

Carbo loading will not help you run faster, but it can help you maintain your pace longer before tiring. If your race or event will last less than 90 continuous minutes, a 10K road race or one leg of a relay race for example, you won't gain any advantage from carbohydrate loading. Eating normally, along with a substantial prerace meal, will ensure that you have enough glycogen on board to complete short-duration events and races.

If you will be on the move or engaged in low- to moderate-intensity endurance exercise for several hours, your fat stores can provide the majority of the energy you need to perform, but only if you have enough carbohydrates on board to oxidize the fat. "Fat loading" with a week to go will not enable you to burn more fat, instead of glycogen, during endurance activities. Eating too much fat (over 30 percent of your total calories) makes it even more difficult to load up on the carbohydrates you definitely need. Aerobic training, of course, teaches your body to prefer fat and spare your limited glycogen reserves, but you can't influence that factor with only a week to go.

Be alert to situations or factors that can put you at additional risk for dehydration the week leading into your long event or race. Running a low-grade fever, being nauseous and vomiting, menstruating, and having a sunburn can promote fluid loss. Other situations that increase your risk for dehydration include traveling by airplane, acclimating to altitude, and working out in hot and humid weather, especially if that isn't your normal training environment. Carry bottled water or a personal water bottle with you throughout the day to remind yourself to drink.

Keep an eye out for the early warning signs of dehydration: flushed skin, heat intolerance, light-headedness, loss of appetite, fatigue, and small amounts of dark yellow urine. Don't wait until you feel thirsty to tend to your fluid needs. Drink caffeine-free, nonalcoholic beverages before you head out to

Table 3.3   High-Carbohydrate, Low-Fat Meals

Waffles with fruit and syrup Bagel Low-fat milk	Chili with beans Rice Lemonade Sherbet
Cereal with banana and granola Whole-wheat toast with jam Orange juice	Grilled chicken sandwich Baked potato Iced tea Frozen fruit bar
Roast beef sandwich on whole grain roll with tomato and lettuce Applesauce Fruit juice Low-fat vanilla milkshake	Pizza with mushrooms Salad with veggies Breadsticks Soft drink
Spaghetti with tomato sauce Garlic bread Garden veggie salad Low-fat frozen yogurt Low-fat milk	Chicken on romaine salad with sliced apples Oatmeal raisin cookie Low-fat yogurt Soft drink
Bean burrito Low-fat chips and salsa Lemonade	Turkey sub Low-fat chips Apple Sports drink
Pasta with vegetables Italian roll Strawberries Iced tea	Rice with vegetables and black beans Garden veggie salad Fruit cup Low-fat milk

train (one to two cups of fluid 15 to 30 minutes beforehand), during exercise (aim for four to eight ounces every 15 to 20 minutes), and afterward (at least two cups for every pound of body weight lost during exercise). You should be able to urinate before and after exercise, and your urine should run clear if you're well hydrated. Drinks containing alcohol or caffeine promote the loss of body fluids, worsening dehydration and fatigue. Alcohol negatively affects how the liver metabolizes carbohydrates, as well.

Remember to consider how travel will affect your diet plan. Most airlines can accommodate special requests if you notify them at least 48 hours in advance (even better, reserve a special meal when you make your airline reservation). Make your visits to airport concession stands worthwhile by choosing healthy low-fat, high-carbohydrate snacks such as frozen yogurt, unbuttered popcorn, bean burritos, baked potatoes, soft pretzels, bagels, fruit juices, milk and smoothies, and fresh or dried fruit. Another smart move is to pack your own supply of nonperishable foods. Depending on the destination and length of your trip, include such items as cold cereals, instant oatmeal, instant breakfast powders, low-fat cookies and crackers, pretzels, dried fruit, prepackaged puddings, granola, breakfast and energy bars, canned fruit or fruit juices, instant soups, a peanut butter and jelly (or honey) sandwich, bottled water, and sports drink powders, including high-carbohydrate and meal-replacement options. If you need it to perform well, bring it with you.

International travel, in particular, can cause unwanted problems. Don't test your immune system once you arrive by experimenting with local "bugs." Drink only bottled water (even for brushing teeth), avoid swallowing shower or pool water, turn down ice cubes made from the local water supply when ordering beverages, and stick to familiar foods if possible. Your best bets are foods that have been well cooked, fruits that can be peeled (bananas, grapefruit, oranges, kiwi, and mangoes), and prepackaged ready-to-eat items. Avoid salads and other uncooked foods that kitchen staff workers handle directly and abstain from milk and milk products if pasteurization and refrigeration practices are questionable.

Day Before the Event

The main goal when it comes to eating the day before your endurance race or adventure centers on topping off your glycogen reserves and avoiding any last-minute pitfalls. This is not the time to be adventuresome. Trying new foods the day before an important race or event can be a risky venture. Jen, an avid runner I met while receiving physical therapy, learned this lesson the hard way. After diligently training for months for the Boston Marathon, including experimenting for the first time with using a sports drink, Jen was on pace to set a new PR when I left her office a few days before the marathon. When I paid her a visit the following week, I was shocked to hear that she didn't finish the race. Her enthusiastic friends and husband had taken her to a new ethnic restaurant the night before, and she awoke with stomach pains and diarrhea. She started the race but ended up dropping out at the eight-mile mark.

Be sure to stick with familiar foods and eat them in normal-size amounts. Graze or eat frequently throughout the day, so you don't feel as if you have to stuff yourself at the evening meal. Your last meal should be high in carbohydrates and contain modest amounts of fat and protein. A pasta dinner is a proverbial favorite, but it's not a magical meal. Choose foods you feel comfortable with or that you believe enhance your performance. I routinely eat pizza before my races, dating back to my first year in college when my coach, Jack Bacheler, the ninth-place finisher in the 1972 Olympic Marathon, recommended it. Other elite athletes dine on baked potatoes, or fish or poultry with vegetables and rice. Choose what works best for you. You have enough on your mind at this point, so your last meal shouldn't be something that causes added anxiety.

Other tips to keep in mind the day before the event:

- Drink plenty of fluids throughout the day (expect to urinate frequently).
- Avoid beans, broccoli, cabbage, radishes, and other gas-causing foods if you suffer from bowel problems.
- Avoid high-fiber foods such as raw fruits and vegetables with thick skins, bran cereals, nuts, and seeds.
- Avoid sugar substitutes like sorbitol and mannitol (in gums, candies, and other foods) which may cause diarrhea.
- Limit alcohol or avoid it altogether.
- Set out, prepare, and pack everything you need. Don't wait until the morning of the race!
- Eat or drink a bedtime snack to squeeze in a few more calories and help you sleep better.

Morning of the Event

You don't want to be stuck in the bathroom when the gun goes off or hold back the group because you're running on empty after only the first hour. The most important step you can take is to eat a light to moderate prerace meal. If you've satisfied your carbohydrate and fluids needs throughout the week, you should be well hydrated and your muscle glycogen stores should be at their peak. Your liver glycogen stores, however, may be substantially depleted, especially if you were tossing and turning all night. Liver glycogen is converted back to glucose to maintain normal blood sugar (the fuel used by the brain) and provide fuel for exercising muscles, especially during prolonged endurance exercise. In other words, eating a meal before you compete helps you make wise decisions while you're on the move, like staying on course or remembering to change shoes between events.

Eating a single carbohydrate-rich meal can quickly restore your liver glycogen reserves to normal. Your job will be to find a happy medium in terms of the foods and the amounts you can tolerate: you don't want to suffer from stomach problems or diarrhea, nor do you want to arrive at the starting line feeling hungry and light-headed. Choose familiar foods that you enjoy. I'll never forget my first international race, an all-women's 10K road race that took place in the United States. The Russian women downed a full breakfast of eggs, toast, and bacon, and they didn't seem to suffer one bit during the race. Obviously, they knew what they were doing. Plenty of opportunities exist for practicing what to eat before an endurance endeavor or race. They're called training days.

Plan to eat one to four hours before start time (you can always go back to bed after you eat), and aim for 50 grams of carbohydrate for each hour before the start. For example, down 150 grams of carbohydrate three hours prior to the race by eating a large bagel (50-60 grams) with jam (13 grams per tablespoon), eight ounces of fruit yogurt (34 grams) and sixteen ounces of fruit juice (50-60 grams). Some athletes feel satisfied for longer if their pre-race meal also contains higher-fat foods, such as peanut butter or cheese. Eat early enough, especially if you'll be exercising or competing intensely, since these meals take more time to empty the stomach. If you eat within an hour of exercising, make it a carbohydrate-rich snack (50 grams of carbohydrate), such as an energy bar (30-45 grams) or instant oatmeal (12 grams) with a medium banana (27 grams) and eight ounces of low-fat milk (12 grams). Be sure to drink ample fluids with your meal. If it's caffeinated, drink an equal amount of a noncaffeinated beverage. Aim for at least two cups of fluid two hours before exercise and another cup as close to the time of the race as practical.

If your stomach is tied in knots on race morning, or you have an ultra-sensitive stomach and simply can-

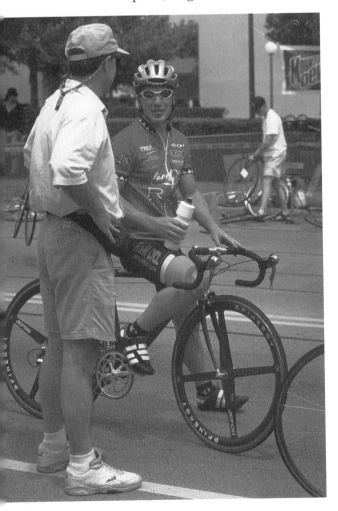

Aim to drink at least a cup of a noncaffeinated beverage as close to the start of the race as possible.

not eat before prolonged exercise, make an effort to eat extra food the day before, including a substantial bedtime snack. Liquid meals, such as breakfast shakes, high-carbohydrate sports drinks, or meal-replacement beverages (for example, Ensure or Boost) empty from the stomach faster than solid foods and leave less residue which may cause discomfort during exercise. Liquid meals are usually well tolerated up to one to two hours before exercise and are handy if you are in transit or have an early start time.

If you shy away from eating before races because you seem sensitive to swings in blood sugar, try experimenting with a prerace meal based on low-glycemic, carbohydrate-rich foods, such as milk, flavored yogurt, whole-wheat bread, bran cereal, pasta, baked beans, apples, and oranges. High-glycemic, carbohydrate-rich foods eaten before exercise, such as honey, white bread, corn flakes, and sports drinks, may cause undesirable reactions in sensitive individuals. Refer back to tables 3.1 and 3.2.

Food and Fuel During the Long Event

The length and intensity of your chosen activity will dictate what foods and fluids you need to consume during your endurance race or event. Stopping to eat a sports bar during a 10K road race doesn't make much sense, but having a bunch on hand for a day-long ski fest does. No matter what your event or race entails, be prepared to battle two major foes: dehydration and glycogen depletion.

Meeting Your Fluid Needs During Endurance Exercise

The loss of body fluids, typically referred to as dehydration, can stop you in your tracks long before your fuel reserves run low. Exercise, especially on a warm day, and you'll sweat, which can mean a loss of two to four pounds of water per hour. As the body's water content drops, blood volume drops, which means less blood is pumped with every heartbeat and less blood is delivered to exercising muscles and the skin. Muscles receive less oxygen, and waste products, such as lactic acid, build up. The body's core temperature rises because less heat is being carried (via the blood) to the skin where it can evaporate as sweat. Your body attempts to compensate by working harder. Your heart rate increases, as much as seven extra beats per minute for each 1 percent loss in body weight due to dehydration.

Athletes of all abilities battle the fatigue associated with dehydration as an elevated body temperature and heart rate take their toll. Studies have shown that athletes slow down by about 2 percent for each 1 percent loss in body weight. For example, a 150-pound runner would slow down by 4 percent after sweating off only three pounds of water (2 percent loss in body weight). At eight-minute pace, slowing down by four percent means an additional twenty seconds per mile. Greater losses, in the range of 6 to 10 percent of body weight, can lead to life-threatening conditions such as heat exhaustion and heat stroke (see chapter 5, Performing Under Extreme Conditions).

Even being mildly dehydrated can affect your ability to make decisions and perform complex skills. Keep that in mind the next time you head out on your bike to bomb down a route with hairpin curves at 45 miles per hour, or negotiate a trail in the dark, or need to get yourself to safety under whiteout conditions. Dehydration also increases your risk for abdominal discomfort and vomiting because it slows the rate at which fluids empty the stomach and move to the intestinal tract for absorption.

Although your risk for dehydration increases the longer you push your body to perform, you need to stay on top of your fluid needs every time you exercise. The closer your fluid intake matches your sweat losses, the better you will feel and perform. Unfortunately, left to their own devices, most athletes don't do a very good job, ingesting only half to two-thirds of the fluid they need. The following fluid-intake guidelines apply in general to all endurance athletes, but you will need to experiment (during training) to find a program that suits the specific needs of your activity or sport. For sport-specific recommendations, see chapters 9 through 15.

1. Follow a predetermined drinking schedule instead of relying on thirst. If you wait until you're thirsty to drink, you've waited too long. Drink four to eight ounces every 15 to 20 minutes or as much as you can tolerate. (Think in terms of gulps instead of ounces. For most adults, one gulp equals roughly one ounce. For younger athletes, two gulps equal roughly one ounce.) Most standard water bottles hold 20 ounces, so aim for one to two water bottles an hour. Try to begin exercise with the largest volume you can comfortably tolerate and continually refill your stomach as a portion of this empties. Larger volumes of fluid (for example, eight ounces) tend to empty from the stomach faster, as do colder fluids. Set an alarm on your watch as a reminder to drink frequently.

Plain water is acceptable for events and races lasting 30 to 60 minutes. Ingesting a flavored beverage, such as a sports drink, however, shouldn't harm your performance and is a plus if it leads you to consume more fluid. If you plan to be on the move for longer than 60 minutes, use a sports drink. Sports drinks designed for use *during* exercise provide modest amounts of carbohydrate (6 to 8 percent) and electrolytes (for example, sodium). The carbohydrates extend your limited glycogen stores. Sodium helps you absorb and retain water and it stimulates you to drink more.

2. Drink early and drink often. Begin drinking immediately to minimize the effects of dehydration instead of trying to reverse it later. Athletes often falsely blame their sports drink for causing stomach upset or diarrhea when dehydration may be the real culprit. Dehydration slows the movement of fluids out of the stomach and their subsequent absorption from the intestinal tract. You can get caught in a self-perpetuating cycle in which you become

increasingly dehydrated because you avoid drinking beverages that seem to cause discomfort. Be especially diligent when exercising in warm weather and during activities that jostle the stomach, such as running. Cold-weather events and sports during which you maintain a relatively stable or horizontal position, such as swimming or cycling, tend to present less risk for developing abdominal pain and diarrhea.

3.   Practice your fluid-replacement strategies in training before you rely on them in important events or race situations. We all sweat at different rates, and the rate at which fluids (and food) empty the stomach varies widely among individuals. Since you need to properly hydrate on a daily basis anyway, practice with the beverages and techniques you intend to use on race day. To tell if you're drinking enough during exercise bouts lasting several hours, monitor your ability to urinate and the color of your urine. (It should be clear to pale yellow.)

Since going without fluid isn't an option, become proficient at meeting your fluid needs without expending a lot of energy. Practice simple techniques, such as drinking on the run. Grab a paper cup and pinch it slightly on the sides to create a funnel from which to drink or add handles to your water bottles. On a bike, grip the handlebar next to the stem when reaching for your water bottle to avoid veering or swerving as you ride one-handed. Endurance swimmers must master drinking while doing a resting backstroke. Adventure racers can conserve energy by sharing water bottles when traveling in single file while walking or running. Reach forward to grab the water bottle from the carrier worn by the person in front of you, instead of struggling to reach around your back. (Obviously, the first person in line must drink from his or her own bottle, but you should be swapping the lead anyway!)

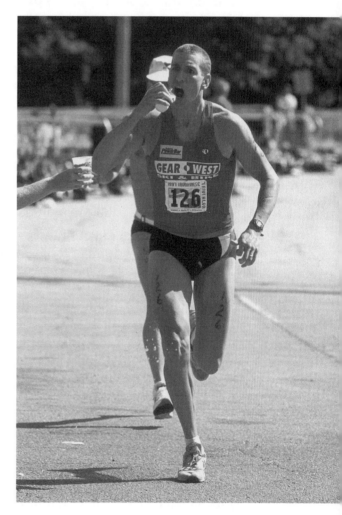

Master the skill of drinking on the run by practicing during training efforts.

Situations in which you need to carry your own fluids (such as events and races with no aid stations, backcountry travel, and ultraendurance events) present an extra challenge. Experiment with hip-mounted water-bottle carriers, fluid belts, sport vests, or fluid-toting bladders worn backpack-style (for example, a Camelbak) to determine what works and what doesn't.

4. Be conscious of the possibility of hyponatremia (low blood sodium) in races or events lasting three hours or more, especially in warm weather. This condition, which causes you to become confused and disoriented, and possibly faint, can arise if you rely only on water or other low-sodium drinks to replace your fluid losses during prolonged exercise bouts. Because the body can lose substantial amounts of sodium, as well as fluid, through sweating, drinking plain water dilutes the remaining sodium in the blood.

The sodium supplied by sports drinks (and foods eaten before or during exercise) is usually enough to protect most athletes from hyponatremia during endurance events and races. If you sweat excessively, have had problems in the heat, or will have access only to plain water, you may wish to experiment with salt or electrolyte tablets. (For more information on preventing hyponatremia and taking salt tablets, see chapters 4, and 5.

You lose appreciably more sodium than potassium (another electrolyte) when you sweat, so taking potassium supplements during exercise is unnecessary and potentially dangerous. Too much potassium in the blood can lead to an abnormal heart rhythm. Most sports drinks contain small amounts of potassium, and foods such as orange juice, bananas, potatoes, dried fruit, tomato juice, and yogurt provide ample amounts.

5. Some other tips to keep in mind:

• Pouring water over your head or body or using sponges can help you feel cooler and provide a psychological boost, but it doesn't help you stay hydrated. Given the option of drinking or pouring fluid over your head—drink it.

• Drinking carbohydrate-containing beverages during intensive exercise or competitions (as well as before and after) appears to lessen the impact of stress hormones on your immune system, which may help protect you against colds and other upper-respiratory-tract infections.

• Your sensation of thirst always lags behind the body's need for fluid. Cold weather further depresses thirst, so adhere to a predetermined drinking schedule when exercising in cold temperatures. You lose a substantial amount of fluid on cold, dry days through rapid breathing (expired air contains water) and sweating, especially if you're working intensely and wearing the proper amount of clothing for the cold. Other confounding factors include exercising at altitude and windy days when sweat evaporates so quickly you may not realize how quickly you are losing fluid.

• Drinking fruit juice and defizzed soft drinks during exercise may increase your risk for nausea, cramps, or diarrhea because of their high sugar content (10 to 12 percent carbohydrate). Some athletes dilute them to half-strength with water or ice. Be sure to try them in training first. If you can tolerate it, fruit juice or a defizzed soft drink could provide a welcome change from sports drinks during long events and races. Be aware that these beverages contain minimal sodium and you may ingest more caffeine than you want with cola drinks.

- If you will be traveling into the backcountry (ski trips, adventure races, trail races, or trekking adventures), check beforehand on the quality and availability of water along the way. No matter how clean the water looks, you need to protect yourself from microorganisms, which can cause significant gastrointestinal problems. Educate yourself on how to use a water filtration device and iodine and neutralizing tablets (in case your filter breaks) to purify backcountry water sources. Water filters and iodine treatment kits are available at stores selling camping or outdoor adventure gear. Water bottles that contain small filters are also available, but they weigh considerably more than a standard water bottle. Be prepared to lug at least two to three quarts of water per person per day if no water is available.

Meeting Your Fuel Needs During Endurance Exercise

As the time you plan to be on the move exceeds 60 minutes, you must pay attention to the body's need for fuel in addition to fluid. Drinking or eating carbohydrate-rich foods during prolonged exercise is crucial on both accounts: maintaining an adequate blood-sugar level and providing a source of fuel for working muscles. Establishing an effective race-fueling routine is the key to being successful in endurance races.

You should have plenty of glycogen stored in your muscles and liver to power you to the finish line of races lasting an hour or less. Eating carbohydrate-rich foods the few days before and at your prerace meal is the best approach for entering the race with full fuel tanks. Staying well hydrated during events or races lasting an hour or less should be your primary concern. Drinking a sports drink isn't necessary (plain water is sufficient). The carbohydrate these drinks provide, however, may give you the extra finishing kick you've been looking for in shorter races.

Traditionally, it was thought that sports drinks wouldn't improve performances in races as short as an hour because you have enough glycogen to last about one and a half to two hours of hard exercise. Researchers have found, however, that taking in carbohydrates and water may be more beneficial than ingesting water alone. One study looked at cyclists who pedaled intensely (80 percent of maximal effort) for 50 minutes and then tried to kick the last several minutes. Cyclists who consumed six ounces of a sports beverage were 6 percent faster than cyclists who consumed six ounces of water. Cyclists who consumed 32 ounces of the sports beverage were an additional 6 percent faster, or 12 percent faster than those who only drank

What Is There to Eat Out on the Trail?

Stacy Allison, the first American woman to summit Mount Everest (September 29, 1988), offers the following advice to day hikers and expedition-bound trekkers alike who set out to enjoy the great outdoors.

- Bring foods you really like. Allison, for example, never leaves home without fancy dark chocolate.
- Bring enough of your favorites to share with others. This builds trust and cements the bonds that form (we hope) between group members during a trip.
- Bring fun foods, like popcorn. There is no better way to make friends or alleviate boredom on days when bad weather keeps you in your tent than sharing a pot of freshly popped popcorn.
- Bring a variety of foods so no one ever goes hungry. Food takes on a whole different meaning on the trail. It can boost morale or cause a whole trip to fall apart.
- Adding spices to your pack adds barely any weight, but they can give new life to the same old foods you normally bring.
- Take seriously the job of staying properly fueled and hydrated. Keep foods and water accessible (not buried in the bottom of your pack), force yourself to eat when necessary (plan at least three mealtimes a day), and try drinking your calories (sports drinks and shakes) when the going gets really tough.
- On extended trips, get everyone to sign off beforehand on the types and quantities of food that the group is taking. The time to find out about likes, dislikes, and possible food allergies is before you leave home.
- Add butter to foods to boost the calorie intake and help foods go down when eating gets really tough, for example, at high altitudes. Allison maintains this is her secret to never losing weight on an expedition.

water. It's worth testing in prerace situations, such as interval workouts or other short, intense efforts, to see if it works for you. If your performance improves, consider if it's enough to offset the time it takes to drink and the potential extra weight if you must carry the beverage.

A properly formulated sports drink (6 to 8 percent carbohydrate plus sodium) should definitely be part of your refueling plan for longer events and competitions. Sports drinks are the most practical way to get the carbohydrates and the fluid you need during exercise exceeding 60 minutes. High-carbohydrate beverages, such as Gatorlode and Ultra Fuel, and liquid food supplements, such as Ultramet and Metabolol Endurance, are generally best used before and after, but not during, exercise. The high carbohydrate concentration of these beverages (along with the fat and protein) means they empty from the stomach more slowly, which increases your risk of dehydration, nausea, cramps, and diarrhea. Ultraendurance athletes use them during long-duration events, though, when the need for calories is almost as high as the need for fluid.

Other carbohydrate-rich foods, such as energy gels and bars, fruit, candy, cookies, bagels, and other solid foods, can be equally effective at supplying carbohydrates during extended bouts of exercise, and they help you feel more satisfied than drinking just fluids. Solid foods, especially those with low water content such as cookies and energy bars, are compact and easy to carry but can be difficult to chew when you're working hard. On top of that, solids take longer to empty the stomach, which could lead to more intestinal problems. Remember, the most important nutrient you need during exercise is water. Solid foods (including semi-liquid energy gels), don't help in that regard, so you will have to drink plenty of fluid along with these foods.

The following general guidelines for refueling during long races and events apply to all endurance athletes. Of course, just as Cannon and Smyers showed us, every athlete will develop their own unique race-refueling strategy. Chapters 9 through 15 provide additional sport-specific recommendations.

1. To delay fatigue, replace carbohydrates throughout exercise before your muscle glycogen reserves become depleted. Don't wait until you begin feeling poorly or can't maintain your pace. Begin supplementing with carbohydrate immediately (within the first 30 minutes) if you know you will be moving for at least 60 minutes or longer. Consume 30 to 60 grams of carbohydrate every hour you exercise. Sports drinks supply fluids and carbohydrate simultaneously. Most supply 14 to 20 grams of carbohydrate (50 to 80 calories) per one-cup serving or 35 to 50 grams per one standard (20-ounce) water bottle (140 to 200 calories).

The longer you're on the move, the more your body will need a readily available supply of fuel of at least 200 to 300 calories per hour. Aim for 60 grams or more of carbohydrate per hour in the latter stages of long (over four hours) events and races. High-carbohydrate foods, such as a banana (30 grams), $^1/_4$ cup raisins (30 grams), energy bar (20 to 50 grams), packet of sports gel (25 grams), or other familiar and well-tolerated solid foods, can help meet your needs (see appendix B for a list of high carbohydrate foods).

Energy gels need to be taken with water; otherwise, they end up as a thick syrup sitting in your stomach. Ideally, to produce an absorbable sports drink that falls into the optimal 6 to 8 percent carbohydrate range, try to drink at least six to eight ounces of *water* with every packet of energy gel you consume. You can carry the contents of three to five gel packets in a small, plastic recloseable container that you can clip onto your shorts or store in a bike jersey pocket until you need it. For backcountry adventures, get a refillable tube (like a toothpaste tube) from a camping supply store that you can fill yourself.

2. Have a game plan going in but be willing to adjust it. Experiment in training, ideally under conditions similar to your upcoming race or event, to get a handle on how to meet your carbohydrate and calorie needs while avoiding intestinal problems. This is truly a trial-and-error endeavor. How much and how frequently you need to eat to maintain a readily available supply of blood glucose for fuel varies widely among individuals. Practice drinking ample amounts of a sports drink (the most you can tolerate) and then supplementing with solid foods (if applicable) as the duration of your event or race increases. If you participate in several sports (for example, a triathlon) you'll need to have strategies in place for each activity. If you're involved with a sport or event that permits support crews, work out a feeding schedule beforehand.

Once you have a defined eating and drinking program in place, be flexible and keep an open mind. Your tastes may change after hours of exercise, during warm weather, or at altitude. You may need to abandon your intention to eat wholesome fruits and sports bars for M&M's and potato chips. Forcing the same routine or giving up on eating altogether usually spells disaster. Listen to your body and eat what you crave or can keep down. Many athletes perform perfectly well eating foods and drinking fluids that fall outside the established guidelines. Getting down some type of nourishment is better than consuming nothing during endurance activities and competitions.

3. Do what you can to protect what is usually an endurance athlete's weak link at some point—the stomach. Build up a cache of tried-and-true foods that are familiar (that is, passed the test in training) and enjoyable to eat during exercise. Keep in mind that solid foods will empty the stomach more slowly than liquids, especially if they contain large amounts of fat or fiber, and are probably more difficult to tolerate during running events and races. Try to drink and eat (if applicable) small amounts continually. Beware of fructose, a form of sugar found in fruit, honey, and products made with high-fructose corn syrup (including some energy bars). Even a small amount can cause some athletes abdominal distress and diarrhea. You may find sports drinks made with maltodextrins (small glucose chains) to be more palatable because they taste less sweet.

Again, pay particular attention to your fluid needs early on. Dehydration wreaks havoc with your gastrointestinal tract and isn't an immediately reversible situation. Don't forget that you should consume energy gels along with plenty of water. In situations when you will not be carrying your own fluid, for example, in road races, consume gels before or at aid stations where water will be available.

4.   Learn to recognize the signs and symptoms of bonking or hypoglycemia (low blood sugar). If you or a teammate (or an athlete you coach) is acting exceptionally irritable, combative, disoriented, indecisive, or lethargic, suspect hypoglycemia. For the quickest relief, stop and ingest rapidly absorbable carbohydrates immediately, such as a sports drink, soft drink or juice, packet of energy gel, glucose tablets, sugar cubes, or candy (gumdrops, jelly beans, and so on). If you only have energy bars or other solid food on hand, eat those instead. Pay extra attention to your food and fluid intake from that point on and keep an eye on susceptible individuals in your group. During exercise in the cold, hypoglycemia impairs shivering, thereby increasing the risk of hypothermia (low body temperature).

5.   In events and races in which you rely on others to finish (relay and adventure races, for example) or for safety and company (treks and ski adventures), make sure everyone takes seriously the responsibility to hydrate and fuel themselves. In other words, pick your teammates and adventure partners wisely. All members of any group should carry fluids and some essential foods in their pockets, fanny packs, or backpacks for convenience and, more important, in case they become separated from the group.

In essence, though, foods and fluids belong to the group and must be given to whoever needs it. Be prepared to share your favorite candy bar; otherwise you may not finish the race or complete what you set out to do. In the same vein, choose your crew or support team wisely. You depend absolutely on these people to arrive on time at appointed sites and to remain unfazed, positive, and supportive even when you're not performing (or behaving) at your best. If you think you have a tough job, try being a crew or support person.

6.   Be mindful of situations when consuming carbohydrate during exercise is particularly important. Relatively speaking, supplemental carbohydrates appear to be more critical during prolonged cycling (two hours or longer) than prolonged running or walking. You may have a harder time maintaining your blood-glucose level when cycling because a smaller active muscle mass uses glucose at a faster rate. Eat often instead of loading up every few hours. Eat by your watch when fatigue or sleep deprivation dampens your appetite. For example, snack every 20 to 30 minutes, aiming for 125 to 200 calories each time (for example, one-two bananas or three-four fig newtons).

Exercising or competing under extreme conditions, such as heat and humidity, cold, and at altitude, also boosts the body's need for carbohydrates and calories. You'll need extra calories to counter an increased metabolic rate at altitude (especially for extended stays), with an emphasis on carbohydrates as your skeletal muscles shift to relying more on carbohydrates than fat for fuel. In cold weather, muscle glycogen, supplemented with carbohydrate-rich foods and fluids, remains the most important fuel. Exercising in the heat (especially if you're not acclimated) increases the rate at which you burn muscle glycogen. (For specific strategies for exercising in extreme conditions, see chapter 5).

7. Develop a taste for a liquid meal-replacement product if you're involved in single-day ultraendurance events, such as a 100-mile running race, or multiday or multistage events, such as a hut–to-hut ski trip or the Race Across America (RAAM) individual and team cycling race. Liquid meals are easier to consume than solid food when you feel exhausted or have no appetite, make good prerace meals, and reduce the need to defecate. Get accustomed to drinking it during long training efforts first. Foods containing moderate amounts of fat and protein can also help satisfy cravings and provide a much needed psychological boost during ultraendurance events.

8. Have a long chat with yourself if you have any doubt about the value of drinking and eating during endurance events and races. Be prepared for the little voice in your head that squawks, "You're wasting time," when you think about slowing down or stopping to drink and eat, especially in the early stages of endurance events and races. Switch over to a new mental tape, the one that says, "I'm increasing my chances of going faster or further or both."

Food and Fuel After the Long Event

Unfortunately, your job isn't done as you flop across the finish line or stagger back to your car. You need to make some small efforts now to rehydrate and refuel to reap some large dividends later, such as a faster recovery from your endurance endeavor. Keep in mind that the effects of dehydration and muscle glycogen depletion are cumulative. If you plan to head back out in several hours, hit the road or trail again the next day, or just want to rejoin the land of the living quickly, you need to pay attention to your fluid and fuel needs even when you least feel like it. Exercising on dehydrated and depleted muscles increases your risk for soft-tissue injuries, and you can make poor decisions when you try to function in a depleted state.

Replacing both fluids and glycogen are the immediate priorities as you set about trying to recover and prepare for tomorrow. (Yes, there is a tomorrow.) Your muscles are most receptive to reloading glycogen in a 15- to 30-minute window immediately following exercise. The blood flow to muscles is enhanced immediately following exercise. Muscle cells can pick up more glucose and are more sensitive to the effects of insulin, a hormone that promotes the synthesis of glycogen (by moving glucose out of the bloodstream and into cells).

You may be able to boost the rate at which your muscles store glycogen, as well as speed up the recovery and repair of muscle tissue, by ingesting protein in combination with carbohydrate at this time. Eating the right balance of protein and carbohydrate (one study used one gram of protein per three grams of carbohydrate) appears to produce a greater secretion of insulin than eating either carbohydrate or protein alone. Along with glucose, insulin also stimulates a greater uptake of protein into muscle cells.

Because it takes at least 20 to 24 hours of refueling with carbohydrate-rich foods to replenish your muscle stores fully, you need to start as soon as you can. Don't neglect your fluid needs either (even doing a good job during exercise, you can only hope to match 80 percent of what you lose by sweating) because you can suffer with headaches and nausea for hours after you finish simply because you're still dehydrated.

The following strategies will help all endurance athletes meet their fluid and refueling needs following a long race or endurance event.

1.   Rehydrate by drinking at least two cups of fluid for every pound of sweat you lose. Weighing yourself periodically in training (before and after exercise) can help you estimate how much fluid you typically sweat off. Sports drinks are probably the most efficient and convenient way to meet your needs because they also provide carbohydrates. Fruit juices, low-fat milk shakes, smoothies, and even nondiet soft drinks will do the trick. Alcoholic beverages are a poor choice, particularly if you're really dehydrated, so if you consume them do so only after you've filled up with adequate amounts of nonalcoholic beverages.

If you haven't urinated within a few hours after an endurance activity or you feel headachy or nauseous, you most likely need to concentrate on taking in more fluid. Be careful not to consume copious amounts of plain water, because you also need to replenish electrolytes, especially sodium. Again, fluid replacement drinks containing sodium are the best option.

Go ahead and satisfy your cravings for salt, especially if you've lost substantial weight during the event. The salt will help you hold onto fluid and stimulate you to drink more.Use salt on foods at meals and include salty foods, such as soup, vegetable or tomato juice, salted pretzels and popcorn, pickles, low-fat crackers, baked goods, spaghetti sauce, and pizza.

2.   After exercise, it doesn't matter whether you eat or drink your carbohydrates, just do so quickly. Aim to consume about half a gram of carbohydrate per pound of body weight (50 to 100 grams for most athletes) within the first 15 to 30 minutes following a long event or race. Because most sports drinks intended for use during exercise (Gatorade, PowerAde, and so on) contain only 14 to 20 grams per cup, make sure you drink enough of them or choose a high-carbohydrate sports drink (50 grams per cup), fruit juice (25 to 40 grams per cup), or, in a pinch, a non-diet soft drink (40 or more grams in a typical 12-ounce can).

The best recovery plan also includes eating carbohydrate-rich foods as soon as you can tolerate them. For example, ease in some postrecovery favorites, such as yogurt, pudding, fresh fruit, a milkshake, an energy or breakfast bar, or a bagel. Aim to consume an additional 50 to 100 grams of carbohydrates every two hours until your next full meal. Some healthy examples include a bagel with jam (about 50 grams), a banana with four fig newtons (about 70 grams), a cup of yogurt with cereal stirred in (about 60 grams) or a baked potato (about 50 grams).

Just as you can't rely on thirst to tell you when you need to drink, don't wait until you feel hungry or your appetite returns to start the refueling process. The longer you wait to eat, the less glycogen you store and the longer it takes to recover. Intense or exhaustive exercise, especially in warm weather, depresses your appetite. You need to anticipate and prepare for a depressed appetite by having foods that you like and can tolerate on hand. A good rule of thumb to follow: drink or eat at least 50 grams of carbohydrate as soon as possible after exercise and then followup with a carbohydrate-rich meal within two hours.

Carbohydrate-rich foods with moderate- or high-glycemic-index ratings (absorbed and digested quickly so they elevate blood sugar quickly) should, at least in theory, enhance glycogen storage after exercise. Examples of moderate- and high-glycemic-index foods include ripe bananas, mangoes, orange juice, sports drinks, cornflakes and muesli cereals, white rice, oatmeal, baked and instant mashed potatoes, cooked carrots, white or wheat bread, jelly beans, and ice cream. (Refer to table 3.1 for more options.)

3. Eating small amounts of protein (15 to 30 grams) along with carbohydrate-rich foods (50-100 grams) appears to help replenish glycogen faster, as

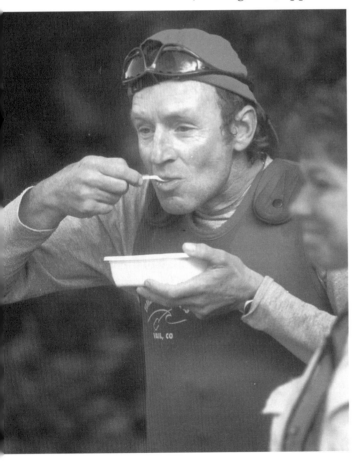

well as help with muscle repair. Tubes of puddinglike protein supplements (10 grams of milk-based protein per tube) are now available for use following exercise, but you can experiment just as easily by drinking a glass of milk or eating a cup of yogurt (eight grams). Including small portions of meat, poultry, or fish at your next meal (three ounces, the size of a deck of cards provides 20 to 25 grams) can also do the trick. For example, a postrace meal of rice with a small portion of chicken, a bowl of cereal with milk, a bagel with a thick slice of cheese and a piece of fruit, or a tuna sandwich with a piece of fruit provides the optimal carbohydrate/protein combination.

For a speedier recovery, consume carbohydrate-rich beverages and foods immediately following a race.

Complete meal-replacement products, such as Ensure and Boost, and other liquid food supplements such as Metabolol II and GatorPro are another convenient option. These products provide a balance of energy nutrients with approximately 40 to 70 percent carbohydrate, 15 to 30 percent protein, and 5 to 25 percent fat. Choose one whose taste you enjoy.

4. Write down what worked and what didn't. Even if you want to forget the whole experience, quickly jotting down some notes now will help you prepare for and succeed in future endurance endeavors. As soon as you can, record fluid and refueling strategies that worked well (for example, one bottle of sports drink and one energy gel per hour) and those that didn't (cookies were too dry or candy bars too hard in the cold to eat). Note how your tastes and cravings changed as the race progressed, any intestinal problems you incurred, your ability to handle the elements, and drinks or foods you want to have available next time.

Supplements for Performance

4

"I remember the first time I had Gatorade. It was in 1968 following a 10-mile road race. I remember sipping it and thinking what the heck is this odd stuff? In those days there was a macho ethnic that said you shouldn't drink during a race because it was a sign of moral and mental weakness. In the 70s I began to drink a bizarre concoction during my marathons—E.R.G sports drink mixed with Pepsi. My brother or a friend would hand it to me at various spots throughout the race—it became my secret weapon drink."

—Bill Rodgers, four-time winner of the Boston Marathon and New York City Marathon

My friend Peter, an avid and dedicated trail runner, performs a ritual every morning and evening. He religiously swallows a tablespoon of a vile-tasting, smelly concoction he affectionately calls bark juice. He hasn't missed a day in the past seven years. Why? Because he's convinced it helps him recover from his weekly training volume of 60 or more miles of running and 150 miles of cycling.

Whether it does or not may be hard to prove. As with many supplements, the scientific evidence doesn't yet exist to rule definitively on what impact, if any, taking a particular substance may have on an athlete's health or performance. What can you do? What should you do? If you rely on your body to perform, I recommend learning as much as possible about the substances you wish to take. With knowledge comes power. On top of that, you'll also need a healthy dose of skepticism and a bit of common sense to sidestep potential minefields when evaluating supplements.

The first part of this chapter presents the most up-to-date information on supplements most commonly used by endurance athletes—some with proven benefits and others with potential benefits for improving your performance. In the second part of this chapter you will learn how to determine if a supplement is safe, effective, and legal to take, and how to better evaluate claims made by supplement manufacturers.

Popular Supplements for Endurance Athletes

The following section contains information on specific supplements that may help you stay healthy and perform better during endurance activities. Before looking to supplements for a boost, however, make sure you have in place a healthy diet and a sound training program.

Beneficial Supplements

I consider the following supplements to be safe when used as directed, backed by enough science to be proven reasonably effective, and legal to experiment with in terms of boosting your athletic performance.

Fluid Replacement Drinks, Energy Bars, and Energy Gels

These items may be the most powerful supplements you have at your disposal. During exercise, you can't last very long without fluid, and you won't get very far without adequate fuel for your muscles. Water is adequate for exercise bouts lasting an hour or less, but a properly formulated sports drink does triple duty by providing fluid, electrolytes, and carbohydrates. As your adventures and races stretch past an hour, your success (from setting a personal record to just plain finishing) can hinge on consuming a fluid replacement drink.

The closer you come to replacing your fluid losses during exercise, the better you'll perform, especially in the heat. An adequate fluid intake helps your heart beat properly, attenuates the rise in body temperature that results from exercise, and delays the onset of dehydration. Study after study has shown that athletes offered either water or a sports drink during exercise will drink a greater amount of the sports drink.

Bars, gels, and sports drinks also provide carbohydrates that help stabilize your blood sugar and act as fuel for your muscles during exercise. To perform at their best during events lasting longer than 90 to 120 minutes, endurance athletes need to consume at least 30 to 60 grams of carbohydrate per hour of exercise. Most sports drinks provide 14 grams of carbohydrate per eight ounces, gels offer 25 grams per packet, and bars (if you can tolerate solid food during your event) range from 20 to 50 grams per bar. Thanks to powders and convenient packaging, you can now refuel easily during most endurance endeavors.

Fluid replacement drinks and sports bars can also be used as part of a carbohydrate-loading regime before

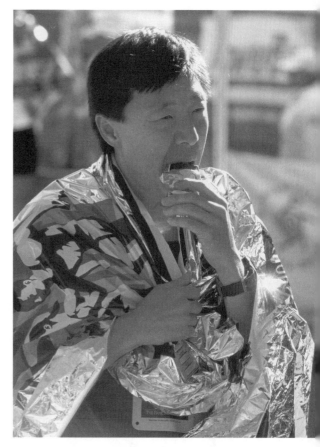

Refuel following workouts and races with easily digestible foods, such as energy bars.

exercise and to help replenish muscle glycogen stores following exercise. Recent research also suggests that drinking carbohydrate-containing beverages in events and races lasting longer than 90 to 120 minutes can bolster the immune system to the physiologic stress initiated by prolonged exercise.

Possible side effects.   May cause gastrointestinal distress, such as nausea and diarrhea, during exercise. May compromise overall nutrient intake if energy bars routinely replace meals and snacks from the Food Guide Pyramid's five food groups.

Advice.   The best fluid replacement drink is the one that you will drink the most of. Experiment during training sessions with different flavors and brands to find products that taste good and sit well with your stomach. Fluid replacement drinks formulated for use during exercise (6 to 8 percent carbohydrate concentration), such as Gatorade, Cytomax, and Race Day, are generally tolerated the best (see table 4.1 for a comparison of the different fluid replacement drinks on the market).

Table 4.1 Comparison Chart of Fluid Replacement Drinks (per 8 oz serving)

Beverage	Carbohydrate type	Calories	Carbohydrate (grams)	Carbohydrate concentration	Sodium (milligrams)
All Sport	High fructose corn syrup	70	20	8%	80
Cytomax	Maltodextrins, fructose, polylactate, glucose	50	10	4%	50
Endura	Glucose polymers, fructose	60	15	6%	92
Gatorade	Sucrose, glucose	60	15	6%	110
Gookinaid E.R.G	Glucose, fructose	46	12	5%	69
Hydra Fuel	Glucose polymers, glucose, fructose	66	16	7%	25
Met-Rx O.R.S.	Rice syrup solids, glucose	70	19	8%	125
PowerBar PERFORM	Glucose, fructose, maltodextrins	60	16	7%	110
Performance (Shaklee)	Maltodextrins, fructose, glucose	100	25	10%	115
PR*Solution	Maltodextrins, fructose	120	30	12.5%	50

Product	Ingredients				
PowerAde	High fructose corn syrup, maltodextrins	70	19	8%	55
Race Day	Maltodextrins, fructose, sucrose	70	17	7%	100
Red Bull	Sucrose, glucose	113	28	12%	215
Revenge	Amylopectin, glucose polymers, fructose	50	10	4%	42
SUCCEED! Ultra	Maltodextrins, sucrose	64	14	6%	trace
Ultima	Maltodextrins	20	5	2%	25
Warp AIDE	Dextrose, maltodextrins, fructose	70	18	8%	80
XLR8	Glucose, fructose, glucose polymers	50	12	5%	40
Compared to:					
Coca Cola	High fructose corn syrup and/or sucrose	100	27	11%	35
Orange juice	Fructose, sucrose	120	29	12%	trace
Water	—	—	—	—	—

During exercise lasting 90 minutes or longer, it's particularly important to consume a sports drink (or water and an energy gel) to prevent precipitous dips in blood sugar. A low blood-sugar level causes the body to release large quantities of stress hormones, particularly cortisol. Elevated cortisol levels profoundly suppress the immune system, leaving you vulnerable to colds and other upper-respiratory-tract infections in the days following the exercise bout.

Experiment with energy bars and gels, too. Reduce your chance of stomach problems during exercise by taking energy gels with plenty of water (ideally, six to eight ounces) rather than a sports drink. To avoid "flavor fatigue" during daylong or multi-day events, develop a taste for more than one flavor of your favorite brand of energy bar or gel. In terms of your training diet, energy bars make handy snacks, but use them to *supplement*, not replace wholesome foods in your diet.

Liquid Food Supplements

High carbohydrate beverages, such as GatorLode and CarboFuel supply a concentrated dose of carbohydrate (40 to 50 grams per eight ounces) to help build muscle glycogen stores before exercise and to replenish these stores following exercise. Other products, such as Ensure, Metabolol II, and EnduroxR4, supply a package of nutrients—carbohydrate, protein, and fat, as well as various vitamins and minerals. Consume them two to five hours before exercise as a low-fiber preevent meal, immediately afterward to enhance recovery, or to provide a concentrated dose of energy, carbohydrates, and nutrients during periods of heavy training or when you need to gain weight. These products can also be easily ingested source of calories and nutrients during ultraendurance events (see table 4.2 for a comparison of some of the different liquid food supplements on the market). Powdered varieties provide portable, convenient nutrition while traveling.

Possible side effects. May cause gastrointestinal problems and dehydration when consumed during exercise, nutrient deficiencies or excesses if routinely used to replace foods in meals, and weight gain from consuming excess calories.

Advice. To recover more quickly from daily training bouts and reduce your risk of injury, get in the habit of replenishing your muscle glycogen stores as soon as possible. Drink either a high-carbohydrate beverage or a meal replacement product within 15 to 30 minutes following exercise, especially if you don't plan to eat a meal within an hour or two. Aim to consume half a gram of carbohydrate per pound of body weight. These products also come in handy as prerace meals and as part of a carbohydrate loading regimen before endurance races lasting longer than 90 to 120 minutes.

Table 4.2　Liquid Food Supplements

Beverage	Serving size	Calories	Carbohydrate (grams)	Protein (grams)	Fat (grams)
Boost	8 oz can	240	33 (54%)	15 (24%)	6 (22%)
Carbo Fuel	3 scoops/16 oz	320	80 (100%)	0	0
Endura Optimizer	2 scoops/12 oz	280	58 (84%)	11 (16%)	0
EnduroxR4	2 scoops/12 oz	280	53 (75%)	14 (20%)	1.5 (5%)
Ensure	8 oz can	250	40 (64%)	9 (14%)	6 (22%)
Ensure Plus	8 oz can	360	50 (57%)	13 (15%)	11 (28%)
GatorLode	2 scoops/8 oz	200	49 (100%)	0	0
GatorPro	11 oz can	360	59 (66%)	17 (19%)	6 (15%)
Genisoy Natural Shake	1 scoop/8 oz	120	17 (55%)	14 (45%)	0
Go	8 oz can/box	190	27 (56%)	15 (31%)	3 (13%)
Metabolol Endurance	2 scoops/12 oz	200	24 (49%)	14 (28.5%)	5 (22.5%)
Metabolol II	2 scoops/12 oz	260	40 (62%)	18 (28%)	3 (10%)
Met-Rx Original	1 packet/16 oz	260	24 (37%)	37 (56%)	2 (7%)
EAS MYOPLEX Plus	1 packet/16 oz	280	24 (34%)	42 (60%)	2 (6%)
OptiFuel 2	3 scoops/8-12 oz	480	100 (84%)	20 (16%)	0
Physique (Shaklee)	4 scoops/ 8 oz	210	38 (73%)	14 (27%)	0
PR*Powder	1 packet/12 oz	190	19 (41%)	14 (30%)	6 (29%)
SUCCEED! Amino	2 scoops/20 oz	150	36 (97%)	1.2 (3%)	0
Sustained Energy	3 scoops/8-12 oz	334	73 (88%)	10.5 (12%)	0
Spiz	4 scoops/20 oz	507	97 (76%)	19 (15%)	5 (9%)
Ultramet	1 packet/12 oz	280	24 (34%)	42 (60%)	2 (6%)
Ultra Fuel	2 scoops/16 oz	400	100 (100%)	0	0

Liquid food supplements are also the easiest and most convenient way to meet your energy needs during ultraendurance events, such as a 100-mile ultrarun or a century bike ride. Experiment in training with any product you intend to consume during an event or race, so you know what to expect of its taste and how it will settle in your stomach. Ingesting both carbohydrate and protein in the latter stages of ultraendurance events may help lessen the breakdown of muscle tissue associated with these endeavors.

Round out a healthy diet with these products, especially if you need extra calories or are trying to gain weight. Homemade milk and yogurt smoothies, beverages fortified with nonfat dried milk powder, or instant breakfast drinks can serve the same purpose. Keep in mind that you need adequate protein, carbohydrates, and calories (along with a weightlifting program, of course) to build lean muscle mass. Excess protein beyond your needs (as supplied by high-protein drinks) will be stored as fat instead of contributing to muscle growth, and it will increase your need for fluid. If you're trying to lose weight, watch out for the calories these products pack.

Finally, keep a supply of meal replacement products on hand to use as backup meals while recovering from exhaustive efforts or races, when traveling, or on busy days when you would otherwise skip meals or eat poorly.

Multivitamin/Mineral Supplement

Take a multivitamin/mineral supplement to bolster a diet that is sometimes less than adequate, especially if you're dieting, are lactose-intolerant (possible riboflavin, calcium, and vitamin D deficiencies), or if you avoid foods because of food allergies. Multivitamins are also appropriate for vegetarian athletes (who run the risk of being low in iron, zinc, and other nutrients) and women who are trying to become pregnant (you need at least 400 milligrams of folic acid daily to help prevent birth defects).

Possible side effects.   Some athletes may rely too heavily on a multivitamin to compensate for a poor diet. Multivitamins may supply too little or too much of key nutrients.

Advice.   Along with taking a multivitamin, work on making better food choices. Vitamin/mineral supplements don't give you energy (calories), fiber, phytochemicals, or yet-to-be-discovered magic bullets that occur naturally in foods. Eating right is still key. Choose a brand with 100 percent of the daily value for most nutrients and be sure it carries the United States Pharmacopeia (USP) stamp of approval to guarantee that it will dissolve properly (but not necessarily be absorbed effectively) in the body. Take your daily multivitamin/mineral supplement with a meal to enhance absorption.

Men and nonmenstruating women may need to consider a supplement with little (10 milligrams) or no iron to avoid iron overload. Most multivitamins contain negligible amounts of calcium (the pill would be too big to swallow), so you may need a calcium supplement too.

Calcium

Besides building strong bones and teeth, calcium helps muscles contract, nerves send messages, and blood clot properly. Consuming an adequate amount throughout life, especially during adolescence and the early adult years, reduces the risk of osteoporosis (a condition characterized by brittle bones that break easily). Calcium may also play a role in alleviating symptoms of premenstrual syndrome and hypertension (high blood pressure).

Possible side effects. May cause kidney stones in some individuals. Some athletes may rely too heavily on a calcium supplement to compensate for poor eating habits.

Advice. Calcium can be found in foods from all of the food groups, so work on including alternative sources if you don't drink milk or eat dairy products (see chapter 1, Best Bets: Calcium). Aim for 1,000 milligrams a day (1,300 milligrams for younger athletes age 9 to 18, 1,200 milligrams for adults over age 50). Peak bone mass is gained between the ages of 16 and 25. The more calcium you deposit into your bones, the more withdrawals you can withstand (as you get older) before you get into trouble.

If you can't get all the calcium you need from your diet, you should take a supplement. To get the best absorption, take your calcium supplements at mealtimes and divide your dose throughout the day, taking no more than 500 milligrams at a time. (Pay attention to the amount of *elemental* calcium listed per tablet.) Don't take more than you need and be careful not to think of your supplement (like Tums or Viactiv soft calcium chews) as candy.

Choose a calcium supplement that contains vitamin D (needed by the body to absorb calcium efficiently) or if you take a multivitamin, check to make sure it contains 200 to 400 IU of vitamin D. Calcium carbonate is generally well absorbed, but choose calcium citrate if you plan to take your supplements between meals. If you take a multi containing iron as well as a calcium supplement, don't take them at the same time if you have problems with a low blood-iron level (anemia). High doses of calcium can impair your ability to absorb iron. If you want to experiment with alleviating mild to moderate premenstrual symptoms, take 1,200 milligrams of calcium a day for at least two to three months.

Iron

Iron is an essential component of the oxygen carriers hemoglobin (found in red blood cells) and myoglobin (found in muscle cells), as well as some of the oxidative enzymes needed to convert food into fuel for working muscles. Inadequate hemoglobin or body-iron stores (ferritin) affect how the body transports and uses oxygen and impairs performance in endurance activities.

Possible side effects. May cause constipation or diarrhea, or contribute to hemochromatosis (iron overload).

Advice. Work at obtaining adequate iron by eating foods rich in heme iron (meat, fish, and poultry) and nonheme iron (plant sources such as dark green leafy vegetables, tofu, dried beans, dried fruit, and fortified foods). Keep in mind that heme iron is absorbed better than the iron from plant foods or supplements. To increase the absorption of the nonheme iron in plant foods, consume these foods with heme-rich foods, such as three-bean chili with a small amount of meat added, or eat foods high in vitamin C along with foods that provide nonheme iron. Drink a glass of orange juice, for example, with a bowl of iron-fortified cereal.

Monitor your iron status through blood tests that measure hemoglobin, hematocrit, and ferritin (iron stores). Female endurance athletes and athletes training at altitude, in particular, may want to supplement with a small daily dose of iron 15 milligrams for teenage and adult females, 12 milligrams for teenage males, or 10 milligrams for adult males to prevent iron depletion during training. Most multivitamins contain iron, so check the label before you take an additional supplement.

If your hemoglobin and iron stores are normal, taking iron supplements will not boost your performance, and it could be harmful. Hemochromatosis, or iron overload, is a genetic disorder affecting as many as one in every 200 people. Hemochromatosis disrupts iron metabolism in such a way that the body absorbs too much iron. The excess iron deposits in the liver, heart, joints, and other tissues, damaging these tissues and potentially increasing the risk for heart disease and cancer. Since this disorder is not routinely screened for, take large doses of supplemental iron only if you've been diagnosed as iron-depleted or anemic by your physician, and then only until your iron status normalizes.

Antioxidants

Antioxidants, such as vitamins C and E, and beta-carotene, protect cells and tissues by working to neutralize the damaging effects of free radicals (by-products of strenuous aerobic exercise, pollution, cigarette smoke, and so on). Consuming supplemental doses of antioxidants might translate into less muscle tissue damage, speedier recoveries, and a bolstered immune system, as well as help prevent some chronic diseases like heart disease. Antioxidants have not been found to directly improve athletic performances.

Possible side effects. Excessive vitamin C (such as 1,000 to 3,000 milligrams) can cause diarrhea and kidney stones in some people. Excessive vitamin E (over 800 IUs for long periods of time) can lead to fatigue, headaches, and diarrhea, as well as impaired immunity. Vitamin E supplements can also interfere with anti-blood-clotting medications. Excessive vitamin A (such as 10,000 to 20,000 IU) can lead to liver damage, cause birth defects, and possibly osteoporosis.

Advice. Antioxidants found in food cannot always be replicated in a pill. Many of these compounds work together and when isolated could produce effects significantly weaker than desired. Your best bet is to eat a diet rich in nutrient-dense fruits and vegetables to obtain beta-carotene (converted to vitamin A in the body) and vitamin C, as well as other antioxidants coming to light. Develop a taste for brightly colored fruits and vegetables such as papaya, cantaloupe, strawberries, apricots, oranges, grapefruit, kiwis, mangoes, sweet potatoes, carrots, spinach, collard greens, broccoli, red peppers, and kale.

Antioxidants work quietly behind the scenes, so don't take megadoses to try to see an effect. Beta-carotene, for example, is only one of 600 carotenoids discovered to date. Be cautious about taking a beta-carotene supplement (if you do, keep it to three milligrams or less), since supplementing with too much of one carotenoid may interfere with the absorption of others. Vitamin A can be toxic, so don't take more than the RDA (5,000 IU).

Consider taking a vitamin C supplement if you participate in ultraendurance events (about 600 milligrams a day for at least one week before the event), which may help protect important immune cells. Meeting the RDA for vitamin E (15 IU for males, 12 IU for females) can be difficult for even the most nutrition-conscious athlete (vitamin E is found in vegetable oils, margarine, nuts and seeds, wheat germ, and whole-grain products). For protective health benefits, consider supplementing your diet with a daily dose of 100 to 400 IUs of vitamin E, especially if you eat a very low-fat diet, train at altitude, exercise in heavily polluted areas, or are at risk for heart disease. (Be sure to check with your physician first and don't take vitamin E supplements if you take anti-blood-clotting medications.) To get the most from your vitamin E supplement, choose one that contains natural vitamin E (also called d-alpha tocopherol or RRR-alpha) rather than synthetic vitamin E (dl-alpha-tocopherol or all-rac alpha).

TIPS FOR AVOIDING A COLD

Your biggest fear may not be hiking through whiteout conditions or descending a steep hill at 40 miles per hour on your bike, but simply the thought of catching a cold. As an athlete, you know that a common cold or other upper-respiratory-tract infection can keep you from even getting to the starting line of your favorite activity. What can you do besides pay homage to vitamin C tablets? Plenty.

1. Eat a well-balanced diet. Keep your vitamin and mineral reserves at optimal levels so your immune system will function at its best.

2. Don't shortchange yourself in the sleep department. Disrupted sleep has been linked to a suppressed immune system.

3. Avoid overtraining and chronic fatigue. When in doubt, leave it out, especially if you feel like you're coming down with something. Give your body a chance to mount an attack without the extra stress generated by intense or prolonged physical efforts.

4. Wash your hands often. Viruses can easily enter your body when you touch germ-ridden hands to your eyes and nose.

5. Avoid large crowds and sick people whenever possible before important events. Consider getting a flu shot if you compete during the winter. You're particularly vulnerable to catching something immediately following a workout or race, so choose your companions wisely!

6. Use carbohydrate-containing beverages before, during, and after intensive training bouts and competitive efforts, which may help lessen the impact of stress hormones on your immune system.

7. Don't try to drop weight quickly before a competitive event. Rapid weight loss stresses the immune system.

8. Keep other life stresses to a minimum. When this isn't possible, recognize that you're vulnerable to colds and infections, and moderate your training accordingly.

9. Experiment with supplements. The popular herb Echinacea may boost your resistance to colds, flu, and other upper-respiratory-tract infections by stimulating certain white blood cells to destroy invading organisms before they become infectious. It's most effective when taken every two hours until symptoms are relieved. Take it for short periods—a few days to a few weeks. Continual use can actually suppress your immune system. (Don't take it at all if you're pregnant, nursing, have an autoimmune disease, or have allergies to ragweed.)

10. Sucking on zinc lozenges (the published research was done with zinc gluconate) may reduce the severity and duration of a cold if you take them at the first sign of sniffles. To avoid zinc overload, don't take them for more than a week at a time. Avoid drinking citrus juices and soft drinks, which can interfere with zinc absorption, one half hour before and after the lozenges. To reduce feelings of nausea, don't take them on an empty stomach.

11. Taking vitamin C supplements will not prevent you from catching a cold but may help you feel better while you have it. Limit yourself to 1,000 milligrams a day, no more than 500 milligrams per dose. Larger doses might trigger diarrhea or kidney stones in some people. Athletes participating in ultraevents may reduce the oxidative stress to their immune cells by taking vitamin C supplements (about 600 milligrams a day for at least one week before the event).

12. If you do come down with a cold, comfort yourself with an 800-year-old remedy. Remember a big bowl of hot chicken soup that can improve coughing and help clear the lungs.

Adapted, by permission, from D.C. Nieman, 1998, "Immunity in athletes: current issues," *Sports Science Exchange*, 69 (11).

Supplements That Might Be Helpful

The following section profiles several popular supplements that may improve your performance in endurance activities, but research is mixed. I consider these supplements reasonably safe (within limits as noted), backed by some science to warrant another look, and legal for endurance athletes to experiment with. Keep in mind that I'm not suggesting nor advocating the use of any particular supplement. The decision to take a supplement always lies with you.

Caffeine

Use of caffeine has been shown to reduce times in marathon and cycling time trials, as well as increase the time trained elite and recreational athletes were able to exercise vigorously—in the laboratory. Theories abound about why this occurs, but caffeine appears to promote the release of free fatty acids from fat stores. Free fatty acids are then readily available for energy, which encourages working muscles to use fat as fuel. This conserves muscle glycogen and allows the muscles to keep working at a high level for longer periods. Caffeine may also stimulate the brain and alter the perception of how hard you are working, thereby making exercise seem easier. The exercise studies on caffeine typically last about two hours so no specific information exists for ultraendurance events.

Possible side effects.   Caffeine may cause dehydration, nausea, and abdominal cramps during exercise. Excessive caffeine (as little as one cup for some people) may cause you to feel dizzy, jittery, headachy, or nauseous, or upon withdrawal, may lead to insomnia, poor nutrient intake if other more nutritious beverages or foods are routinely passed over, calcium loss from bones, impaired iron absorption, problems trying to conceive, and a possible failure of a drug test in competition.

Advice.   Potential performance-enhancing benefits from using caffeine exist for endurance athletes because the longer the event or race, the more important fat is as a fuel. You'll really need to experiment with caffeine as a performance aid, though. Some people feel no lift at all, and the physical side effects outweigh the benefits for others. Try it in training first (ingest caffeine three to four hours before exercise) under various conditions. Don't wait until the morning of your big event. Caffeine acts as a diuretic, so don't skimp on your non-caffeinated, nonalcoholic fluids.

To decrease your tolerance to caffeine and receive the maximal boost, habitual caffeine users may need to reduce or abstain from caffeine for three to four days prior to competition. Avoiding caffeine withdrawal can be tricky, though. During a race, don't underestimate the potential side effects of caffeine (from drinking caffeinated sodas, for instance) such as dehydration, nausea, and abdominal cramps, as these conditions already occur with high frequency during endurance races.

If you're an elite athlete subject to drug testing following competitions, be aware that excessive caffeine levels (12 micrograms or more per millimeter of urine) are considered performance-enhancing by the International Olympic Committee. According to the U.S. Olympic Committee's handbook, an average-size person "would have to consume six to eight cups of coffee in one sitting and be tested within two to three hours" to produce a positive test. Athletes metabolize caffeine at very different rates, though, and some medications (such as Vivarin, No Doz, and Tylenol) and supplements contain appreciable amounts of caffeine, so your caffeine intake can add up. Be careful not to combine caffeine with other stimulants such as ephedrine (found in supplements containing ma huang or Chinese Ephedra), which can lead to an irregular heartbeat.

Don't abuse caffeine. On a daily basis, milk, juice, and sports drinks make far healthier choices than tea, coffee, soda, and chocolate-covered espresso beans. Caffeine can leach calcium from your bones, so boost your calcium intake with at least two extra tablespoons of milk or yogurt for every cup of coffee you drink. If you have problems with iron-deficiency anemia, drink your caffeinated beverages between meals so the caffeine doesn't interfere with your absorption of iron. For women trying to conceive, consume as little caffeine as possible and continue to restrict yourself while pregnant (two cups or less per day) to reduce the risk of miscarriage or an underweight baby.

Glucosamine and Chondroitin Sulfate

Synthesized by the body, glucosamine plays a major role in building and repairing joint cartilage, as well as inhibiting the breakdown of existing cartilage. Chondroitin reportedly helps joints remain fluid and also inhibits enzymes that break down cartilage. Short-term (four to eight weeks) controlled trials have found glucosamine sulfate as effective as ibuprofen in relieving pain and increasing range of motion in people with osteoarthritis, a degenerative joint disease.

Possible side effects.   May cause gastrointestinal discomfort and diarrhea in some people. May give some athletes a false sense of security that a supplement will heal or cure an exercise-induced injury.

Advice.   Glucosamine appears to be safe, but no long-term studies have been done on either supplement or the combination together. Don't be fooled by claims that glucosamine or chrondroitin sulfate can cure osteoarthritis. The evidence doesn't exist, especially since glucosamine apparently can't influence the repair of cartilage when little or no cartilage remains. If you decide to try these substances for relief of everyday aches and pain or a more serious injury, the commonly recommended dose is 500 milligrams three times a day. Just don't neglect or abandon well-established treatments for athletic or overuse injuries, such as stretching, massage, physical therapy, strengthening exercises, orthotics, and so forth.

Glycerol

This substance may help reduce dehydration and fatigue during exercise by prompting the body to store more water than possible by ingesting plain water alone (glycerol attracts and holds water like a sponge). Some studies have shown these benefits: greater fluid retention, lower core temperatures during exercise, and improved performance during prolonged exercise. Other studies have shown no physiological benefits or positive effects on performance. Research is lacking on the effects of ingesting large doses over a prolonged period.

Possible side effects.   May cause headaches, nausea, vomiting, bloating, dizziness, and muscle stiffness.

Advice.   Experiment with a commercially prepared sports drink that contains glycerol or mix a premeasured amount (such as Pro-Hydrator) with water or a sports drink as directed. Don't exceed the recommended amount—the dosages are based on body weight (see the package label for exact amounts). If you're pregnant or have diabetes, high blood pressure, or kidney problems, check with your physician first. Glycerol's potential benefits increase the farther the distance you intend to race and the hotter and more humid the weather. It's unlikely you'll see any benefit with races lasting less than one hour.

To hyperhydrate, consume the glycerol-fluid mixture 90 minutes to three hours before an endurance event. Experiment in training before using it in competition. Keep notes on how long it takes you to drink the mixture comfortably, how long you feel it takes to clear your stomach, and if you feel bloated, how long the feeling lasts. Be aware that you will still need to replace your fluid losses as much as possible by drinking water and fluid replacement drinks throughout the race.

Branched Chain Amino Acids (BCAAs)

BCAAs (leucine, isoleucine, and valine) are located primarily in muscle, and they can be broken down and burned for energy during prolonged exercise (over two hours) as muscle glycogen levels fall. Supplementing with BCAAs may improve performance by preventing muscle protein breakdown and damage or by delaying the mental fatigue that arises in the latter stages of prolonged exercise when blood levels of BCAAs fall. Findings of research studies are promising but inconclusive on the effect of BCAAs on performance.

Possible side effects.   Large doses may cause gastrointestinal distress. Routine consumption might interfere with the absorption of other amino acids into the body.

Advice.   Supplementing with BCAAs to alleviate mental fatigue during exercise is promising for endurance athletes. In studies to date, however, carbohydrate-containing beverages have been found just as effective in improving performance as drinks containing both carbohydrates and BCAAs. To capitalize on potential benefits, experiment with supplements, powders, or sports drinks that contain added BCAAs during prolonged exercise, when blood levels of BCAAs decrease and you're most likely to be in a glycogen-depleted state. BCAA supplementation appears to be safe, but the effects of long-term use, if any, are unknown. Don't overdo it because large doses can contribute to stomach upset.

You can maintain your muscle mass most effectively by consuming enough calories and adequate protein each day. Protein-rich food sources, which provide 10 to 15 grams of protein per serving (meat and milk in particular), provide ample amounts of BCAAs as well. A sound training program and a carbohydrate-rich diet will also help spare your protein stores from being converted to fuel during exercise. Ingesting large doses of individual amino acids on a daily basis could influence the absorption and metabolic balance of other amino acids, so choose supplements or powders that provide a full complement of amino acids. Don't be duped by the large numbers on labels. For example, 10,000 milligrams of amino acids may sound like a lot, but this is only 10 grams of protein, an amount you can easily get (for a lot less money) by drinking a glass of milk.

Salt (Electrolyte) Tablets

Traditionally given to athletes exercising in the heat to prevent muscle cramps, salt tablets can help endurance athletes maintain an adequate sodium level in the body during prolonged activities, such as marathons, ultraruns, and triathlons. Sweating causes you to lose electrolytes, primarily sodium. You can lose as much as 1,000 milligrams of sodium for every two-pound sweat loss.

Electrolyte deficits, particularly of sodium, can result from repeated training bouts in extreme conditions (heat and humidity), when you're acclimating to a hot climate, and during ultraendurance events, especially if you consume only plain water. Hyponatremia (a low blood-sodium concentration of 135 milliequivalents per liter or less), a potentially dangerous condition that can arise during prolonged exercise, can result from excessive loss of sodium (through sweating), excessive intake of plain water, or both.

Possible side effects. May cause nausea, vomiting, and dehydration.

Advice. Moderately salting your food (a half teaspoon of table salt provides 1,200 milligrams of sodium) and choosing salty foods in the few days prior to competition, as well as consuming a sports drink that contains sodium during exercise will be more than adequate most of the time. Use caution if you decide to experiment with salt tablets during exercise. Save them for intensive or prolonged exercise (that is, ultraendurance events) in extreme conditions. Be sure to try them in training situations first.

No definitive guidelines exist but start with the recommended dose (one tablet per hour depending on the weather and how heavily you sweat) and be sure to consume plenty of fluid at the same time. Otherwise, your body draws water away from your muscles and into your stomach to dilute the tablets, negating the effect of taking them. Choose a buffered variety to reduce the risk of nausea and vomiting. Salt tablets don't increase your thirst like salty foods do, so don't overdo it. Most supplements supply 200 to 350 milligrams of sodium per tablet.

MCT Oil

Consuming high-fat foods during exercise provides insufficient fuel for working muscles because of the extended time required to digest and absorb regular fats. Medium-chain triglycerides (MCTs), on the other hand, a unique form of fat characterized by shorter-than-normal fatty acids, are digested and burned for fuel at a much faster rate, similar to carbohydrates. Consuming MCTs during endurance events and races may enhance performance by sparing the body's limited glycogen stores. Other purported benefits of consuming MCTs, such as an increase in metabolism, less weight gain, and a lower body-fat level have been demonstrated only in animals, using relative doses of MCTs that humans could not reasonably consume.

Possible side effects.   Large doses (more than 30 grams) can cause intestinal discomfort, such as cramping and diarrhea, and MCT is unsafe for athletes with diabetes or liver function problems. Essential fatty acid deficiencies can arise if MCTs are the sole source of fat in the diet.

Advice.   MCT oil is expensive ($25 to $30 per quart) and may be diluted with water or other ingredients. Try to find a product containing only MCT oil. Start by stirring small doses into a carbohydrate-containing sports drink or experiment with a commercially prepared sports drink containing MCTs, such as SUCCEED! Increase your intake gradually, as large doses can cause gastrointestinal problems, including cramping and diarrhea. Don't wait until race day to experiment with MCT oil. If you need extra calories while training, supplementing with MCT oil is a possibility. Just don't rely on it as the sole source of fat in your diet, due to MCT oil's lack of essential fatty acids.

Glutamine

As the most abundant amino acid in the body, glutamine plays a key role in maintaining a healthy gastrointestinal tract and immune system. Glutamine reserves (particularly in skeletal muscles) are depleted in times of stress, such as infection, surgery, trauma, and possibly even exercise. Prolonged strenuous exercise, running a marathon for example, depresses blood levels of glutamine, with several hours of recovery needed to restore proper levels.

Typically synthesized by the body, glutamine may become "conditionally essential" during illness and acute stress when the body can't make enough to keep up with its needs. Low glutamine levels have been measured in athletes suffering from overtraining syndrome. Glutamine supplementation may help improve athletic performance by helping the body build and maintain muscle mass, decreasing muscle damage and recovery time, strengthening the immune system, and stimulating the accumulation of muscle glycogen.

Possible side effects. Supplementation may give athletes a false sense of security or lead them to abandon lifestyle factors that may prevent poor health or overtraining syndrome. Free-form L-glutamine is unsafe for athletes with kidney or liver dysfunction.

Advice. No standard dose exists but research suggests potential benefits with five to 20 grams a day. Experiment with meal replacement powders or nutrition bars containing glutamine mixed with other amino acids to aid absorption. To obtain an adequate dose, glutamine should be listed as one of the first five protein ingredients, as many companies do not list the exact amount the product contains.

Don't let glutamine's emerging role as an indicator of exercise stress and overtraining lead you to abandon other healthy practices. Low blood levels of glutamine appear to be linked with the overtraining syndrome but do not necessarily cause it. Supplementing with glutamine isn't a substitute for time off from training, a healthy diet, adequate sleep, or learning how to manage stress appropriately.

Cijuiwa (Endurox)

This popular herb is used in traditional Chinese medicine to treat fatigue and bolster the immune system. Early information focused on mountain climbers using cijuiwa to improve their ability to work at high altitudes and low oxygen conditions. Limited human research has produced striking results and indicates that cijuiwa (Endurox) may increase fat metabolism and delay lactic acid buildup by shifting the energy source during exercise from carbohydrate to fat. Purported benefits include less muscle soreness, delayed onset of exercise-induced fatigue and exhaustion, speedier recoveries, and the ability to work more efficiently for a longer time.

Possible side effects. Cijuiwa appears to be a safe herb, but could cause an athlete to fail a drug test in competition.

Advice. Cijuiwa is marketed extensively under the name brand Endurox. The commonly used dose in the few studies conducted was 800 milligrams. Be aware that no studies have looked at long-term use. Further studies need to be done to see if cijuiwa actually improves performance, especially in highly trained individuals. Scientists have had difficulty reviewing many of the scientific articles because they are published in Chinese.

Cijuiwa does not contain caffeine, nor does it produce any stimulant or anabolic steroid effects. If you're a competitive athlete subject to drug testing, however, remember that all supplements bear some risk. Botanicals or plant-based supplements carry a higher risk of containing a banned substance because of impurities and a lack of standardized quality control practices.

Creatine Monohydrate

Creatine supplementation helps the body increase and rapidly replenish its stores of readily available energy (phosphocreatine and ATP)—the primary fuels needed for short, high-intensity efforts such as sprinting and lifting weights. For endurance athletes, creatine's ability to increase muscle strength and help buffer lactic acid buildup in the blood and muscles could improve the quality of interval workouts and other training efforts, which could ultimately translate into improved race performances.

Possible side effects. Creatine can cause weight gain (from tissues holding onto extra water), dehydration, and an increased risk of muscle cramps, tears, and pulls.

Advice. Humans need approximately two grams of creatine a day. Animal foods, such as meat, poultry and fish, are rich sources of creatine. Our bodies also synthesize creatine from nonessential amino acids at the rate of approximately one gram a day. As far as endurance athletes are concerned, creatine supplementation has been shown to have no effect on maximal aerobic capacity ($\dot{V}O_2$max), nor has it been shown to improve endurance. Some researchers believe, however, that creatine supplementation might indirectly improve an athlete's ability to perform in endurance events. Creatine supplementation may lift an athlete's lactate threshold (the speed or intensity above which lactic acid accumulates in the blood, which correlates with the percentage of your aerobic capacity at which you are able to perform), thereby allowing more intensive interval-type training. By facilitating strength and cardiovascular improvements in this manner, creatine supplementation could improve your overall performances in endurance events.

Short-term creatine supplementation (up to eight weeks) appears safe, but the American College of Sports Medicine recommends that all athletes check first with a physician. Be aware that even though studies fail to support an increase in muscle cramps and pulls with creatine supplementation, anecdotal information from athletes abounds! Dehydration may be the culprit, so athletes taking creatine need to consume more fluids than usual during training and competition. The safety of more prolonged creatine supplementation has not been completely established.

Two loading techniques that purportedly induce less water retention (and thus less weight gain) than the traditional 20-gram per day strategy include six grams per day over five to six days (half-gram or one gram doses) with a maintenance dose of about two grams a day, or three grams a day over 30 days. Supplementing with creatine will not build muscles or improve performance on its own. Coordinate creatine supplementation with your training schedule by starting just before you begin a period of high-intensity training. Keep in mind that 20 to 30 percent of people fail to respond even when creatine is taken correctly and training is appropriate.

Taking Supplements: What's Behind the Hype?

Taking supplements is nothing new. For centuries, athletes have attempted to improve their performance by eating just the right foods or taking dietary supplements or other ergogenic (performance-enhancing) aids. Endurance athletes are no exception. Unfortunately, more often than not, supplements don't deliver on their promises. The response I hear most often from athletes is, "Big deal, what's the harm in trying?" First, investing time, energy, and money on supplements that don't work is, well, not a very good use of your time, energy, and money. On top of that, it could prove harmful to your health, hurt your performance, or get you disqualified from competition.

Of course, if you're like the athletes I meet, you don't intend to harm yourself or your performance when you jump on the latest nutrition bandwagon. Rather, you rationalize that taking supplements compensates for a less-than-ideal diet or lifestyle, or you believe that you have special nutrient needs resulting from strenuous exercise. If you're highly competitive, you may see supplements as helping you avoid colds and injuries, as well as giving you that little extra competitive edge. Let's face it: you're not out there to lose.

Unfortunately, the extraordinary drive endurance athletes possess to improve and excel (you know, the drive that keeps you going that last hour) can leave you particularly vulnerable to the lure of dietary supplements. The supplement industry capitalizes on this weakness by spending millions of dollars to market the latest promise of the day, including vitamins, minerals, herbals, botanicals, amino acids, and other substances such as phytochemicals, extracts, and glandular concentrates and metabolites. On top of that, it's easy to be swayed by the opinions of those who perform better than we do, so advertisers target us by using successful athletes and coaches to represent products. To make matters worse, you probably have at least one friend or teammate who swears by how well a particular supplement is working. This influence, coupled with the fact that you may not have had a nutrition course since ninth grade, makes it easy to see how myths regarding nutrition supplements are perpetuated.

Just the Facts Please

Be aware that supplements fall into a special category that lies somewhere between foods and drugs. Although supplements are now required to carry a supplements facts label and an ingredient list similar to the nutrition facts

A DoubleDeca Triathlon:
The Ultimate Time for Liquid Food?

Meet Chet "The Jet" Blanton, a 40-year-old endurance athlete who works in a running store in Hawaii and coaches on the side. He certainly isn't famous for eating an ideal diet—in fact, he abhors fruits and vegetables and dines at Taco Bell at least once a day. In the ultraendurance arena, though, Blanton is more than impressive. He's one of only four people to finish the DoubleDeca Triathlon, held in Monterey, Mexico, in October 1998—48 miles of swimming, 1,120 miles of cycling, and 524 miles of running. While I can hardly advocate a daily diet based on meal-replacement products, Blanton's success in the DoubleDeca provides a prime (albeit, extreme!) example of the usefulness of liquid food supplements during ultraendurance events.

At noon on October 31, 1998, Blanton, who doesn't really like to swim, began the first of 760 laps in a 50-meter pool (two lengths counting as one lap). Fifty-two hours later (including half a dozen 30-minute catnaps), he finished. Fired up after completing his time in the pool, he was on his bike an hour later circling a 1.2-mile loop through a local park that would be his home for the next 26 days. Averaging 175 miles a day, Blanton squeezed 5 hours of rest and 5 hours of sleep around 14 hours of biking. Twelve days and 20 hours later, he threw his bicycle away (literally), and 9 minutes later began to run. He spent 12 hours a day running and walking the 1.2 mile-loop, resting 7 hours and sleeping 5. He covered his last mile in 6 minutes and 28 seconds, for a total of 13 days and 4 hours. His total elapsed time for the event was 28 days and 6 hours—9 days behind the winner (Lithuanian Vidmantas Urbonas, who finished in just under 19 days.) Two weeks later, Blanton ran the Honolulu Marathon in 3 hours and 48 minutes.

To what does Blanton attribute his success and remarkably quick recovery? Spizerinctum (a Southern expression meaning pep or energy) or "Spiz"—a liquid food supplement that packs 500 calories, 97 grams of carbohydrate, and a healthy dose of antioxidants, vitamins and minerals, glutamine, and electrolytes into one 20-ounce serving. Developed by a cardiopulmonary physical therapist and a dietitian, Spiz is the "food" of choice among top cyclists competing in the grueling Race Across America—a bike race where individuals and teams cycle 2,900 miles from California to the East Coast. (Top teams cross the finish line in less than six days, with the top individuals following close behind two days later.)

Blanton drank Spiz around the clock, along with a fluid replacement drink during exercise. In fact, for the first 13 days of the DoubleDeca, he ingested nothing but Spiz. On day 14, he enjoyed a vanilla milkshake and nibbled on fries and a cheeseburger. By the end of the swim and bike segments, Blanton had lost only a pound. After losing his appetite during the run and dropping nine pounds in four days, he returned to drinking a minimum of

20 ounces of Spiz every two hours. He regained four pounds and went on to finish with no problems (except for blisters on his feet). He treated himself to pancakes and egg burritos a few times during the race, but essentially he relied on Spiz to provide the 6,000+ calories he ingested daily.

Blanton is now chasing a new goal—a world record for the most Ironmans in one year. His goal is 30. Don't worry: he's not looking for a training partner, and he has plenty of Spiz on hand.

label found on food packages, dietary supplements do not have to meet the same tough standards regarding health claims, manufacturing processes, and product safety that apply to all food additives and drugs.

Keep these facts about supplements in mind, as written in the 1994 Dietary Supplement Health and Education Act (DSHEA), as you reach for the latest "magical potion."

Fact number one: Proof that a supplement works is not required. In other words, the stringent guidelines set by the Food and Drug Administration (FDA) for drugs and food additives do not apply to supplements.

Fact number two: Supplement manufacturers, as well as the companies that sell supplements, do not have to prove that their products are safe. Don't be fooled just because supplements look like drugs or "pills" that the FDA has thoroughly tested and approved.

Fact number three: Supplement manufacturers can put health claims on their labels. Health claims on supplement packages must be "truthful and not misleading." Unfortunately, these terms continue to be defined. In other words, as long as a claim does not promise that the supplement will prevent or cure a disease, almost anything goes. For example, claims that do not relate to disease, such as "helps you relax," "for muscle enhancement," "for common symptoms of PMS," or "maintains a healthy circulatory system," are allowed without prior FDA approval. Remind yourself to read the small print on product labels and ads that states "This statement has not been evaluated by the Food and Drug Administration. This product is not intended to diagnose, treat, cure, or prevent any disease."

Fact number four: Supplements do not have to conform to any manufacturing standards. In other words, each company can decide for itself how to prepare and package its supplements, leaving the potency and quality of dietary supplements up in the air.

Do Your Homework

Okay, now that you realize that taking supplements requires a consumer-beware approach, where should you turn for guidance and sound advice?

The supplements facts label is certainly a good place to start. Look here to find a complete list of the ingredients found in the supplement (including the breakdown of "magical formulas"), the nutrients these ingredients provide, and how these amounts compare with established daily values (DVs). You can also determine which part of the plant is used in an herbal or botanical supplement. Checking the bottle for a USP stamp of approval lets you know the supplement will dissolve properly in your body, but it doesn't tell you how effectively it will be absorbed (see figure 4.1).

You won't want to rely solely on the label or the health claims plastered all over the packaging. Unlike conventional foods, no standard serving sizes exist for dietary supplements. Dosage amounts and schedules have been left to the discretion of manufacturers (the people who want to sell the product), so you need to remember this age-old advice: more is not always better. Some nutrients and substances don't have established recommended daily intakes, so you'll need to stay alert for current information from reputable sources on safe doses.

Is it Legal, Safe, and Effective?

When it comes to deciphering health claims, a healthy dose of skepticism and a bit of common sense can help steer you through the maze. You want to consider if the supplement in question is legal, safe, and effective. Common sense tells you that securing this information requires looking past the promotional literature, advertisements, and anecdotal reports put out by the

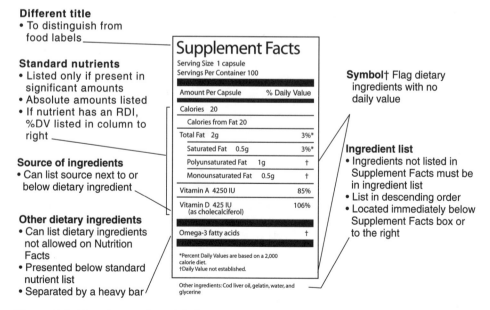

Figure 4.1 Supplement facts label.

Reprinted, with permission, from *SCAN'S PULSE*, Fall 1998, Vol. 17, No. 4, official publication of Sports, Cardiovascular, and Wellness Nutritionists (SCAN), The American Dietetic Association, Chicago, IL.

manufacturers. Because of gaps in the DSHEA, companies commonly exaggerate claims and rely on deceptive marketing techniques to sell products. Typical approaches used include presenting information that may not be accurate or that has been taken out of context; failing to provide scientific research when asked (it's still under way or not available to the public); relying on testimonials from athletes and authority figures (for example, "research scientists"), which are most likely paid endorsements; and conducting and reporting their own research without having it published in journals where other scientists have a chance to evaluate it. Incidentally, obtaining a patent means that the product is unique, not necessarily safe or effective.

If you're a top-notch competitive athlete subject to drug tests, you'll want to make sure you don't take a prohibited substance that can disqualify you from further competitions. You can do this by contacting the National Collegiate Athletic Association or the United States Olympic Committee (see Selected Resources). From an ethical standpoint, you may also be interested in this information, as were many of the "purists" I met in the mountaineering community while I lived in Boulder, Colorado.

U.S. Triathlete Disqualified for Banned Drug

What you don't know *can* hurt you. Lee DiPietro, the 15th-place female at the 1998 Hawaii Ironman World Championship in Kailua-Kona, Hawaii, was disqualified and suspended from competition as a result of a positive test for banned substances. The penalty was imposed despite her unintentional use. DiPietro ingested a natural dietary supplement during the latter part of the race without realizing that it contained the banned substances ephedrine and pseudoephedrine. Officials at the hearing noted that it is an athlete's personal responsibility to ensure that they do not ingest a prohibited substance. No exceptions are granted for unintentional violations of the doping-control rules. Under these rules, penalties included disqualification, forfeiture of any prize money, and a three-month suspension from competition.

Statement from Lee DiPietro: Let this serve as a warning to athletes about so-called natural supplements. Although many safe natural supplements are on the market, there are some that contain banned substances. This past October, while competing in the Ironman, I made the mistake of my life. In the days preceding the race, I had been sick and to make matters worse was confronted with female problems two days before Ironman. In a moment of self-doubt, I changed my regime and put a supplement in my special needs bag to be taken in the last five miles of the run. Had I only stuck with my routine and just taken my usual supplement, Endurox, I never would have had a problem. At the end of the race, I was drug tested and much to my horror was informed that there was a banned substance (ephedra, or pseudophederine) in my test results.

After calling the USOC, I discovered that the "all-natural supplement" I ingested contained a banned substance. Triathlon rules state that it is the responsibility of the athletes to know what they're taking. It never occurred to me that what I was taking would contain such a substance.

As an athlete, I felt that the reputation I have built over the past 10 years would be destroyed. As a mother of two boys (ages 15 and 11), I was worried how public disclosure of this would affect them and the rest of my family. I was also greatly concerned that I let down my sponsors and was anxious about how the news would be accepted. Luckily, I have had tremendous support from my family, friends, and sponsors. At the hearing, USA Triathlon agreed that this was an unintentional ingestion of a banned substance, but their rules do not allow for flexibility, and ultimately it is the athlete's responsibility. USA Triathlon imposed a 90-day suspension with public disclosure.

As an athlete, you must know what you're taking. Ironically, I have since discovered that when I ingested this supplement, I was so dehydrated that the supplement would have taken much longer to enter my system and the effects of it would probably have only worsened my state of dehydration, rather than helped me. For this reason, it is also extremely important that athletes are aware of what they are ingesting and what effect it will have on their performance. Although this has been a horrendous experience and a tough lesson to learn, I hope that it will open other athletes' eyes to question whatever they are ingesting and verify with the USOC (800-233-0393) that it does not contain any banned substance.

Reprinted, by permission, from The United States Olympic Committee. 1999. U.S. triathlete disqualified for banned drug. *Inside Triathlon* [Online], February, 9 paragraphs. Available: http://www.greatoutdoors.com/insidetri/1999/feb.html.

You may not like what you hear though. You'll find that some ingredients, such as DHEA and ma huang (Chinese Ephedra), are specifically banned. Other than that, you're on your own when it comes to dietary supplements. Because no one can guarantee the purity or potency of all the supplements available, anything you take is at your own risk.

The reminder "let the buyer beware" should be printed on every nutrition supplement package. Why? When it comes to the possible side effects of using a supplement long-term, you may be part of an ongoing study for the supplement manufacturer! Don't assume you can resolve safety issues by buying high-priced versions or sticking with "natural drug-free" herbal remedies. To begin with, you may not even be getting what you pay for. For example, one study found 60 percent of 64 "pure" ginseng products worthless because they were so watered down with cheaper herbs.

Herbs fall under the same regulations in the United States as do other dietary supplements, which means they may not be adequately tested to determine how safe or effective they are, especially if taken for longer periods than experts recommend.

For the most part, herbal dosages are recommendations from manufacturers or based simply on historical use. By the way, the dosage listed usually applies to men, so children and women will likely need less. As with all supplements, don't be afraid to call the manufacturer and ask about clinical trials, manufacturing practices, and their use of standardized extracts. Remedies composed of a single herb are generally considered safer than herbal mixtures. Be sure to consult with your doctor about any herbal products you use, especially if you're pregnant or trying to become pregnant, have a health problem, or take prescription medications.

Now the big question: how can you tell if a supplement does what it claims to do? In other words, will you have more energy, lose weight, run faster, jump higher, and throw farther? Now is the time to pull out that healthy dose of skepticism I mentioned earlier and remember the counsel, "If it sounds too good to be true, it probably is." Be leery of general, broad claims that promise to positively affect a complicated, multifaceted process in the body, such as "slows aging" or "speeds up your metabolism." Also be alert to "miracle," "secret," and "effortless" effects. Does it make sense, for example, that you could eat all you want and lose weight at the same time? When "scientific" mumbo jumbo appears, read it more closely. For example, aren't you a bit curious about the percentage of people who "may" be deficient and why you "may" be deficient rather than "are" deficient? Contact the manufacturer for more information about alleged benefits and request copies of, or references to, scientific articles reviewed in reputable medical journals.

Bottom Line

I'm not saying that supplements can't work—for some people, some of the time, to some degree. After all, when it comes to the human body and enhancing athletic performance, the science often falls into a gray area. Just keep in mind that we each represent an experiment of one, which may help explain why you don't notice any appreciable benefits from a supplement that a training buddy (or an elite athlete profiled in this book) raves about or you don't seem to get the same boost from an old favorite you've taken for years.

You may also simply *believe* that a product works. Perhaps you started taking a supplement during a period of natural improvement due to other factors such as improved training or better mental preparation. Maybe you simply experience a psychological lift (known as the placebo effect) when you take a certain product. This mental boost alone can be enough to power you to a greater performance. Of course, if prudent scientific evidence exists (such as using sports drinks during exercise to maintain your blood sugar), or you're diagnosed with a nutrient-specific deficiency (iron-deficiency anemia, for example), then taking a supplement will most likely help.

Keep the definition of the word *supplement* in mind. A supplement should add to or fill out a sound diet and training program. Even if certain substances are shown to be of some benefit in improving athletic performance, keep the gains in perspective. Your inherited talent, mental attitude, training methods, eating habits, and equipment choices all play a far greater role in your success than could any dietary supplement. Maybe you even excel in spite of something you take! You can't go wrong covering all these bases before you seek out a safe, legal supplement.

Finally, make sure you're willing to pay the price for taking supplements—literally and figuratively. I know it's tempting to take supplements for a chronic health problem or for an injury that standard medical treatments fail to solve. Be prepared, however, to feel disappointed and even less hopeful every time you invest in a supplement that doesn't do what it claims to do. You may even become less motivated to seek any kind of help. If you continue to exercise and rely solely on a supplement to cure your illness or injury, you must consider the opportunities you lost to try something else, such as another treatment plan, further medical help, or simply rest and time off. Even if you're just looking for an edge, don't let taking supplements keep you from doing what you might really need to do, such as revamping your training program or learning some basic cooking skills so you can prepare healthier meals.

Performing Under Extreme Conditions

"I never leave home without plenty of water, enough snacks to keep me going until my next meal, and a package of soup mix to help me rehydrate at the end of the day. This way I'm always prepared to deal with whatever I encounter—be it hot weather, freezing temperatures, or altitude sickness."

—Karen Berger, hiked America's Triple Crown—the Appalachian (2,158 miles), Pacific Crest (2,660 miles), and Continental Divide (3,000 miles) Trails

You've probably heard the saying, "when the going gets tough, the tough get going." Obviously, they were referring to endurance athletes. Who else would be dedicated (or crazy) enough to push their bodies to the limit for a T-shirt or a belt buckle? And I mean push—through snowdrifts, haze shimmering off sun-baked asphalt roads, and thin air found on high mountain ridges.

Often held under mind-boggling conditions, endurance events ultimately come down to a battle with Mother Nature. She sets the rules, and anything goes. Be prepared to broil, pant, and freeze, sometimes all in one day. To persevere (or just plain survive) you must be able to handle unusual conditions. Heat, humidity, cold, and high altitude challenge the best of athletes. Whether you desire to compete in endurance sports or you simply enjoy hiking, mountaineering, or skiing, this chapter provides nutritional strategies that will help you deal with extreme environmental conditions.

Temperature Regulation

How is it possible to go from freezing temperatures to 90 degrees without breaking a stride? Thank your body's thermostat—the hypothalamus. Located at the base of the brain, the hypothalamus receives signals from two sets of thermoreceptors. Central receptors sense changes in the temperature of your blood as it circulates through the hypothalamus; peripheral receptors monitor the temperature of your skin and the environment around you. Because your hypothalamus has a predetermined temperature, or set point, that it seeks to maintain, you must deal quickly with fluctuations in body temperature.

When your body temperature rises, your hypothalamus signals into action the sweat glands and blood vessels in your skin. Your blood vessels dilate, or open wider, bringing more blood and the heat it carries to your skin, where the heat can escape to the environment. At the same time, your sweat glands produce more sweat. As this moisture evaporates, it pulls heat from the skin. If your body temperature falls, your blood vessels constrict, so less heat is lost across the skin. You also begin to shiver, which raises your metabolism and generates heat. Several hormones, such as thyroxine (from your thyroid gland) and epinephrine and norepinephrine (from your adrenal glands) can also increase your metabolic rate, thereby increasing the amount of heat you produce internally.

Extreme cold and heat limit your ability to exercise, particularly if you're trying to compete. For example, in hot weather your working muscles and skin compete for a limited blood supply. Your muscles need blood and the oxygen it carries to keep working. Your body, however, must divert blood to the skin to bring the heat generated by working muscles to the surface to keep you cool. At some point, neither your muscles nor your skin receive enough blood flow to function optimally. In cold environments, trouble sets in when you dissipate heat faster than you produce it. In either case, you can exacerbate the situation by not paying close attention to your fuel and fluid needs.

Performing in Extreme Heat

From a physiological standpoint, you encounter the most severe stress possible when you exercise in the heat. You must deal with the heat gained from the combination of physical exertion and the hot environment. Nevertheless, you still rely primarily on the evaporation of sweat to shed excess heat and remain (relatively) cool. Although sweating is a vital thermoregulatory mechanism for removing heat, it comes at a price. Dehydration results if you don't take in enough fluids to keep pace with your sweat loss. An average-size individual (110 to 165 pounds) might lose one and a half to two and a half quarts of sweat, or 2 to 4 percent of his or her body weight, each hour during an intense effort on a hot, humid day. Fluid losses of as little as 2 percent of body weight (for example, a weight loss of three pounds for a 150-pound athlete) can impair performance.

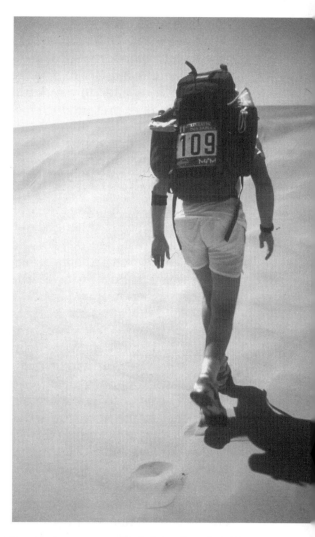

To complete an event like the Marathon de Sables— a 150-mile foot race across the Sahara Desert, participants must first acclimatize to the extreme heat.

To provide a cooling effect, sweat must evaporate, not just drip off your skin. That's why humid conditions hinder your athletic performance. High humidity prevents cooling so less sweat evaporates because the air is already saturated with water. Consequently, you seriously increase your risk of heat illness when faced with the dual challenge of exercising in heat and high humidity. For example, exercise physiologists estimate that a marathoner who typically runs a marathon in two and a half hours will be almost five minutes slower over the same distance when the thermometer hits 80 degrees.

Exercising in hot weather decreases your economy, or efficiency. In other words, you use more fuel to perform at a particular pace or intensity compared with exercising under cooler conditions. As you become progressively dehydrated from failing to take in enough fluids to match your sweat losses, your blood volume falls and your heart compensates by beating faster. Working muscles receive less blood flow and less oxygen in the heat (as blood is rerouted to the skin for cooling purposes), so they use more muscle glycogen and produce more lactic acid. This helps explain why a given effort in the heat leaves you feeling more fatigued and exhausted than the same effort in cooler weather.

Heat Acclimatization

The body does acclimatize to heat after approximately 7 to 14 days of training in warm conditions, although how quickly you adapt and to what extent is highly individual. The physiological adaptations that occur better prepare you for future exercise bouts in the heat. Within the first few days, you begin to sweat earlier and at an increased rate. (Remember, sweating allows you to eliminate excess heat and hold down your internal body temperature, so more blood flows to your working muscles.) Various hormonal messages will signal your sweat glands to reabsorb valuable electrolytes such as sodium and chloride. Sweating triggers the release of other hormones, which stimulate your kidneys to excrete less sodium and reabsorb more water. Thus, your body attempts to compensate for fluid and minerals lost through heavy sweating by reducing their losses in urine. After you are acclimated to the heat, you reduce the rate at which your muscles use glycogen during exercise in the heat by as much as 50 to 60 percent.

Don't underestimate the importance of making small adjustments when training in the heat, such as wearing light-colored, loose-fitting clothing, seeking out shady training routes, and taking longer rest breaks. While training in the swamplike conditions of Washington, D.C. (often 80 degrees and 85 percent humidity at 6:30 A.M. during the summer), I managed with early morning runs or I headed to the pool for water-running sessions instead. When weather patterns change abruptly or you travel to a warmer climate, reduce your pace and training volume for at least a few days. If you're competing, lower your expectations of what you can reasonably and safely accomplish.

Dehydration and Heat Illnesses

The dangers of exercising in the heat include severe dehydration, heat cramps, and potentially more serious conditions such as heat exhaustion, heat stroke, and hyponatremia (sodium depletion).

Dehydration

Besides throwing your thermoregulatory mechanisms off track, dehydration reduces your strength, power, endurance, and aerobic capacity. Many endurance athletes I meet believe they need to be less careful about replacing fluids as they become acclimated to the heat. In fact, you need to drink more to offset your enhanced sweating response. As you become progressively dehydrated, you negate your improved ability to tolerate heat. Dehydration may also be behind the gastrointestinal woes so many marathoners and ultrarunners suffer from.

Think of dehydration as a fierce competitor that won't let go. When you become dehydrated beyond 2 percent of your body weight during exercise, your heart rate and body temperature rise and your performance begins to suffer. Fluid losses of 3 to 5 percent of your body weight can significantly impair your performance, and losses that total more than 5 percent of your body weight are dangerous. There is no way to adapt to dehydration, so don't even try.

Meltdown Man

Although there are many anecdotes regarding the travails suffered by those who become dehydrated when exercising in the heat, perhaps one of the most highly publicized and horrifying encounters befell Australian Mark Dorrity, often referred to as the Meltdown Man. In the Australian summer of 1988, Mark and a few friends began an 8K run at 2:30 in the afternoon when the ambient temperature was in excess of 38 degrees Celsius (100 degrees Fahrenheit). In fact, the fun run in which the men were supposed to take part had been postponed from 2:30 until 5:30 in hope of cooler temperatures. Well in the lead near the end of the run, Mr. Dorrity, 28 years old and in good physical condition, suddenly collapsed and was in such obvious trouble that he was transported directly to a hospital. Upon admission, his body temperature was 42 degrees Celsius (107.6 degrees Fahrenheit). A tracheotomy was immediately performed to ensure the pulmonary ventilation that his impaired respiratory system could not maintain. Because his immune system was subdued and his blood-clotting mechanisms were impaired by his high body temperature, an opportunistic infection set in, a result of a scrape sustained on his left leg when he initially collapsed. Over the next few days, the muscles of his left leg turned a khaki color and had the stringy texture of overcooked meat. This accelerated rhabdomylosis [degeneration of skeletal muscle tissue]—overenthusiastically and inaccurately referred to as meltdown in the Australian press—caused acute renal failure, requiring months of dialysis. Twenty-seven days after admission, the leg was amputated at the hip. Mark remained comatose for 132 days before regaining consciousness and beginning years of convalescence.

Reprinted from R. Murray, 1995, "Fluid needs in hot and cold environments," *International Journal of Sport Nutrition* 5, S62-73; Meacham, S. Resurrection of the meltdown man. *The Sydney Morning Herald-Late Edition*, November 8, 1990, p. 67; O'Grady, S.E. How a fun run meant meltdown for Mark Dorrity's body. *The Sydney Morning Herald-Late Edition*, March 8, 1988, p.1.

Heat Cramps

If you've ever suffered from heat cramps or watched someone else do so, you won't soon forget the experience. Severe cramps hit the skeletal muscles most heavily used during exercise. For endurance athletes, that means abdomen, calf (lower leg), quadriceps (front of the thigh), and hamstring (back of the thigh) muscles. During my first adventure race, our three-person team had to kayak, mountain bike, trail run, and conquer various obstacles together along the course. We encountered a hot (over 90 degrees), sunny day in Portland, Oregon. Unfortunately, our star athlete, although blessed with a competitive spirit, was low on physical conditioning and had just stepped off a plane from England, where he had been working for the last year. An hour in the kayak and two more on the bike didn't seem to faze him, until he hopped off the bike. He collapsed to the ground with severe cramps in both quadriceps. Having survived two hours of single-track mountain biking, I was not about to miss the chance to put my running background to good use. With the help of a sports drink and electrolyte tablets, we got him up and running. We managed to pass more than 10 teams on that final leg and finish in the top 25 teams overall.

You don't necessarily have to be dehydrated to experience heat cramps. Low levels of minerals involved in muscle contraction such as sodium and chloride, are most likely the major cause of heat cramps. You put yourself at risk if you sweat heavily for several hours and rehydrate with only plain water. To prevent heat cramps, acclimate to hot and humid conditions as much as possible, be liberal with the salt shaker in your daily diet, and rely on sports drinks rather than plain water for prolonged, strenuous exercise in the heat.

Heat Exhaustion

Heat exhaustion, or the inability to continue exercising in the heat, results from dehydration. You might recall photographs of then-President Jimmy Carter attempting to race the hilly Catoctin Mountain Park 10K run on a hot, humid September morning. Ashen-faced, staggering, and dazed, he was forced to drop out slightly past the halfway mark even though he had trained for the race. When you suffer from heat exhaustion, your cardiovascular system simply can't meet the simultaneous demands of sending blood to your active muscles and your skin. This happens when your blood volume drops because of the excessive loss of fluid or minerals from sweating. Your thermoregulatory mechanisms are still working, but you can't dissipate heat quickly enough because too little blood (and the heat it carries) goes to your skin.

Signs of heat exhaustion to watch for during exercise include extreme thirst, headache, weakness, dizziness, heat sensations on the head or neck, abdominal cramps, chills, goose bumps, nausea, and vomiting. You may also hyperventilate (breathe rapidly and deeply), act confused, and possibly even faint. The risk of suffering heat exhaustion increases if you're exercising at or near your maximum capacity, are dehydrated, aren't physically fit, or are not yet acclimated to the heat. Athletes suffering from heat exhaustion should stop all activity immediately and seek a cooler environment (get in the shade or an air conditioned area if available). If you're coherent and conscious, consume fluids, preferably beverages that contain sodium such as sports drinks, fruit drinks, or soup. Force yourself to drink, even if you're feeling nauseous.

Heat Stroke

If left untreated, heat exhaustion can deteriorate to a potentially life-threatening disorder called heat stroke. Characterized by severe hyperthermia, when the body temperature rises to dangerously high levels (exceeding 104°F), heat stroke can permanently damage your central nervous system or even kill you. During heat stroke, the thermoregulatory mechanisms of the body fail due to excessive heat buildup and excessive dehydration. Symptoms include vomiting, diarrhea, disorientation, convulsions, and unconsciousness. You may stop sweating altogether and your skin will feel hot and dry. Rapid cooling of the entire body is crucial, accomplished by applying wet towels and fanning the person, applying ice packs, or immersing the person in a cold stream.

Don't be lulled into thinking that it needs to be the hottest day of the year for heat stroke to be a possibility. Incidents of heat stroke have been reported in cool to moderate environments (55 to 82°F). Several factors that may increase your risk of heat stroke include being overweight or in poor physical condition, advanced age, lack of sleep, alcohol or drug use, having a sunburn, not being acclimated to the heat, and suffering a previous heat injury.

Hyponatremia

Athletes (especially women) competing in endurance and ultraendurance events in the heat and humidity are at particular risk of developing hyponatremia, or a reduced blood-sodium level below the normal range of 136-143 mmol/L. Hyponatremia generally results from losing large amounts of sodium (for example, through prolonged sweating), drinking excessive amounts of plain water during or following prolonged exercise, or both. Research on triathletes competing in the Hawaii Ironman triathlon, for example, found that almost 30 percent of the finishers were hyponatremic.

Your blood-sodium levels drop as you replace the fluid lost through sweating, but not the sodium, by drinking large amounts of plain water. In fact, the sodium concentration in your body becomes diluted. If you develop a headache while exercising and become nauseous, lethargic, confused, or disoriented, seek medical attention. In severe cases, athletes lapse into unconsciousness, develop epileptic-like seizures, and may stop breathing or suffer cardiac arrest. A woman who collapsed at mile 24 of the 1998 LaSalle Banks Chicago Marathon, held in October, later died due to hyponatremia. If the ultraendurance event you compete in features weigh-ins, be aware that gaining weight while exercising can indicate you are overhydrated and at an increased risk for developing hyponatremia. Eating salty foods in the days prior to the event and consuming beverages containing sodium before, during, and after prolonged exercise, such as sports drinks and soup or broth, is usually sufficient to ward off or slow the progression of hyponatremia.

Nutritional Strategies for Beating the Heat

Let's assume you are physically fit, heat acclimated, well rested, and well fueled for whatever endeavor you choose to undertake in the heat. What else can you do to maximize your chances of performing well?

1. *Start out with a full tank.* Common sense should tell you that if you set out to exercise without being adequately hydrated, things will only get worse, especially in the heat. Don't rely on thirst to prompt you to drink enough. Feeling thirsty is actually a sign that you're already dehydrated! Consciously remind yourself to drink during the day by carrying a water bottle with you (especially during air travel) or leaving one in plain view, such as on your desk. Drink beverages with all your meals and snacks and match every cup of coffee you consume with a glass of water. Being in an air-conditioned environment all day doesn't let you off the hook, since it may make acclimatizing to the heat more difficult.

Many athletes walk around in a chronically dehydrated condition, especially if they train in the heat more than once a day or complete long exercise bouts on successive days. Weighing yourself before and after exercise is an easy way to monitor how well you handle training in the heat. Any weight loss following exercise represents fluid lost as sweat or urine. If you progressively lose weight over the course of a few days, you're most likely dehydrated. Replace every pound lost during daily exercise with at least two cups (16 ounces) of fluid as soon as possible, or better yet, try to consume that amount of fluid while you exercise. Incidentally, you should be able to urinate before and after you exercise. If you're unable to do so or your urine is dark yellow, work on drinking more throughout the day.

2. *Stick to a predetermined drinking schedule during exercise.* As discussed in chapter 3, drink early and drink often. Some athletes sweat off two quarts of water per hour in hot conditions. Aim for four to eight ounces of water or a sports drink every 15 to 20 minutes. Set your watch alarm as a reminder. Freezing bottles beforehand or using an insulated bottle helps keep liquids cool and refreshing. Young athletes dehydrate quickly, especially on warm days, so make sure each child has his or her own water bottle and schedule

mandatory fluid breaks. Drinking on a predetermined schedule is mandatory on warm, windy days or hot days with low humidity when you may not be as aware that you're sweating.

Research has shown that athletes exercising in the heat who are given free access to water replace only one-half to two-thirds of their fluid losses. Sports drinks can help you drink more because they contain electrolytes that boost your drive to drink. Experiment with different flavors and concentrations (mix up a more dilute drink on really hot days). The more you like the taste, the more you'll drink. With practice, you can increase the amount you're able to handle during exercise. You can also find relief from the heat by pouring cool fluid over your body, using sponges, or passing through sprinklers, but . none of these practices can substitute for ingesting fluids.

3. *Be your own pack mule.* Although it helps to know the location of every water fountain in town, get in the habit of carrying fluids with you during warm weather. Depending on the activity you're involved in, experiment with handle devices that slip over or attach to water bottles, fanny packs that hold one or two water bottles, and bladders (a pouchlike container with a long plastic drinking tube that is worn backpack style). These items are available at outdoor and sporting goods stores, or specialty shops that cater to cyclists, runners, and skiers.

In any case, don't worry about turning into a tortoise. The benefit of having ready access to fluid far exceeds any negative consequence of carrying extra weight. For example, drinking at regular intervals promotes sweating—your primary avenue to lose heat. Be sure to pack a water filtration device or iodine tablets if you're venturing into the backcountry.

4. *Don't underestimate the power of salt.* Even if you're heat acclimated, you can lose large amounts of sodium and chloride through extensive and repetitive sweating (200 to 400 milligrams of sodium per pound of sweat), along with the sodium typically excreted in urine. (White rings on your clothing or streaks on your skin following exercise are visible signs of sodium loss.) You can exacerbate this loss if you consciously limit your salt intake. If you're a normal healthy adult, your body has several sophisticated mechanisms for regulating how much sodium you take in and retain, so you don't have to restrict your intake.

When faced with hot weather, especially seasonal changes, add salt to the foods you eat (one-half teaspoon provides 1,200 milligrams) or consume sodium-rich foods such as bouillon, canned soup or beans, cheese, tomato or vegetable juice, pretzels, salted crackers, and other low-fat snack foods. The sodium in these foods and in the sports beverages you drink before and during exercise will help you retain water and avoid a sodium deficit, as well as boost your drive to drink. In fact, of all the electrolytes, sodium appears to be the most critical when it comes to restoring and maintaining fluid balance.

The Beauty of a Bladder Hydration System

Whether you're traveling by foot, bike, ski, snowshoe, or kayak, you need to hydrate or you'll die—figuratively, if not literally. Many of the problems encountered during endurance activities, such as nausea, headaches, heat illness, and altitude sickness, often occur from not drinking enough. Bladder hydration systems encourage you to drink by making fluids readily accessible. You don't have to come to a stop, miss a step, or tie up your hands while reaching for a water bottle. Bladders also allow you to carry large quantities of fluid comfortably. A 50-ounce bladder is equal to two large water bottles, and a 70-ounce bladder equates to three large bottles. The granddaddy of all bladders can hold 100 ounces, the equivalent of four large water bottles. Bladder hydration systems come in various styles and forms, designed specifically for different sports and activities. Worn alone or as part of a pack, sport vest, or hip-mounted belt, a bladder hydration system can efficiently distribute the weight of the fluid without interfering with normal movements.

Fully insulated bladders help liquids stay cool as temperatures rise, and you can add ice to some models. During winter, keep your hydration system bladder and hose from freezing by wearing a layer of clothing on top of it. Keep the drinking hose under cover until it's time to drink. Drinking small amounts at regular intervals should keep the contents from freezing. In severe cold, blow air into the tube and force the liquid back into the bladder or experiment with winterizing adaptation kits available from some manufacturers.

Keep your bladder system clean and free from mold and bacteria by rinsing it with warm water following every use. For more thorough cleaning, use a biodegradable dishwashing detergent and a bottlebrush to clean the tube. You can buy bottlebrushes at a local hardware store or supermarket, or you can buy a cleaning kit from the manufacturer. To sanitize your bladder, add a teaspoon or two of household bleach to a full bladder. Shake vigorously, and then rinse the bladder and tube well with hot water. Don't overkill potential germs. You can make yourself sick from using too much bleach or not rinsing well enough with hot water. Use a paper towel to towel dry the inside of the bladder and then prop the sides open with a paper towel or similar item and hang to air dry. If you're bothered with residual tastes and odors, fill the bladder with water, add two teaspoons of baking soda, and let it sit over night. Rinse well and dry as explained earlier.

Ingesting salt or electrolyte tablets (which contain primarily sodium) during exercise may be an option in some cases. No definitive guidelines exist, but don't overdo it. Generally, don't take more than one tablet (200 to 350 milligrams of sodium) per hour of exercise and take it with plenty (six to eight ounces) of water. Some athletes may need two tablets an hour during long, hot races. If you don't take in enough fluid, water is drawn into your intestines to dilute the ingested salt. You may experience nausea, vomiting, or diarrhea, so don't wait to experiment in an important race or event. Try them in training sessions first.

If you plan to carry electrolyte tablets with you, store them in a plastic bag or waterproof case because they can disintegrate if they contact any moisture, such as sweat. Most athletes can get enough salt in their daily diet, so only use salt (or electrolyte) tablets during prolonged exercise in extreme conditions or if you plan to exercise for three or more hours in the heat and will have access only to plain water.

5. *Prepare for a decrease in appetite.* It's not uncommon for athletes to drop a few pounds in the summer due to a reduced appetite. Concentrate on drinking some of the calories you need to refuel with, especially immediately following exercise. Lemonade, fruit juices, milk shakes, yogurt, instant breakfast drinks, fruit smoothies, and complete meal-replacement products go down fairly easily.

You may need to consume more carbohydrates than usual to keep your muscles well stocked with glycogen, at least during the time when you are acclimating to the heat. Ease in other high-carbohydrate foods, such as bagels, cereal, and energy bars, as soon as you can tolerate them. Resist the urge to wait until your appetite returns because you'll miss the window of opportunity (15 to 30 minutes) that exists after exercise to best replenish your muscle glycogen stores. Eating solid foods will also help replace the other electrolytes you lose through sweating (in much smaller amounts than sodium), such as potassium. You should be able to keep up with your losses easily if your diet includes potassium-rich foods such as juices, fruits, vegetables, milk, and yogurt.

Be aware that hot conditions and intense exercise can doubly suppress your appetite. If you're in for a long day of exercise, such as all-day hike or an adventure race that may even stretch past a day, you will have to force yourself to eat. Eating anything is better than eating nothing, so don't be worried if you survive on the same few foods.

6. *Experiment with glycerol.* Glycerol, a hyperhydrating agent, acts like a sponge in the body, soaking up and holding on to extra water. Now available as a sports supplement, glycerol is to be ingested with water or sports drinks before exercise to help reduce or delay dehydration (see chapter 4, Supplements for Performance). Experiment with it in training before using it in an important event or competition because it can cause nausea or vomiting and you may feel heavy and bloated. Although glycerol enhances fluid retention, it may or may not improve your performance. Try it in long races held in hot, humid conditions, such as marathons, ultraruns, and half and full-length Ironman triathlons, which carry the greatest risk of dehydration.

Performing in Extreme Cold

Thanks to year-round sporting activities and advances in performance clothing, you may find yourself out in the cold for long periods of time. No matter what sport you're involved in, you'll be better prepared to withstand the rigors of exercising in a cold climate if you're well hydrated and well fueled.

Cold Acclimatization

Exercising in cold weather may be something you grin and bear or it may be something you relish. Although it is possible to acclimate to the cold, the process is not well understood and it appears to be harder to accomplish than warm-weather acclimatization. Generally, very fit athletes and those with slightly higher body-fat levels tolerate cold-weather exercise most comfortably.

As anyone who lives and trains in the cold can attest, psychologically adjusting to the cold may be what counts the most. Whether it was growing up running in the snowbelt of upstate New York, surviving ice and snowstorms while attending Georgetown University in Washington, D.C. (a city with few snowplows), or tolerating seven winters in Boston and two more in Colorado, I simply *know* I can handle the cold.

Dehydration and Hypothermia

Exercising in the cold brings its own set of challenges. Endurance athletes must be aware of two potential problems: dehydration and hypothermia.

Dehydration

Although you may not believe it, dehydration can hinder your ability to perform in cold weather similarly to when you exercise in the heat. Do you ever wonder why you would possibly have to make a pit stop in the middle of a snowstorm? Blame it on cold-induced diuresis. When you venture out into the cold, the peripheral blood vessels that carry blood to your skin and to regions of your body such as the ears, hands, and feet constrict to conserve heat and maintain your core temperature. This peripheral vasoconstriction causes your blood pressure to rise, including the blood pressure in your kidneys, which induces you to urinate and lose fluid.

You also lose a considerable amount of fluid exercising in the cold as your respiratory passages warm and humidify incoming cold, dry air (the air you exhale is saturated with water). This could cause a loss of as much as one quart of fluid daily! On top of that, fluids are often not readily available during cold-weather exercise. You either simply don't feel as thirsty or crave fluids when you exercise in the cold, you struggle with keeping it from freezing, or you consciously restrict your intake to avoid the logistical problems or discomfort associated with making pit stops in the cold.

And although Jack Frost is nipping at your ears and toes, you don't stop sweating. Anytime your body temperature rises sufficiently, you sweat. If you tend to overdress when you exercise in the cold, you can sweat profusely, especially during intense efforts. Researchers estimate that if you wear clothing with insulating properties equivalent to four business suits, your sweat losses could reach two quarts per hour during moderate to heavy exercise in freezing conditions. So it's easy to see why athletes become dehydrated during cold-weather exercise.

Hypothermia

Hypothermia, a decrease in your body's core temperature below 97°F, occurs when you lose more heat than you produce. Early warning signs include shivering, euphoria, and confusion. Often accompanied by dehydration and exhaustion, hypothermia can progress to lethargy, weakness, slurred speech, disorientation, and combative behavior as the core temperature continues to fall. Left untreated, a hypothermic person may stop shivering, become progressively delirious, and lapse into a coma.

You don't have to scale the world's tallest mountain in the dead of winter to be at risk for hypothermia. It's a real danger anytime you exercise in cool or cold weather as hypothermia can develop in relatively mild temperatures (50 to 65°F). Be alert for the signs of hypothermia in the following high-risk situations: whenever the weather changes quickly (for example, in spring and fall or at high altitudes), during windy days, if your event involves swimming or passing through water, and during the second half of long races, such as marathons and triathlons, when you may fail to generate enough heat due to a slower pace combined with losing heat through wet clothing (from sweat, rain, or snow).

You may be able to generate enough heat during exercise as long as you keep moving but face trouble when you stop. I encountered hypothermia while climbing Mont Blanc, the tallest of the Alps (15,771 feet) on a sunny August morning in relatively mild wind conditions. Unfortunately, I don't remember the spectacular views of Italy and France from the top, because I was too busy shivering uncontrollably. Caught up in the moment (and not wishing to slow our French guide), I kept on record pace to the summit (5,000 vertical feet in four hours) without any major stops to adjust clothing or eat anything beyond the candy we carried in our pockets. I was in trouble as soon as we reached the top and I stopped generating heat from kicking steps into the snow with heavy double boots. Luckily, I'm still around to tell you how to avoid this scenario!

Hot Chocolate Smoothie

Here is a rich, thick beverage you can eat or drink.

1 tablespoon plus 1 teaspoon of sugar

1 tablespoon plus 1 teaspoon of cocoa powder

1/4 cup of powdered milk

1 tablespoon plus 1 teaspoon of potato starch (used as a thickener; find at your local supermarket or an Asian market)

At home: combine all ingredients and place in a zip-lock bag.

On the trail: place ingredients into an insulated mug, water bottle, or thermos. Add 1 cup of boiling water, stir well, cover, and let stand 5 minutes. Makes one 8-ounce serving.

Nutritional Strategies for Beating the Cold

Mom's advice to have a bowl of stick-to-your ribs oatmeal before you head out into the snow makes a lot of sense, not because the temperature has dropped (you can compensate by dressing appropriately), but because you're less efficient moving over slippery surfaces. In other words, you expend more energy (calories) performing most outdoor activities in a cold climate as compared to a temperate climate. For example, the simple act of walking on snow requires almost twice as much energy as traversing the same route on dry ground at the same speed. You also burn more calories due to the extra weight of heavy boots and winter clothing, which can increase your energy needs by 5 to 15 percent. No universally accepted standard exists for figuring your caloric needs in the cold, but the U.S. Army sets a goal of 4,500 calories a day (for the average male).

Your ability to think clearly and avoid injury and hypothermia decreases when you don't consume enough carbohydrate to replenish your glycogen stores and keep your blood-sugar level steady. Take a look at the scientific basis behind the common adage, "Never ski tired." As you deplete the glycogen in your fast-twitch muscle fibers, you lose muscular strength, and consequently, power. You rely to a large degree on your fast-twitch muscle fibers to correct and control your movements while skiing (and during similar activities), so your ability to execute a series of perfect telemark turns late in the day may hinge on stopping to refuel with a midafternoon snack.

Along with your muscles' need for carbohydrate, your brain relies exclusively on glucose (a simple carbohydrate) for fuel. If your blood sugar falls below a critical level, your judgment and ability to perform skilled maneuvers will severely deteriorate, which could result in injury or death. (Skiers often lament ignoring their desire to call it a day and then being injured on their last trip down the mountain.) Uncontrollable shivering (the body's attempt to raise its core temperature) uses carbohydrate, and if severe, can deplete your glycogen stores as well. Exercising in cold water also uses muscle glycogen at a somewhat higher rate than in warmer conditions.

When it comes time to consume the calories needed for cold-weather exercise, athletes and experts alike continue to debate the merits of a carbohydrate-rich diet versus a diet higher in fat. This debate likely endures because people who live in cold regions often appear to favor high-fat (higher protein) foods. Keep in mind, though, that the relative use of carbohydrate and fat for energy varies widely among individuals. Your fitness level and degree of cold acclimatization, the intensity of the exercise, and the severity of the cold all factor in. For example, the more fit and acclimatized you are, the more fat you burn, which helps spare your limited glycogen reserves. Studies on energy metabolism in the prolonged cold are limited, but the findings do suggest that we metabolize both fat and carbohydrate at a higher rate in the cold. The bulk of the calories you

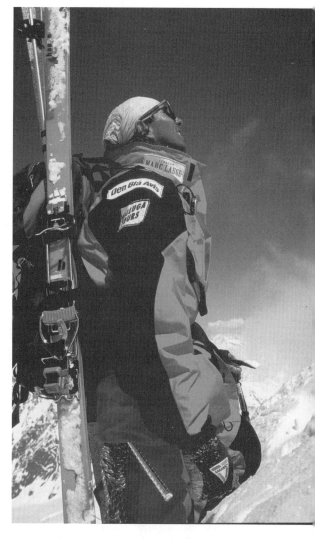

Drink plenty of fluids and refuel at regular intervals to improve your ability to tolerate the cold.

consume during cold-weather exercise, however, should still come from carbohydrate-rich foods because the increase in carbohydrate metabolism is substantially larger than that of fat.

When it comes to improving your ability to tolerate the cold, look at both the source of your calories and the timing of your snacks and meals. Despite conventional wisdom, a high-carbohydrate diet has been found superior to a high-protein diet in improving cold tolerance, and a high-fat or a high-carbohydrate diet has essentially the same effect when meals and snacks are consumed every four hours. A high-fat diet may be superior, though, when snacks and meals are eaten more frequently, for example, every two hours. (However, adequate amounts of carbohydrate must still be consumed to replace muscle glycogen and prevent excess fatigue.) The best advice I have for athletes looking to stay out in the cold (especially for prolonged adventures that involve overnight stays): be in good physical condition, wear the proper clothing, and eat *enough* calories (regardless of the source) to maintain your body temperature.

Assuming you're properly clothed, venturing out into the cold doesn't increase your requirement for any specific nutrient per se. Extra weight from heavy cold-weather clothing and packs and negotiating difficult terrain, however, will increase your calorie needs. We tend to feel less thirsty in cold weather, however, and that can make it logistically difficult or uncomfortable to eat. Without consciously and deliberately fulfilling your fluid and fuel needs, prolonged exercise in the cold can deplete carbohydrate reserves to the extent that hypoglycemia (low blood sugar) and hypothermia (low body temperature) occur. Here's how to give yourself the best chance to perform well in the cold.

1. *Rise and dine.* The mere act of eating revs up your metabolism and generates heat (although not nearly enough to warrant throwing away your long johns). At the very least, warm and nourishing foods provide a psychological boost. If rich in calories, they'll also help you meet your anticipated calorie needs. If you're heading out for a single, short bout of cold-weather exercise, you don't need to worry as much. But hours of continuous exercise can really boost your calorie needs. For example, depending on your body size, pace, pack weight, and terrain, you can expend 3,000 additional calories (or more) during a six-hour hike with a full backpack—on top of your normal daily needs.

Fuel up before you set out or you'll dig a big hole by lunchtime, even if you do snack along the way. And I don't mean a Starbucks Grande and a biscotti. Carbohydrate-rich foods provide the fuel of choice for hard-working muscles. Dress up oatmeal, a classic send-off, by stirring in raisins or other dried fruit, brown sugar, honey, or a scoop of peanut butter. If oatmeal isn't high on your list of favorite foods (it's not even on mine), opt for a peanut butter sandwich or just-add-water products that take only minutes to prepare, such as individual serving cups of chili, couscous with lentils, mashed potatoes, or grits. My breakfast of choice before a long hike, for example, includes a "cup" of macaroni and cheese (230 calories—71 percent from carbohydrate, 14 percent from protein, and 14 percent from fat). If you're worried about gastrointestinal woes, try drinking your calories instead. An ultrarunner friend swears by a couple cans of Ensure before he hits the trail. Instant breakfast and meal-replacement drinks provide another option.

2. *Drink before you're thirsty.* As is true for exercising in any conditions, don't rely on thirst to trigger your need for fluids. Dehydration is often coupled with hypoglycemia and both impair your performance and set you up for hypothermia. You must have access to a source of safe water or other acceptable fluids. A good rule of thumb is that you need a minimum of two quarts per person for a daylong (six-hour) event.

Suggested Menu Items for Cold-Weather Adventures

Whenever you push your limits, you need to eat high-quality foods to replace calories, carbohydrates, and other nutrients, especially if you're exercising in the cold. Although energy bars and gels can certainly fill the bill some of the time, here's a list of foods that you may want to consider on your next cold-weather adventure. The foods you select, obviously, will depend on your activity, tastes, length of time outside, and other practical considerations, such as how much you can carry and how long it takes to prepare the food.

Milk

powdered milk, cocoa mixes, powdered breakfast drinks

Grains

instant whole-grain cereals (oatmeal, Wheatena), granola (eat hot or cold), instant grits, rice, mashed potatoes, couscous and bulgur, quick-cooking pasta and bean products, instant ramen noodles, bagels, pita bread, tortillas, crackers, cookies (especially fruit-filled), rice pudding, breakfast bars

Fruit

fresh fruit—apples, oranges, grapes, and so on; dried fruit—raisins, apricots, banana chips, apples, prunes, dates, pineapple, cherries; fruit leathers, freeze-dried dessert products

Vegetables

freshly cut and peeled (packaged and ready to go), dehydrated, or freeze dried

Protein

peanut butter, nuts, seeds; cured meats—ham, sausage, and so on, dried meat sticks and jerky; assorted cheese; powdered hummus; powdered eggs; no-cook refried beans, canned turkey, chicken, tuna, and shrimp; prepackaged, freeze-dried, or dehydrated entrees

Snacks

chocolate, candy bars, cookies, gumdrops, hard candies, licorice, instant pudding, trail mixes

Beverages

fruit juices and drinks, lemonade, apple cider, herbal teas, coffee, cocoa, fluid-replacement drinks, powdered drink mixes, no-cook soups

Others

margarine, butter powder, seasonings, condiments (honey, sugar cubes, and so on)

Adapted from D. Benardot, 1993, *Sports nutrition-A guide for the professional working with active people,* 2nd ed. (Chicago: American Dietetic Association).

If possible, pour drinks hot into an insulated water bottle (even closed-cell foam secured by duct tape will help) or a sturdy thermos in the morning. Keep fluids from freezing by stashing your container near your body, for example, in a breast jacket pocket rather than your backpack, or strap on a bladder hydration system designed or winterized for cold-weather adventures. Depending on your activity, instant fruit or fluid-replacement drinks, herbal teas, apple cider, cocoa, and soup make good choices. (Be aware that tea provides no calories unless it's spiked with sugar or honey.) Stay away from strongly caffeinated drinks or alcohol because they cause you to urinate. And although you may feel warmer when you first drink alcohol, it doesn't increase your body's core temperature. In fact, it causes you to lose heat by opening the blood vessels to your skin.

Eating snow is a poor option, too. The energy you expend warming the snow can lower your core body temperature enough to induce hypothermia. If you want to obtain water by melting snow, be prepared to spend two precious commodities—your time and your fuel. It takes approximately five cups of snow to obtain one cup of water. Be sure to bring it to a rolling boil (keep an eye on it; five minutes isn't necessary) to kill waterborne microorganisms. If you're on the move, speed up the process by packing snow into your water bottle while it still has liquid in it. Filter or chemically disinfect any melted snow or water that you don't bring to a rolling boil. Despite your best intentions, eating snow or drinking untreated water may be your only option to ward off dehydration and enable you to keep moving in an emergency. Look for clean snow or running water free of contaminants from animals or other humans.

3. *Feed the furnace.* To generate heat, you need to keep moving, and to keep moving, you need fuel. Shovel in the carbohydrates (at least three grams per pound of body weight per day) to keep your tank full and bring on the fat so you can deal with the cold and meet your elevated calorie needs. Choose foods that pack a lot of wallop, especially if you're spending prolonged periods of time in the cold (like overnight) or you're limited as to what you can carry.

On longer excursions, such as four to nine-day excursions, figure on at least two pounds (precooked weight) of food per person per day. Don't skimp on protein but don't overdo it. Carbohydrates and fat are superior to protein when it comes to providing fuel for muscles and improving your cold tolerance. The bottom line when exercising in the cold is to maintain your body temperature by eating enough calories, regardless of the source. Bring a small reserve of extra food in case you get lost or your adventure takes longer than expected.

Be sure to test your favorite foods under various conditions before relying on them in the cold. You won't be the first athlete to find that a favorite energy or candy bar turns into a rock when the temperature drops. It may help to store it in an inner pocket where it soaks up body heat. Remove unnecessary

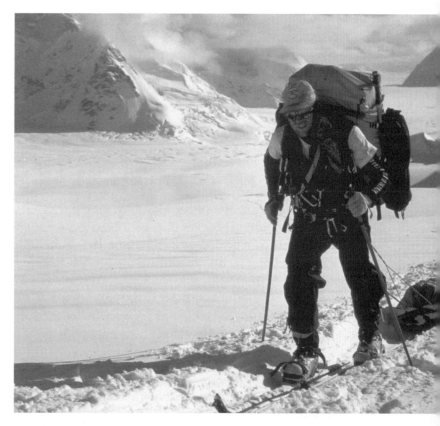

Exercising in extreme conditions requires you to consume additional calories due to the extra clothing, heavy gear, and slippery footing.

wrappings and packages from food to save time and reduce the weight you have to carry. To save removing your mittens or gloves, chop, slice and dice foods, such as energy bars and cheese, before you leave home, and repackage into plactic food storage bags.

Snack or break for minimeals on a regular schedule. Don't wait until you're too wet, tired, or cold to think about your next meal. Make sure you actually down the calories. Because I like to travel light and fast while hiking, I often found myself carrying the food I intended to eat in my hands for a long time, rather than ingesting it. I now have to consciously make myself stop and eat. Plan ahead by anticipating the terrain, weather and other elements you will most likely encounter.

If you're out for hours at a time or it's extremely cold, you may be able to improve your cold tolerance by snacking on high-fat foods every two hours while exercising. Aim for 500 calories per snack. For example, try a peanut butter and jelly sandwich made with two tablespoons of peanut butter or gorp with two to three ounces of peanuts mixed with the same amount of raisins. If you plan to sleep in the cold, try another 500-calorie snack immediately before retiring to your sleeping bag. You may sleep better and your extremities, such as fingers and toes, may stay warmer through the night.

4. *Mind your iron stores.* You may be more susceptible to the cold if your iron levels are low. Researchers have found that iron-deficient women were able to produce heat but had difficulty retaining it to maintain their body temperature. Men suffering from iron deficiency, although not studied, probably respond in a similar manner. Have your serum hemoglobin, hematocrit, and ferritin (stored iron) checked before you pop any supplements. There's no evidence you can enhance your cold tolerance by taking excess iron if you're not deficient.

Performing at High Altitude

If your favorite activity or competitive event has lost its challenge, try doing it at altitude. Rapidly changing weather and less oxygen to draw on for physical efforts, coupled with having a headache, queasy stomach, and a lack of appetite, can make things far more interesting. Mother Nature may rule when it comes to the weather, but you can stay in the game by acclimating, drinking adequate fluids, and making wise food choices.

Altitude Acclimatization

Travel too quickly to higher elevations and you may develop a headache, experience difficulty breathing, suffer from general malaise, weakness and nausea (even vomiting), lose your appetite and have trouble sleeping. Welcome to the world of acute altitude or mountain sickness (AMS). Experts estimate that 6.5 percent of men and 22 percent of women will suffer from this malady when traveling above 6,000 to 8,000 feet (1,800 to 2,400 meters). The underlying mechanism remains unclear, but carbon dioxide accumulating in tissues and fluid seeping into the brain are likely culprits as your body adjusts to less oxygen than it is accustomed to. Why women tend to suffer more from AMS than men do remains unclear.

What else is happening as you gasp for air and your working muscles scream for oxygen? Initially, you breathe more rapidly in an attempt to extract more oxygen out of the air. Your plasma (watery portion of your blood) volume drops to increase the concentration of red blood cells (oxygen carriers) in your blood, and your heart kicks into overdrive to deliver more blood (and thus more oxygen) to active muscles. If you stay long enough, at least 10 to 14 days, your body begins to acclimate and make adjustments that are more permanent. Your plasma volume returns to normal, and your muscles begin to extract more oxygen from the blood, thus reducing the workload on your heart. Stay even longer (four to eight weeks) and you'll end up with more red blood cells, which will really help you compensate for the thinner air. By the way, the percentage of oxygen in the air (20.93 percent) remains constant regardless of the altitude. What varies is the atmospheric (barometric) pressure—it decreases as you ascend, thus decreasing the partial pressure of oxygen in your bloodstream. A substantially reduced pressure gradient between the oxygen in your blood and the oxygen in your active tissues hinders the transfer of oxygen from the blood to the tissues. Less oxygen being delivered to working muscles translates into reduced performances for endurance athletes.

Dehydration and Glycogen Depletion

Dehydration and glycogen depletion remain your nemeses at high elevations. The air holds little water (especially if it's cold), which increases the amount of water you lose through respiration and sweating, even though you may not be aware of it.

Exercising at altitude, particularly extended stays at high altitude (9,000 feet and above), also influences the body's metabolism. Upon acute exposure to high altitude, the body's basal metabolic rate, or the energy it needs to maintain the processes that support life, rises as much as 30 percent. This means you need more calories just to maintain your body weight. You also require more energy to fuel your high-intensity exercise efforts, such as carrying a heavy pack up a steep grade, compared with the same work done at sea level. A shift takes place in your muscles, too, as they begin to rely less on fat and more on carbohydrate (glucose) for fuel. An increased reliance on glucose while at altitude may be advantageous because exercising muscles use carbohydrate more efficiently (in other words, it requires less oxygen) than they do fat. Fortunately, carbohydrate-rich foods seem more palatable at altitude than protein and high-fat foods.

Spend several days to a few months above 14,000 feet (4,300 meters) and you can expect to lose weight. The higher you go and the longer you stay determines how difficult you will find it to maintain a balance between the calories you take in and those that you expend. Initially you can drop a few pounds of water as you acclimate. Your appetite may lag behind also, especially if you suffer with AMS, so your food intake may be low for several days. Of course, if your adventure involves a lot of physical activity at high altitudes, you will be expending a substantial amount of calories that need to be replaced daily. Fortunately, you may be able to largely avoid losing weight (at least up to 16,500 feet or 5,000 meters) by making sure you have access to a variety of tasty foods. Researchers followed eight healthy male Caucasians at the Italian Research Laboratory in Nepal (16,650 feet or 5,050 meters) to test this theory. After one month in comfortable surroundings with a wide choice of palatable foods available, the men did not experience significant change in weight, body-fat percentage, circumference of arms or legs (measures of muscle mass), or performance on strength and vertical-jumping tests.

On the whole, digestibility and absorption of nutrients does not appear to contribute to weight loss unless you're at extreme altitudes (above 23,000 feet or 7,000 meters), in which case your digestive tract may lose some of its absorptive capacity. Of course, at that altitude, you may experience a few other problems too! Most of the weight you lose after prolonged exposure to altitude is simply loss of body fat and muscle mass. The cause is a combination of taking in too few calories—because of physical discomfort, lack of appetite, and limited food choices—and expending more calories, including an elevated resting metabolic rate.

A sizable portion of altitude-related weight loss, up to 70 percent, is a loss of muscle mass. In elite mountain climbers, researchers have documented losses that decrease the thigh cross-sectional area by 15 percent over a two-month period at altitudes above 18,000 feet (5,500 meters). Detraining may be a partial cause of this muscle loss. If you arrive in top condition, you may lose muscle due to a relative lack of exercise while you acclimate, recover from hard days, and wait out weather delays. On the other hand, acute hypoxia (lack of oxygen) may directly affect protein metabolism by decreasing your ability to synthesize new protein.

Nutritional Strategies for Handling High Altitude

If possible, give yourself a chance to acclimatize when traveling to a higher altitude than you're accustomed to. Arrive at least two weeks before a competitive event. If that's not possible, compete within 24 hours of your arrival to minimize the effects of AMS. On hikes and expeditions when you plan to spend the night, ascend slowly, in stages. A good rule to follow over

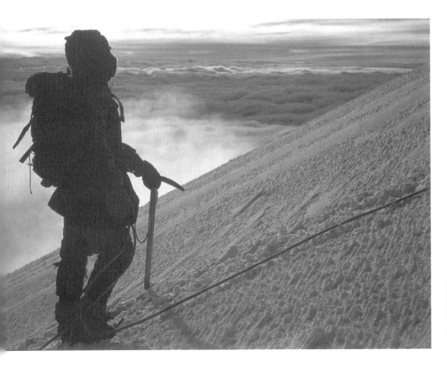

Minimize acute altitude sickness by drinking adequate fluids and making wise food choices.

10,000 feet (3,000 meters) is to climb only 1,000 feet (300 meters) per day. To limit your weight loss, bring a variety of palatable food and try to limit the time you spend at extreme altitude. Beyond that, here's how to enhance your performance at altitude.

1. *Ignore your lack of appetite.* Just because you're nauseated or don't feel like eating doesn't mean you're off the hook. With less oxygen going to your brain and stomach, you can expect to lose your appetite, especially the first few days as you acclimatize. Unfortunately, active muscles can't wait that long. Food is fuel, so the more you eat, the more you'll be able to do. Plus you'll feel better and enjoy the experience more. On my trip to Kilimanjaro, Africa's tallest peak (19,340 feet), I could definitely tell which group members were experiencing AMS just from their lack of mealtime conversation!

Don't worry about chowing down on exactly the right thing. Just be sure to bring a variety of appetizing foods with you because your tastes often change at altitude. In other words, don't rely solely on a pack full of gels and energy bars. (At the very least, bring several flavors to ward off "flavor fatigue.") Foods you love at home typically have the best chance of being eaten when you're up high. Keep in mind that sweet-tasting foods, in particular, can become overwhelming at altitude. I was caught off guard by the complete lack of appetite that can strike at high elevations as I hiked up to 15,000 feet on Kilimanjaro. Partial to sweet-tasting, red-colored sports drinks at sea level, I couldn't even look at my favorite drink, never mind stomach it. Finding a canister of lemon-lime powered sports drink in the bottom of my pack saved the trip. (Butterfinger candy bars and potato chips helped me reach a new "high," too.) Eat small, frequent meals to keep your energy up and help combat nausea.

2. *Load up on carbohydrates and fluids.* Fill up on carbohydrates (at least 60 percent of your total calories) because they require significantly less oxygen for metabolism and are generally better tolerated than high-fat foods at altitude. You have about 1,600 to 1,800 calories of glycogen (stored carbohydrate) in your liver and muscle tissue. If you don't constantly replenish this supply with foods rich in simple and complex carbohydrates (for example, bread, cereals, grains, pasta, fruit, vegetables, powdered milk, candy, and sugar), you'll end up exhausted and less able to tolerate the effects of being at altitude. On top of that, your body will use valuable protein stores as energy instead. Keep snacks handy and munch often on carbohydrate-rich choices such as bagels, pita bread, instant pudding, fresh and dried fruit, carrot sticks, pretzels, gorp, granola or breakfast bars, fig newtons, candy, and energy bars and gels.

Exercising at altitude increases the rate at which you lose water, so your fluid intake must increase to match this loss. By the time you reach 10,000 feet you might need four to five quarts or more a day. Energy drinks provide both calories (in the form of carbohydrates) and fluid. Other good choices (besides plain water) include instant fruit drinks, reconstituted powdered milk or meal-replacement drinks, hot chocolate, and soup. Avoid alcohol completely because it contributes to both dehydration and nausea. The oft-repeated advice that urine runs clear when you're well hydrated holds true at any elevation.

3. *Cook simple fare while on the trail.* Preparing even routine foods at altitude can be tedious, so get everyone in the group to pitch in. Don't weigh yourself down with foods that take a long time to cook, such as beans, brown rice, and elbow or shell pasta. Concentrate on instant mashed potatoes, couscous, thin pastas, low-fat ramen noodles, quick-cooking rice, dehydrated foods, and freeze-dried foods. Be sure to estimate how many cups of hot water and fuel you'll need to prepare these items. To save time and energy, pack whole meals together ahead of time and label them with the dates you will eat them. Soak dehydrated foods during the day in an extra water bottle to shorten their cooking time.

Don't worry if you don't prepare gourmet fare. That's not the goal. A simple spice kit can beef up ordinary fare. Of course, you could always buy a bigger pack and bring your whole kitchen. I met a woman at base camp (10,000 feet) on Mount Rainier who brought a fresh lemon and a kitchen knife to slice it just so she could flavor her drinking water!

4. *Eat iron-rich foods and supplement as necessary.* If you live and train at moderate altitudes (3,000 to 8,000 feet, or 1,000 to 2,500 meters) or you're planning an extended trip to high altitude, be sure to consume plenty of iron-rich foods on a regular basis. Meat (especially red meat), fortified breakfast cereals, dark leafy greens, dried beans and peas, dried fruit, and prune juice make good choices. You want to take advantage of your body's desire to build new red blood cells. Iron is a crucial component of hemoglobin (housed in red blood cells), the prime carrier of oxygen in blood. Female athletes must pay particular attention to their iron status while training at altitude. The need for supplementation can be easily determined though routine blood tests (see chapter 8: Hitting the Wall).

5. *Explore the merits of vitamin E.* Vitamin E, a powerful antioxidant, helps keep cell membranes healthy. Without enough of it, your red blood and muscle cells are destroyed more rapidly by oxidative damage from free radical molecules. Exercise raises your need for vitamin E, and exercise at high altitude probably raises it even more. Eat a training diet containing whole-grain products, wheat germ, vegetable oils, green leafy vegetables, nuts and seeds, and liver and eggs (yolks) to ensure an adequate intake of vitamin E. Supplementation may help for intense, prolonged exercise at high altitudes, although no firm recommendations currently exist. A reasonable dose for most physically active people at sea level is 100 to 400 IU per day. Taking large doses is mostly harmless, but some individuals report flu-like symptoms when taking more than 400 IU daily for prolonged periods.

Developing a Lean and Strong Body

6

"Female athletes often think they need to look a certain way to be an athlete. It took me years to realize that I am an athlete no matter what I look like! My body weight is irrelevant. I weigh more than a lot of the guys on my team. In fact, they tease me all the time about being so muscular, but the added muscle and strength I gain from weight training is crucial to my success as an adventure racer. I went from weighing 125 pounds (25 percent body fat) and wearing a size 10 to 145 pounds (13 percent body fat) and a size 6."

—Cathy Sassin, second-place, 1998 Raid Gauloises Adventure Team Race

Do you jump on and off the scale all day long or play the body-check comparison game every time you toe the line? Athletes participating in endurance events typically fall into two categories when it comes to body weight: those who wish they had less weight to carry around, and those trying to gain weight by bulking up with muscle. In either case, you're wise to aim for a lean, healthy body through a combination of solid training and healthy eating habits. You will perform poorly and may even do serious harm to your health, however, if this quest turns into an unhealthy obsession.

The Issue of Weight

If you're like most of the athletes I meet, you've probably tried to lose or gain weight at one time or another, most likely in hopes of performing better. Although most of us readily accept our height, we often spend far too much time and energy on trying to manipulate our body weight. The important thing to remember is that your weight is influenced by more than what you eat and how much you exercise. Your sex, age, and height, as well as the thickness of your bones and your ratio of muscle to fat all affect how much you weigh. Obviously, many of these factors are genetically predetermined and out of your control.

If you're using a typical bathroom or locker-room scale to monitor your weight, accept its limitations. Your bathroom scale cannot differentiate between fat weight and muscle weight. Besides, body weight is not static, remaining constant from day to day or even throughout a single day. Think of your body weight as a vital sign, like your blood pressure or body temperature, which can vary throughout the day. To gain useful information from the scale, weigh yourself nude in the morning, once or twice a week, after emptying your bladder and before you exercise or eat breakfast. Monitoring your weight over time (during a specific phase of your training, for example) can be valuable. An otherwise unexplained drop of several pounds over a few weeks or months, for instance, may help explain poor performances.

Daily weigh-ins, on the other hand, provide information only on shifts in body fluids and are influenced by many factors. Sweating during exercise and vomiting or diarrhea due to an illness will temporarily decrease your weight, whereas you may appear to gain weight (literally overnight) due to water retention related to hormonal changes or your carbohydrate intake. If you still want to weigh yourself daily, put your time and energy to good use by weighing yourself before and after exercise to monitor your fluid losses. To rehydrate, drink at least two cups of fluid for every pound lost.

As a serious-minded athlete, don't put too much stock into standard height-weight tables or even the more recent weight guidelines from the National Institutes of Health that are based on body mass index (BMI). BMI is calculated with a formula that considers body weight relative to height. It does a better job of predicting a person's body-fat percentage than simply looking at body weight by itself. Health professionals developed BMI to help find people at risk for obesity-related diseases such as diabetes, coronary heart disease, and some cancers.

Many athletes and even regular exercisers, however, may show up on the charts as overweight (BMI of 25.0 to 29.9) or obese (BMI of 30.0 or above) even when they're not. You can blame your lean body mass, or muscles, which are denser and thus heavier than fat. If you're working out regularly and are really fit, don't worry about your BMI. Healthy bodies come in all shapes and sizes. What's important is your fitness level, not your weight.

Body Composition and Performance

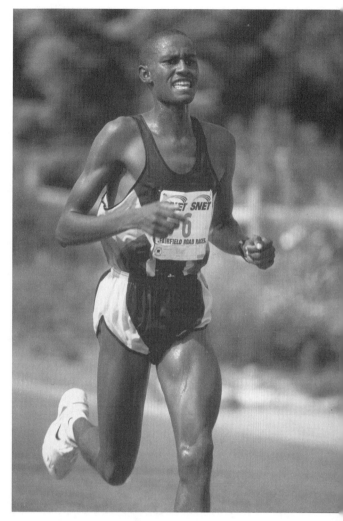

Ignore the scale. Many of the best athletes weigh more than you expect—muscle is denser than fat.

Rather than relying solely on a scale to evaluate the effectiveness of your diet and training programs, take a look at your body composition. Simply put, the body is divided into two compartments, fat mass and fat-free lean body mass. You can distinguish the amount of body weight due to fat (expressed as percent body fat) from the body's nonfat tissue, or lean mass (bones, muscles, organs, and connective tissue) using various techniques of body-composition analysis.

Generally, leaner athletes, or those with lower percentages of body fat, perform better on tests of speed, endurance, balance, agility, and jumping ability. For endurance athletes in particular, excessive body fat can be undesirable. It translates into extra weight that you must transport for extended periods. The ideal body composition varies from sport to sport. In general, body-fat levels of elite endurance athletes, such as marathoners and triathletes, range from 5 to 9 percent in men and 8 to 15 percent in women.

Keep in mind that these levels are what studies show, not what all endurance athletes must strive for or necessarily attain. Doing whatever it takes to whittle your body fat down into these ranges doesn't guarantee that you'll enter the elite ranks.

In fact, shaving your body fat level too low can be unhealthy and detrimental to your performance. Your body needs some essential fat to function—at least 3 to 5 percent for men and 8 to 12 percent for women (female athletes require higher body-fat levels to protect menstrual and child-bearing functions). If you choose to monitor your body-fat percentage, be realistic. The goal is to achieve an appropriate body-fat level that allows you to perform at your best without harming your overall health. As with weight, the top performers within any sport will vary in body-fat percentage. For example, in the early 1980s, I was involved in a comprehensive study of elite female distance runners. Most of the women were running well at body-fat percentages between 10 and 12 percent. The top collegiate 10K runner and the world's leading female marathoner at that time, however, were both significantly higher than that range!

Methods of Assessing Body Composition

Several different techniques are available for assessing body composition. The following section provides information, including the advantages and drawbacks, of the most common methods available to endurance athletes. Body fat can't be measured directly, only estimated by one of these methods and even the best methods have errors of 3 percent or more. In other words, if you're told you have 10 percent body fat, you could have anywhere from 7 to 13 percent.

Underwater (or Hydrostatic) Weighing

This method requires you to expel all the air from your lungs and then be weighed in a special tank while totally immersed under water. The difference between your weight on land and your weight in water is used to estimate your body density. From that your body-fat percentage can be extrapolated. This is definitely a time when being found dense is okay, as denser bodies have less fat! If you're interested in underwater weighing, check out a local sports medicine center, hospital with a wellness department, or a university with a physical education or exercise physiology program.

Underwater weighing is the gold standard, or the technique of choice, when it comes to assessing body composition, and all other methods are compared to it. Much of the success of this method, however, depends on the athlete's ability to expel as much air as possible. Also, underwater weighing can be expensive (up to $100 a test) and time-consuming, and the formulas used may be less appropriate for some populations (such as older and non-Caucasian athletes).

Air Displacement (Bod Pod)

This new technique relies on the same whole-body measurement principle as underwater weighing: the overall density of the body can be used to determine the percentage of fat and lean tissue. You sit in an enclosed capsule (the Bod Pod) for about one minute as computer sensors determine the amount of air displaced by your body. Estimating body-fat percentage using the Bod Pod is fast, does not require you to get wet, and appears to correlate closely with hydrostatic weighing. More studies are needed on competitive athletes, though, and since very few facilities can afford a Bod Pod, this option can be expensive and may not be available in your area. Check research laboratories and athletic facilities serving professional and collegiate athletes.

Bioelectrical Impedance Analysis

Bioelectrical impedance analysis (BIA) involves having a low voltage (undetectable) electric current passed through your body via electrodes attached to your hand and ankle. Your lean body tissue (primarily your muscles), containing most of your body's water and electrolytes, conducts the current faster and more easily than adipose or fat tissue. The faster the current travels through your body, the less body fat you have.

Although quick and non-invasive, BIA can be inaccurate when used with athletes. It tends to overestimate body-fat percentages in lean individuals, and results are easily swayed by fluid shifts in the body caused, for example, by dehydration from exercising or fluid retention due to a menstrual cycle. To get accurate and reliable measurements, you must be well hydrated (although avoid eating and drinking four hours prior to the test), and it's best to avoid exercising for 12 hours before the test.

The same advice applies if you purchase a scale-like device based on BIA designed for home use (like the Tanita body-fat scale). You need to take readings at the same time of day, when you are in a hydrated state (with an empty bladder). Avoid getting on the scale when you are most likely to be dehydrated—early in the morning or late at night, following exercise, after a sauna, or within 24 hours of consuming large amounts of caffeine or alcohol.

Skinfold Caliper Test

A skinfold caliper test involves using hand-held calipers to pinch and measure the thickness of fat located right under the skin. Typically three to seven sites are measured, for example, the abdomen, back of the arm, thigh, hip, and back of the shoulder. These measurements are plugged into a formula to estimate percent body fat. This simple, noninvasive, inexpensive technique can provide very accurate and reliable readings, but only if the measurement taker is skilled and has lots of practice. Skinfolds are not the most valid predictor of body fat but the measurements can be used to monitor or indicate changes in body composition over time.

Using a Tape Measure

You can do essentially the same thing as skinfold tests by using a tape measure. This method requires no fancy scientific formulas, just taking precise measurements. Simply measure selected points on your upper arm, chest, waist, hips, thighs, and calves to the nearest eighth of an inch with a tape measure and record these readings. You won't be calculating a specific body-fat percentage. Over time, though, as you repeat the measurements, you will be able to see your body respond as you adopt healthier eating habits or undertake a new training program.

If losing weight is your goal, for example, monitoring the amount you "lose" (with your measurements getting smaller over time) can be gratifying and reassuring. If you lose fat and gain muscle at the same time, your weight as registered by a scale may not change at all. Female athletes who intensify their training or begin a strength-training program often struggle with this fact. A pound of muscle (think of it like a brick), however, takes up less space than a pound of fat (think of cotton balls), so a tape measure will more accurately reflect changes in body composition than a scale.

Determining a Healthy Body Composition

Many athletes I counsel want to know what they should weigh, especially those who are new to a sport or embarking on a challenging physical endeavor for the first time. I remind them that determining an exact weight or body-fat percentage isn't necessary or even desirable. Strive to keep your weight within an optimal *range*, within a few pounds for example, during a competitive season. Living on salad and rice cakes while training twice a day to reach or maintain a specific weight should be a clue that your weight goal is unrealistic.

Remember that your weight and body-fat percentage will vary throughout the year depending on the amount and type of training you are engaged in. Measuring your body-fat percentage is better than knowing only your weight, but it's still just a number. Don't give a single reading too much credence. Rather, use several readings taken over time to monitor changes in body composition. Since these changes can take time to detect, most athletes won't benefit from having their body-fat percentage estimated more than twice a year. To make it most worthwhile, keep accurate notes on the type and volume of training you were involved in at the time of each measurement.

Instead of focusing on your weight, concentrate on setting up a sound training program and establishing healthy eating habits. These two factors will help carry you over the long haul. The weight you end up at is your optimal healthy weight—one that you can realistically achieve and maintain, perform well at without compromising your health, and still have enough energy left to enjoy life. You may not like what this healthy weight turns out to be, but that's another issue!

Changing Your Body Composition

I find that many athletes struggle when it comes to achieving a healthy weight. Some need to gain weight, while others want to lose weight (or body fat). Whether you maintain, lose, or gain is primarily a matter of energy balance. You'll maintain your weight if you consume roughly the same amount of energy, or calories, that you expend. To gain weight, you'll need to consume more calories than you burn off. To lose weight, you must expend more calories than you take in. In other words, you'll need to eat less and exercise more, or ideally, do both. It sounds simple, but in reality the process can be quite complex. You're dealing with the human body after all, not a machine.

Strategies for Losing Weight

Before embarking on a plan to lose weight, be sure that you really need to. Don't assume that your performance will automatically improve if you lose weight or assume that every time you weigh more on the scale you've gained fat. Determining your body-fat percentage or taking skinfold measurements can be particularly useful before you attempt to lose weight, especially if you're an athlete sporting a stocky, muscular build or a female who tends to look heavier because you carry weight on your hips and thighs. In any case, if your body fat is at a reasonable level, you won't gain anything from dieting or starving yourself to reach a new low on the scale.

You may instead need to concentrate on accepting your inherited body type or, if you're a coach or trainer, on accepting the body types of the athletes you work with. One of my collegiate teammates, the best female cross-country runner in her state as a high school senior, is a perfect example. Tall with a lean upper body, she carried all her weight on the lower half of her body. Despite completing a successful high school career at a certain weight, our coach decided she would perform better in college if she lost five pounds. Living on salad, air-popped popcorn, and a small dinner (accompanied by a scoop of ice cream as a reward for making it through the day), she did lose the five pounds. But she was constantly battling an upper-respiratory infection and even pulled some intercostal muscles (between the ribs) from coughing so hard! She never fully recuperated and ran poorly all year.

Second, I always remind people trying to lose weight not to excessively restrict calories or attempt to follow a very low-calorie diet. These methods of losing weight are not an option, especially for a serious athlete. If you lose more than a pound a week (two pounds for males), you're not losing fat—you're losing water, muscle glycogen, and lean muscle mass. Your competitors are the only ones who benefit from this type of weight loss. Athletes who are chronically dehydrated and operating with low glycogen stores find it difficult to maintain their usual training pace, fatigue earlier in workouts and competitions, and suffer more injuries. It's also difficult to be in peak mental shape if you're depressed, anxious, weak, or preoccupied with food.

The long-term consequences of losing weight rapidly can be costly: loss of muscular strength and power, electrolyte disturbances due to dehydration, increased susceptibility to colds and other illnesses, iron deficiency anemia, amenorrhea (loss of menstrual periods), low bone density (due to hormonal imbalances and the lack of calcium), ketosis (an undesirable state the body enters when it must use its fat to fuel the brain), and potential kidney problems. You may ultimately end up losing training time or even missing competitions, so don't try to lose weight during your competitive season or when you need to deliver a peak performance.

Repeated attempts to manipulate body weight or body fat below a level that is normal for you are counterproductive. Significant metabolic changes result from chronic dieting or the loss of critical fat stores. For example, if you restrict your caloric intake too drastically, your body resists your attempts to lose weight by immediately dropping its resting metabolic rate—that is, your body will require fewer calories to carry on essential vital functions and will store excess calories as fat. Because your body has no way of knowing how long this "starvation" will last, it attempts to protect itself by adapting to fewer calories.

Although this reduction in resting metabolic rate probably isn't permanent in most people, it may play a role if you lose and gain weight repeatedly. It appears that the body receives messages via brain signals and hormones that help it become more efficient at extracting energy from food and storing it as body fat. Consequently, perpetual dieters often find it progressively harder to lose weight and must eat even fewer calories in the future to induce further weight loss. Muscles burn calories (fat doesn't) and lean muscle tissue is lost every time you diet, especially when you drop pounds quickly. So, as your muscle mass decreases, your body requires fewer calories to remain at the same weight.

Set a realistic weight-loss goal. You can't lose body fat over night. Focus on achieving a weight you can maintain at this point in your life through exercise and healthy eating habits. Perhaps you've added children to your family or picked up additional hours at the office that cut into your training time. If this is the case, don't assume you can weigh what you did in college or even what you weighed last year!

Forget about diets and short-term fixes too. As long as you believe a quick, easy way to lose weight is waiting for you right around the corner—the next miracle diet, a promising new supplement—you'll never fully commit to changing your eating habits. Keeping that in mind, read on for some guidelines on how to lose weight sensibly.

Strategy #1. Keep a food diary

A food diary serves the same purpose as a training log. It can help you or someone with a trained eye (like a registered dietitian) decipher your current eating habits—what works for you and what doesn't. As in the exercise in chapter 1, simply write down everything you eat or drink from the time you get up in the morning until you go to bed. It also helps to record the reason you are eating. For example, are you eating because you are hungry? Bored? Nervous about an upcoming race?

Writing down everything you eat can help you stay committed to your long-range goal of losing weight sensibly. One study followed 38 dieters who had been on a weight-loss program for a year through the "danger zone"; for example, two weeks before Thanksgiving until two weeks after New Year's Day. The 25 percent of participants who consistently recorded all the foods they ate during this period managed to lose seven more pounds! The other 75 percent who weren't so vigilant gained back an average of three pounds.

The very act of writing down your daily choices, not exactly what you record, is what counts. Self-monitoring forces us to be accountable for our daily actions. For example, you can't as easily ignore the fact that you nibbled through a jar of peanuts while meeting a deadline at work if you write it down. You can also glance at a food diary to see if you're eating enough of the healthy foods you need. Leave your food diary in a visible place as a visual reminder (for example, on your desk or in your kitchen) or record what you eat in your day planner or training log.

Strategy #2. Reduce your current intake by no more than 500 calories a day

Losing one pound a week requires you to create a deficit of 3,500 calories, or 500 calories a day, by exercising more and eating less. Drastically reducing the amount you eat isn't realistic for most athletes. Dieting all day by skimping on breakfast and lunch and then beating a path to the refrigerator from dinner until bedtime doesn't work. Starving yourself while working out as hard as you can isn't something you can keep up for long either.

Trimming the amount of calories you currently consume by small increments (such as 200 to 300 calories for an athlete consuming 3,000 calories) shouldn't suppress your metabolism and it helps protect against the loss of too much lean muscle tissue. You'll also still have plenty of energy to train at a high level, which is essential if you want to keep the weight off permanently. Your family, officemates, and training buddies will appreciate this approach, too, as you won't feel deprived and become a complete bear to live with.

Once you've met your nutrient needs (keeping the Food Guide Pyramid in mind) look for ways to trim extra calories. You may be suffering from portion distortion. Due to the "super-sizing" of America, an average bakery bagel now provides 320 calories—the equivalent of eating three to four slices of bread! Paying attention to serving sizes can be an easy way to reel in your calorie intake. Mega-sized cookies, muffins, and sodas may appear to be a good buy, but can you afford the 500 to 800 calories they provide?

If you eat out frequently, watch your intake of high-fat foods. Inquire about how foods are prepared before ordering them to detect hidden fats, such as cream sauces, olive oil, and cheese. And then ask yourself how many times you begin meals by eating a whole basket of bread! If the restaurant won't honor special requests, such as serving the salad dressing on the side and having the skin taken off chicken, find a new restaurant. Getting a handle on how many calories you drink throughout the day can be helpful too. Cutting back on soda, alcohol, sports shakes, and even juice, may be all you need to do.

Keep in mind that losing weight is best done in stages. Once you lose a few pounds, let your body get used to your new weight, then decide whether you're feeling weaker or stronger before trying to lose more. Incorporating even small changes into new habits takes time and effort. Stop and assess how you are doing at maintaining the healthy changes that got you to a lower weight. Can you realistically continue them? Will you be able to do more? You may find that you'd be better off directing your efforts elsewhere, into your training or accepting your body type, rather than continuing to try to lose more weight.

Strategy #3. Eat enough real food

Don't throw the Food Guide Pyramid out the window because you're trying to lose weight. You still need to consume foods from all five food groups, just like everyone else. Many female athletes I know wouldn't dream of sitting down and eating a real lunch, a sandwich and a glass of milk, for example. Instead, they nibble their way though the day racking up calories from mini chocolate bars, candy, energy bars, nonfat frozen yogurt, oversize bagels and muffins, and soda or juice drinks.

If you find yourself constantly eating out of a box, in your car, or while standing up, consider that these unfulfilling actions may be sabotaging your efforts to lose weight. You're more likely to feel full and experience less guilt or denial if you simply plan to eat meals (of at least three food groups) and snacks (aim for one to two food groups). You'll likely eat fewer calories too.

You may lack skills in the cooking and domestic department. I met one college athlete who lived off campus and was responsible for his own meals. He routinely boiled four hotdogs for lunch, followed by four more for dinner! If you're like me and can't afford to hire a personal chef, invest some time and energy into learning basic cooking and meal-planning skills. Keep a variety of nutritious, easy-to-prepare foods on hand so you won't have to rely on takeout and fast foods. Watch how much soda and alcohol you drink. These beverages contribute calories and little in the way of nutrients. You don't want them to crowd out low-fat milk and fruit juices, which are more nutritious.

Strategy #4. Concentrate on eating your calories when you need them most during the day

Have you worked out today? Have you eaten today? Because most of us perform the bulk of our training, our work, and our family obligations between nine and six (even earlier if you train first thing in the morning), why do most of us insist on eating the majority of our calories after six o'clock? Our muscles and our brain cells thrive on having a steady, constant supply of fuel available. To avoid becoming too hungry and devouring everything in sight, divide your calories up throughout the day. Plan to eat a meal or healthy snack every three to four hours so your blood sugar doesn't dip too low. Otherwise, you'll be racing for the nearest vending machine or fast food outlet.

Be creative with your eating schedule. Even if you're trying to lose weight, you still need to be well fueled before you head out the door, and you still need to replenish your glycogen stores following exercise. For instance, if you train after work, eat less at lunchtime and save some calories for an afternoon snack closer to your workout time. A sports drink or energy bar after you finish can take the place of that second helping or extra dessert at dinner. You can diet by eating reasonable size portions (a good reality check is the serving size listed on the label), selecting lower-fat items, and by eating fewer calories at night when you don't really need them.

Strategy #5. Keep some fat in your diet

The fat you eat in foods doesn't inevitably reappear as body fat. You can still obtain a desirable level of body fat if you snack on half a bagel spread with peanut butter or drizzle salad dressing over your greens. Besides supplying energy and essential fatty acids, fat allows your body to absorb and use fat-soluble vitamins.

Fat also heightens the flavors of food, curbs cravings, and helps you feel full. Without some fat in your diet, it's easy to overeat in the carbohydrate department. How many times have you passed on eating a hamburger because it's too fattening only to find yourself plowing through a box of fat-free cookies a few hours later? The fact remains that excess calories will be converted into body fat, whether those calories come from fat, carbohydrates, or protein.

Eating a diet that contains an appropriate amount of fat, at least 20 percent of total calories or $1/2$ gram per pound of body weight, is not overdoing it. The key is to concentrate on eating the right kind of fat. Nuts and "natural" nut butters (those not processed with partially hydrogenated fats), seeds, avocados, and oils such as olive, canola, and flaxseed, are rich in heart-healthy monounsaturated fat. Of course, even these heart-healthy fats supply calories, so watch the amounts you consume.

Fats that you don't need in your diet are saturated fats and partially hydrogenated, or trans, fats. To reduce the saturated fat in your diet, choose low-fat dairy products and lean cuts of meat. Limiting traditional "fatties" such as fried food, fast food, and processed foods containing partially hydrogenated vegetable oils such as stick margarine, snack foods, and bakery goods will help keep the amount of trans fat you consume under control.

Strategy #6. Complement your aerobic training with anaerobic or strength training.

Don't fall into the trap of believing that you must train at a slow pace to burn fat and lose weight. Although it's true that exercising at lower intensities (aerobic exercise) uses a higher percentage of fat than high-intensity exercise (anaerobic exercise, such as interval or speed work), it's not that simple. Exercise does more than just help you burn fat. It helps create a calorie deficit in the body; in other words, it helps you expend more calories than you consume. Remember that to lose a pound, you need to create a deficit of 3,500 calories, either by eating less, exercising more, or some combination of the two. No matter what fuel you burn during exercise, the body can pull from its fat stores at a later time to make up for the calories expended during exercise.

The amount of calories you burn during exercise depends on many factors—your body weight, the type of exercise you do, the intensity, the duration, and whether you are a novice or a trained athlete. As an endurance athlete, you're most likely focusing on putting in the miles. But strength or resistance training and higher intensity exercise, such as intervals, tempo workouts, and fartlek training (breaking your normal pace up with fast bursts), can help you lose weight, as well as boost your performance. Don't forget that during exercise you burn both fats and carbohydrates for energy. Given the same time period, lower-intensity exercise uses a greater percentage of fat, but it also burns fewer total calories than higher-intensity exercise. During faster paced activities, a greater percentage of calories come from carbohydrate than from fat, but the overall amount of calories you use is higher. What matters most is the total number of calories used, not the percentage of fat-to-carbohydrates. Higher-intensity exercise helps you lose weight because it uses more calories per minute.

Think about it this way: a large percentage of a small number can be smaller than a small percentage of a large number. For example, a 150-pound cyclist averaging a leisurely 12 miles per hour may burn 380 calories an hour, with about 70 percent of the energy derived from fat. The same cyclist may burn approximately 780 calories per hour riding at 18 miles per hour, with fat providing about 50 percent of the necessary fuel. However, 70 percent of 380 is 266, and 50 percent of 780 is 390, so the more intense ride burns over 100 more fat calories. More important, because few people have unlimited time to exercise, riding more intensely burns 400 more calories in the same period (780 versus 380).

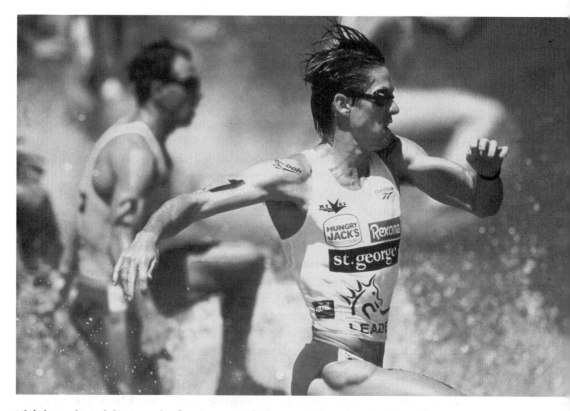

High-intensity training or racing burns more calories per minute than low-intensity exercise.

Trained athletes burn more fat for two reasons. They use fat sooner during exercise (training helps you store more fat within muscles for easy access), and they have the ability to work at higher intensities (thanks in part to an elevated lactate threshold) than recreational athletes, thus burning more calories and proportionally higher amounts of fat. Of course, you can't just go flying out the door and start training frantically every day in an attempt to lose weight. You'll burn very few calories from the couch if you come down with an injury.

Working at lower intensities until you can handle more intense workouts helps you avoid injuries and prepares the body for future stress. As you work up to handling higher-intensity workouts, duration becomes a greater factor in losing weight not to burn more fat, but to burn more calories. In other words, you need to exercise longer to make up for the lower number of calories used per minute. Consider increasing your training volume by adding more miles to your weekly training program. Or simply become more active during the day, such as taking the stairs instead of the elevator and walking instead of driving to complete errands.

Visiting the weight room while trying to lose weight is especially beneficial. Strength training builds muscle mass, which boosts your resting metabolic rate. This means you'll be burning more calories throughout the day, even when you're not exercising. Weight training also helps ensure that the weight you lose is from body fat, not muscle.

Strategies for Gaining Weight

Gaining weight can be an advantage if speed, power, leverage, or mass come into play in your sport or activity. Of course you most likely want to gain lean muscle tissue, not fat. Adding muscle mass can increase your strength-to-weight ratio, which ultimately increases your strength and power, enabling you to perform at a higher level. Depositing extra body fat does little to enhance power or strength. On the other hand, some endurance athletes find that carrying a little extra padding may help them fend off illness and better weather the rigors of hard training.

Like those athletes trying to lose weight, you need to be realistic about the amount of weight or lean body mass you can gain. Adding a few pounds before you head off to an ultrarun or adventure race is one thing, but expecting to transform your physique is a whole different ball game. Your genes, gender, diet, training program (including the amount of strength training you're willing to do), and motivation all count. Look at the other members of your family, especially your parents, to get a clear picture of your potential. If you're a well-trained athlete or simply a "hard gainer," you may find it difficult, if not impossible, to gain weight without substantially increasing the amount of calories you eat or cutting back on your exercise.

The bottom line, of course, is that to gain weight you must consume more calories than you expend. In general, you'll need to eat an extra 500 calories a day to gain about one pound of lean muscle in a week. Don't look to supplements as a substitute for hard work and good nutrition. No magic nutrients exist that promote substantial gains in strength and muscle mass. (See chapter 4 for a complete review of creatine and other supplements that are touted for their potential to enhance lean muscle mass in athletes.) Keep the following guidelines in mind as you attempt to gain lean muscle mass.

Strategy #1. Calories and strength training count the most

Contrary to popular opinion, your calorie intake, not the amount of protein you consume, has the most impact when it comes to gaining muscle. Bulking up, or building muscle, requires you to have enough calories on board to meet your energy demands, as well as support the growth of new tissue. If you don't take in enough calories, the protein you consume will be used to satisfy your energy needs instead of building new muscle tissue. You must also commit to a well-designed strength or weight-training program. Just eating extra calories or protein, or ingesting vitamins or other supplements, won't magically do the trick. Strength training helps muscle cells become more efficient at using available protein to synthesize new cells.

If you're training and eating appropriately, most of the weight you put on will be muscle. Of course, if you simply overeat (literally consume more calories than you burn off), then the extra calories from any source—carbohydrates, protein, or fat—will help you gain weight by increasing your body fat.

You may need to make eating a higher priority to ensure that you're getting enough calories. Eat frequently throughout the day and eat meals even if you don't feel hungry. Plan ahead by buying and keeping healthy snacks on hand at home, at the office, and in your car. You can also boost your calories by choosing heartier versions of foods, such as granola over cornflakes and split-pea soup instead of vegetable broth. Eating larger-than-normal portions of healthy foods, such as another helping of baked beans or an extra sandwich, will also add calories. If you're crunched for time or planning to exercise shortly, drink your calories. Liquid meal products, homemade liquid meals such as milk shakes and fruit smoothies, and even juice, can be easy ways to down additional calories.

Strategy #2. Choose carbohydrate and protein-rich foods to meet your higher calorie needs.

Special protein powders or weight-gainer supplements aren't necessary when you're trying to put on muscle or gain weight. Simply eating more protein, such as meat or eggs, won't necessarily translate into more muscle either. Most athletes have trouble gaining weight because they lack calories or enough carbohydrates in their day-to-day diet, not because they lack protein. Besides, although it's true that you need extra protein when you're involved in a strength-training program, most athletes will consume enough extra protein from the additional food they eat to boost their calories. Carbohydrate-rich foods should still supply the majority (60 percent) of your calories. Your body relies on carbohydrates to fuel your weight-training sessions, as well as the endurance activities you participate in. Consuming adequate carbohydrate also replenishes your muscle glycogen stores so you can continue to train daily.

To meet your protein and carbohydrate needs simultaneously, follow the food pyramid's recommendation to eat a variety of foods. Meat, poultry, fish, eggs, cheese, and tofu all supply quality protein (as well as fat, obviously) but virtually no carbohydrates. Few foods, though, are composed of one nutrient: milk (regular and soy), yogurt, cottage cheese, dried beans, and lentils are good sources of both protein and carbohydrates. Vegetables and other carbohydrate-rich foods like pasta, rice, bread, and cereal contain relatively small amounts of protein, but it really adds up if you are having large portions.

To remind yourself of the importance of eating enough carbohydrate and protein, include a protein-rich food (from the milk group or the meat and beans group) with your carbohydrate-rich meals and snacks. For example, melt cheese on a bagel, add tuna, chicken, or a hard-boiled egg to a salad, top pasta with a meat sauce, and eat baked beans over rice or on top of a baked potato. Adding a strength-training program to an already ambitious training schedule will increase your body's need for protein initially, so pay particular attention to your food choices when you first hit the weight room.

If you're still concerned that you're not eating enough protein, consider sports shakes or complete meal replacement powders. These products offer a more complete nutritional package than straight protein powders or supplements. They're relatively expensive, so you might consider saving them for travel or for days when a busy schedule would otherwise result in missed meals. If you don't have a milk sensitivity, you can add nonfat dried milk powder to homemade shakes or smoothies, or stir it into oatmeal, soup, cooked rice, and other dishes. It's a high-quality, inexpensive protein supplement (a quarter cup provides about 11 grams of protein) without the unproven additives that many other supplements provide.

The World of Disordered Eating

Are you convinced that your life, or at least your performances, would improve if you could just lose a few pounds? Do you feel compelled to jump on and off the scale to check your weight at least once a day, maybe more, hoping to win the battle at last and step off happy? Do you find yourself preoccupied with controlling what you can or can't, should or shouldn't, must or must not, will or won't eat today? If you answer yes to any of the above, it's a safe bet you are dissatisfied with your body as it presently is. If you're a female, you're not alone. At least one-third, and maybe as many as two-thirds, of all female athletes display abnormal eating behaviors. Male athletes can go to battle with their bodies, too. Just think about wrestlers, rowers, and jockeys.

Eating disturbances run the gamut, from poor eating habits to severe eating disorders like anorexia and bulimia nervosa. You don't have to suffer from a full-blown eating disorder, however, to do yourself a lot of harm. Many athletes fall into the world of disordered eating. Here, you'll find less serious but more common eating disturbances, such as excessive and unhealthy dieting (for example, trying to eat little or no fat or seeing how long you can go without eating), and unhealthy weight-loss practices, such as fasting or exercising excessively to counterbalance having eaten "forbidden foods." Unfortunately, because these abnormal eating behaviors are so prevalent, especially among female athletes, we often accept them as normal.

Disordered Eating Among Endurance Athletes

Numerous studies suggest that athletes suffer a high risk of developing disordered eating habits, as well as full-blown eating disorders. Athletes most at risk include those involved in "appearance" sports (such as gymnastics or skating), sports in which low body weight is considered advantageous (distance running and cycling), and weight-category sports (wrestling and rowing). A recent study of elite British teenage runners is a typical example. Seventeen of these 35 girls are believed to have suffered some form of eating disorder. Only four progressed through the ranks and made it to the senior national team.

Of course, eating disorders are not confined to female athletes. Males, in general, do suffer less from eating disorders than females, representing only 10 percent of all diagnosed cases. Anorexia nervosa, however, is more likely to occur in male athletes than other males. Moreover, male athletes can become just as addicted to exercise, even in the face of illness or injury, as some female athletes do. Current statistics may underestimate the problem, though, as few studies to date on male athletes have used the well-established criteria set forth by the American Psychiatric Association to diagnose varying degrees of eating disorders. On top of that, since eating disorders are perceived as a feminine disease, male sufferers typically seek help less.

Male athletes can be just as preoccupied with their body size and shape as many women are. One study examined eating, weight, and dieting practices in 162 competitive collegiate rowers: 82 heavyweights (56 women, 26 men) and 80 lightweights (17 women, 63 men). Lightweight rowers have weight restrictions as part of the sport. The findings (based on self-reported anonymous questionnaires) reveal that while female rowers exhibit more

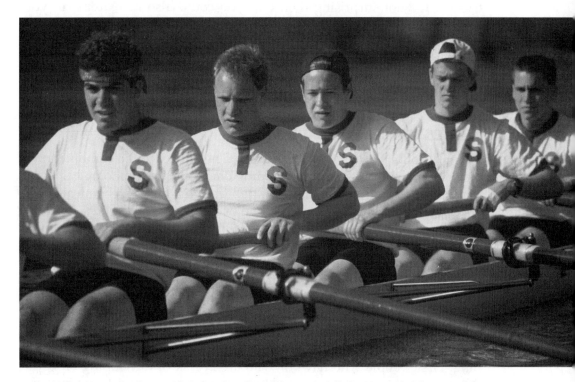

Male athletes can also be at risk for eating disorders, especially in sports that have weight restrictions.

disordered eating behaviors overall, male rowers suffer with significant eating and weight concerns, too.

In this sample, roughly 12 percent of males (and 20 percent of females) reported having binge eating episodes at least twice a week. Binge eating is defined as the discrete consumption of large amounts of food coupled with a sense of loss of control and followed by emotional distress. Moreover, male rowers reported cutting weight (intentional rapid weight loss) more times per season than females (4.3 times versus 0.4 times) and they reported the frequent use of extreme methods to lose weight. Fifty-seven percent reported fasting (compared to 25 percent of females, and 2.5 percent reported vomiting (compared to 13 percent of females). Male lightweights, in particular, are at risk for potential psychological and medical problems. They reported greater weekly and seasonal fluctuations in weight, cut weight more frequently, and were most likely to fast to lose weight compared to heavyweights or lightweight females.

As an athlete, male or female, committed to doing well in endurance sports, you're probably used to doing things in the extreme. For example, rising religiously at five o'clock to train before putting in a full day at work, compiling a decade-long streak of never missing a training day, or spending a rainy Saturday running 30 miles instead of going to the movies with friends. It's not surprising then that you could also be extreme in your attitudes and beliefs about body weight and eating behaviors, variables that certainly hold the promise of improving your performance. Being competitive and compulsive (perhaps you've even been referred to as obsessive) contributes to your success as an athlete, but it's also the very personality type that can lead to an eating disorder.

Causes of Disordered Eating

Eating disorders are complex in nature. They arise from a combination of factors: family problems, long-standing emotional or psychological issues, major life transitions (for example, puberty), possible biochemical imbalances, and societal pressures to be thin or have the perfect body. An eating disorder serves a purpose as an unhealthy coping mechanism. A person manipulates food and their body as a way to cope with feelings and emotions that they don't know how to deal with in a healthy way.

Simply being involved in a particular sport, by itself, rarely causes an eating disorder. We know this to be true because not every athlete who participates in a "high-risk" sport develops an eating disorder. Experts in this field have two theories to explain the high incidence of eating disorders associated with certain sports, such as gymnastics and long-distance running. First, people who have or who are at risk of developing an eating disorder seem to gravitate toward these sports and, second, being involved in these sports triggers, or precipitates, the development of an eating disorder in a predisposed individual.

People who develop eating disorders typically share some underlying traits: they often feel unworthy or inadequate, have an intense need to be accepted, suffer from depression, anxiety or other psychological illness, and lack the skills to cope with emotions and personal issues. Athletes, even the great ones, can suffer with these issues, too. Being involved in an endurance sport can further complicate the picture. You have a heightened awareness of your body (including perceived imperfections), and as a driven and disciplined competitor, you believe that you can always achieve more and do

What Is Anorexia Nervosa?

Self-starvation and excessive weight loss are the primary indications of anorexia nervosa. It is believed to affect between .5 and 1 percent of women, usually in late adolescence and early adulthood (15 to 24 years of age). Signs and symptoms include

- refusal to maintain weight at or above a minimally normal weight for height and age,
- intense and irrational fear of weight gain or becoming fat, even though underweight,
- distorted body image (for example, feel fat even when emaciated or believe one area of the body is too fat even when obviously underweight),
- in females, loss of three consecutive menstrual periods when otherwise expected to occur, and
- extreme concern with body weight and shape.

The possible health complications of anorexia nervosa range from mild to severe enough to be life threatening. They include

- slow pulse and low blood pressure,
- hair loss,
- severe loss of body fat and muscle wasting,
- chronic fatigue,
- anemia,
- amenorrhea (loss of menstrual periods) and infertility problems,
- stress fractures or osteoporosis,
- overuse injuries,
- inability to concentrate and depression,
- insomnia,
- irregular heartbeat or other abnormalities, and
- laxative dependence.

better (the "win-at-all-costs" attitude). On top of that, you may feel a loss of control over your daily activities as well as your goals. Besides pleasing yourself, parents and family members, friends, teachers, and bosses, you must also answer to coaches, teammates, sport associations or governing bodies, and perhaps even the media. Athletes suffering with eating disorders typically speak of their weight as the only thing in life they can control. Ironically, these athletes end up being controlled by the very thing they desperately want to take charge of.

Common Warning Signs

Some common warning signs exist that signal when eating and weight-related concerns dominate and rule an athlete's life. These warning signs include: a marked increase or decrease in weight not related to a medical condition; intense preoccupation with weight and body image (that is, frequent comments about weight or shape); compulsive or excessive exercising beyond purposeful training; development of abnormal eating habits (refusing to eat with others, maintaining a list of forbidden foods, engaging in bizarre food rituals such as moving food around the plate with utensils without actually taking a bite, and so forth); self-induced vomiting (bathroom visits after meals); periods of fasting; abuse of laxatives, diet pills, or diuretics; and amenorrhea. A vegetarian eating style may also be a red flag for eating disorders, particularly among young, athletic women (see chapter 7).

Weight-preoccupied athletes tend to be highly self-critical, appear anxious, irritable, or depressed, and often withdraw from people and activities they normally enjoy. Fatigue or denial of obvious fatigue, dizziness, chills, abdominal discomfort upon eating, insomnia, shin splints, and stress fractures are all typical day-to-day complaints. Bulimia, a secretive cycle of binge eating and purging, can be harder to identify because an athlete doesn't typically lose excessive amounts of weight or experience amenorrhea as do athletes suffering with anorexia. Some signs that do indicate bulimia— "chipmunk cheeks" (from swollen glands), bloodshot eyes (from the force of vomiting), knuckle scars, and worn-off tooth enamel (discovered during dental visits).

If you or someone you know suffers from anorexia or bulimia nervosa, understand that it's a serious medical condition that can have fatal consequences. An estimated 1,000 women die each year of anorexia nervosa. Another study found that 53 percent of patients with anorexia nervosa also have osteoporosis—a condition characterized by brittle bones that fracture easily. Obviously, many of these behaviors or signs, by themselves, do not prove the person is suffering from an eating disorder. Nevertheless, because the best chance of recovery lies with early intervention, it's wise not to ignore a potential problem. For more information on national organizations that provide help, see Selected Resources.

Anorexia Athletica

It may seem like many of the athletes you coach, train with, or compete against are excessively concerned with their eating habits and weight. This may not be healthy, but it doesn't mean they all have eating disorders. Athletes often eat distorted and nutritionally poor diets simply because they lack knowledge about what to eat. A growing body of evidence suggests, however, that more and more athletes (especially females) are suffering from a less severe or subclinical eating disorder called anorexia

What Is Bulimia Nervosa?

Bulimia nervosa is characterized primarily by a secretive cycle of binge eating followed by purging. It affects between 1 and 3 percent of adolescent and young women. College-age women are particularly at risk; it's estimated that one out of every five (20 percent) suffer from bulimia.

Signs and symptoms include

- repeated episodes of bingeing (rapid consumption of large amounts of food in discrete period of time) and purging, two or more episodes a week for three months or longer,
- feeling out of control during a binge,
- purging after a binge (by self-induced vomiting, use of laxatives, diet pills, diuretics, excessive exercise, or fasting) to avoid weight gain,
- frequent dieting, and
- extreme concern with body weight and shape.

The possible health complications of bulimia nervosa range from mild to severe enough to be life threatening. They include

- swollen glands and sore throat,
- dental and gum disease,
- inflammation or tears of the esophagus,
- fatigue,
- electrolyte imbalances and dehydration,
- menstrual irregularities or amenorrhea,
- constipation or diarrhea,
- laxative dependence,
- irregular heartbeat or other abnormalities,
- depression or social withdrawal, and
- insomnia.

athletica. Although they may not meet the strict medical criteria of being anorexic or bulimic, they nevertheless have serious eating problems and body-weight concerns. Dieting and maintaining a low body weight start out as the means to an end, improving athletic performance, but somewhere along the line losing weight becomes itself the goal.

Currently, researchers are looking at this phenomenon in female athletes, but considerable carryover applies to male athletes. One male recreational-level triathlete I counseled was weighing himself several times a day, although he appeared to be at a healthy weight. When questioned about it he replied that he was assessing whether his training program was working, but eventually he expressed his true concern. He desired to lose five pounds from around his midsection. He was irritable and tired all the time from restricting himself to three small meals a day, although he worked a full day and trained daily. He repeatedly proclaimed, "If I didn't have to eat, I wouldn't." After spending time with him, it became apparent that losing weight had taken precedence over his future performances, as he now lacked the desire and energy to maintain his weekly training program.

Female athletes suffering from anorexia athletica have an intense fear of gaining weight or becoming fat although they're underweight (5 to 15 percent below what's normal for their height) or have an extremely low body-fat level. These women generally don't suffer from the severe emotional distress seen in anorexics and bulimics. Nevertheless, they view their bodies in a distorted way. They maintain their below-normal weight for at least a year by restricting the amount of calories they eat (about 80 percent or less of what they expend), severely limiting food choices or food groups, and exercising excessively (beyond what is necessary for success or as compared with other athletes of similar fitness levels). Periods of binge eating followed by various purging methods, such as self-induced vomiting and the use of laxatives, are also typically part of the picture.

Surprisingly, the majority of these athletes manage to maintain their weight (albeit low) although they eat far fewer calories than they expend. It's too early to tell for sure, but it appears that the combined effects of chronic dieting and exercise may induce the body to conserve energy (calories) or become more efficient at using what energy is available. This could spell trouble in the future if these athletes resort to more extreme dieting measures to maintain their weight or lose more. What's even more important—recent research on elite female endurance athletes shows that prolonged dieting is the most important trigger for developing a full-blown eating disorder.

We're not sure about all the implications of anorexia athletica. Although it's evident that many athletes can perform well initially—after all, that's the allure of losing weight—we know it's impossible to do so forever. Even in the short term, you may be compromising your true potential. If you're chronically low in energy and other nutrients, you're more likely to suffer from dehydration and electrolyte imbalances, chronic fatigue, anemia, and upper-respiratory-tract infections, and you'll recover more slowly from injuries, including stress fractures.

The Female Athlete Triad

Female endurance athletes with abnormal eating behaviors are at risk for developing a syndrome of interrelated problems known as the female athlete triad. Individually, each of the three conditions—disordered eating, amenorrhea, and osteoporosis— is worrisome; combined, they can really do some damage to your health. The triad usually begins when you consume fewer calories than your body needs to function properly. Some female athletes end up with an energy deficit by inadvertently expending more calories than they consume due to a strenuous training program. Many times, however, athletes restrict calories in a deliberate effort to lose weight, especially body fat, in hopes of improving their performance. Disordered eating, or unhealthy eating patterns as previously discussed, such as skipping meals, eating as little fat as possible, or occasional bingeing and purging, typically set the stage.

In response to consuming too few calories, the ovaries produce less estrogen and menstrual periods become fewer and less regular (or don't begin at all in young athletes). A lack of menstrual periods before age 16 or a loss of regular cycles for at least three to six consecutive months is called amenorrhea. Researchers aren't sure why some female athletes develop amenorrhea and others don't. Besides consuming too few calories, other factors may play a role. For example, the loss of too much body fat or perhaps the loss of specific fat stores (such as on the hips, buttocks, and thighs), excessive exercise, or a diet high in fiber-rich plant foods because fiber can affect hormonal levels in the body. Even emotional stress can cause some women to lose their periods. What's obvious, though, is that you don't have to suffer from a full-blown eating disorder to induce amenorrhea; abnormal eating habits can be enough.

One of the real dangers with amenorrhea is how it affects your bones. Hormonal disturbances, such as low estrogen levels, accompany amenorrhea and interrupt the way bones normally grow and develop. Without enough estrogen, especially in your teens and twenties, you lose bone rapidly instead of "banking" it for the future. You can be in your 20s and have the bones of a 70- or 80-year-old woman! Unfortunately, this loss is usually irreversible. Because your bones are less dense, you now run a higher risk of suffering stress fractures and other soft-tissue injuries. You're also set up to develop osteoporosis earlier in life. Amenorrhea can also interfere with your ability to become pregnant in the future and possibly even put you at a higher risk for heart disease.

Athletes, parents, and coaches should know that the American College of Sports Medicine considers amenorrhea to be the most recognizable symptom of the triad. While amenorrhea can be caused by certain medical conditions, such as hypothyroidism (an underactive thyroid), female athletes often view the absence of periods as a benign side effect of hard training. Until you determine the cause of amenorrhea, it should raise a red flag. The same advice applies to stress fractures, another easily recognizable sign of the triad. Adjusting your eating habits and training program can help prevent further bone loss and extend your career.

Male athletes can be at risk for osteoporosis as well. Consuming too few calories, especially in conjunction with endurance training, can lower testosterone levels. Insufficient testosterone, besides reducing fertility and your sex drive, puts your bones at risk.

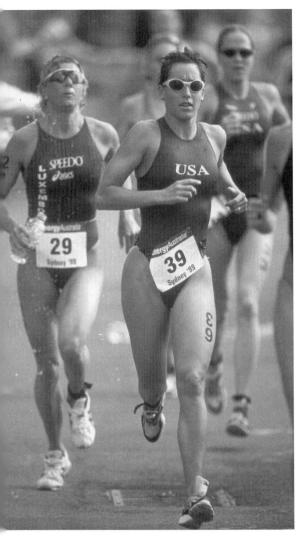

Be aware of the female athlete traid. Disordered eating, amenorrhea, and osteoporosis can damage your health and compromise your ablility to exercise.

Seeking Help

What should you do if you or a training partner, teammate, or someone you coach is struggling with weight and body-image problems? Don't wait for medical problems to prove you right. Seek help immediately from someone you trust who is qualified to provide help. A sports medicine physician, a registered dietitian specializing in sport nutrition, or a sport psychologist or therapist specializing in eating disorders are all good bets. The more serious the eating disorder is, the more likely a team approach (physician, nutritionist, and therapist) will be needed to promote recovery.

Be sure you approach friends, teammates, or athletes under your guidance privately and in a tactful manner. Don't mention their weight or tell them to "just eat normally." Rather, express your concern about their health and what you see as they train and perform. For example, mention their inability to complete workouts, poor concentration at work or school,

Do You or Someone You Know Struggle With Disordered Eating?

You don't have to suffer from a full-blown eating disorder, such as anorexia or bulimia nervosa, to do yourself harm. Abnormal eating habits alone can impair your health, performance, and quality of life. To get a handle on your attitudes about food and your body, answer the following questions honestly.

Do you eat when you're not hungry or wait until you're extremely hungry to eat?

Do you frequently diet or avoid certain foods or food groups?

Are you aware of the calorie content of the foods you eat?

Do you eat until you are physically uncomfortable?

Do you find yourself excessively preoccupied with food, dieting, your body image, or your weight?

Are you terrified about being overweight or gaining fat?

Do you feel guilty, disgusted with yourself, or out of control when you eat?

Do you avoid social situations because you fear food or your eating behaviors?

Are you uncomfortable eating in front of others?

Do you think about burning up calories when you exercise?

Do you feel that food controls your life?

The more yes answers you gave to the preceding questions, the more you need to consider seeking help from a qualified professional, such as a mental health expert or a registered dietitian, for unhealthy eating behaviors.

or frequent colds and nagging injuries. Don't judge or criticize their behaviors. Concentrate on the emotional struggle they are caught up in. Your goal or responsibility is not to change their behavior but to get them into treatment.

Don't be surprised that the help you offer is turned down or goes unanswered. Athletes caught in the throes of an eating disorder cannot simply give up their distorted beliefs or change their behavior overnight. They must first learn to communicate their feelings and needs in a healthier manner and they must develop new coping skills to deal with emotional conflicts. Routinely express your concerns and offer to accompany them to seek medical help or attend a support group. Many athletes find approaching a sport nutritionist, even for a simple nutrition checkup, to be a nonthreatening first step. If the person refuses to seek professional help during a negotiated time span, share your intention to approach someone else, such as a coach, parent, or spouse, if this is appropriate. Obviously, coaches can insist that an athlete get a medical checkup before continuing to train or compete.

If you've been amenorrheic for more than three months, make some lifestyle changes to protect your long-term health. Reduce your training by 10 to 20 percent, increase the calories you consume, and gain a modest amount of weight (2 to 3 percent of your body weight, or as little as five pounds can make a difference) until you regain a normal menstrual cycle. Resistance training can help strengthen your bones too. If you've been amenorrheic for a year or longer, a bone-density scan will let you know where you stand in regard to bone loss. If you're unwilling to make lifestyle changes or making changes doesn't help your menstrual periods return (especially if you have a history of stress fractures or you've been amenorrheic for six months or longer) consider estrogen replacement therapy. Oral contraceptives are generally the recommended method.

When it comes to your diet, work on smoothing out erratic eating habits into a schedule of wholesome meals and snacks. If you find yourself constantly obsessed with food, it's probably because you're trying to eat too few calories. If you've been avoiding eating meat, particularly red meat, you may want to reconsider. It's unclear why meat seems to protect women's menstrual periods, but it does. Aim to include two to three small servings (three ounces each or the size of a deck of cards) of red meat per week. Remind yourself that fat is an integral part of any athlete's diet and eat at least 20 percent (45 to 60 grams for most active women) of your calories from fat. You need extra calcium and vitamin D at this point (1,200 to 1,500 milligrams of calcium and 400 to 800 IU of vitamin D daily), so choose foods rich in calcium and vitamin D. Add a supplement to make up the remainder. Keep in mind that taking calcium supplements alone won't prevent osteoporosis, but they can help you build (up to age 30) or maintain your bone mass once your menstrual periods resume.

Preventing Eating Disorders in Athletes

Prevention is the real key when it comes eating disorders and athletes. If you're involved with athletics in any way, you need to send a clear message that health issues always take precedence over sports performances. For example, treat an athlete struggling with weight and body-image problems as you would an injured athlete. Provide the same medical help and guidelines for participation. Be sure to promote the message that food is fuel and that a serious athlete respects his or her body by eating the necessary calories and nutrients. Emphasize strength and stamina, not "ideal" body weight.

Body-image problems and disordered eating go hand-in-hand. Take a closer look at your attitudes regarding weight and body shapes. Do you constantly diet to try to obtain an unrealistic perfect figure? Are you perpetuating the oldest myth in the book that the thinner you are, the faster you'll be? Do you use terms such as good and bad to describe foods or to describe yourself after you've eaten them? If you must weigh yourself (or athletes under your guidance), do so in private and set a healthy weight range that includes a minimum weight as well as a maximum weight.

Women, in particular, need to realize that we are genetically different, including how much weight or body fat we are predisposed to carry. Concentrate on building your self-esteem. Start by accepting your body type and shape. If you're an athlete who struggles with disordered eating, it's unlikely you'll ever completely lose the pressure to want to look different. You can, however, work on how it influences your current behaviors, and more important, the rest of your life.

Endurance Eating for Vegetarians

7

"My efforts are to impact or take advantage of animals as little as possible. It's a myth that athletes must eat red meat to build muscle. I care about my body and want to eat a 'cleaner diet.' I think vegetarianism is a healthier alternative. I feel perfectly happy and healthy [eating a vegetarian diet] and that is what is right for me."

—Laurie Brandt Hauptmann, four-time winner of the Leadville Trail 100 Mountain Bike Race

Endurance sports and vegetarianism have much in common. Both endeavors require you to be both an artist and a scientist. Guidelines do exist for each discipline, but there's more than one way to get the job done. And although you can certainly jump recklessly into either venture, a little planning goes a long way when it comes to achieving success.

If you choose a vegetarian sports diet while training for and competing in endurance and ultraendurance events, you can obtain all the nutrients you need. However, you must be as committed to meeting your nutritional needs as you are to fulfilling your athletic goals. As a vegetarian athlete you must put more thought and planning into your daily food choices to incorporate alternative sources of key nutrients such as calcium, iron, zinc, and protein. Otherwise, your health and performance will suffer. By reading this chapter, you will become more knowledgeable about the nutritional issues associated with a vegetarian diet and how to best meet your nutrient needs from plant sources. Non-vegetarian athletes will also benefit by learning how to incorporate more plant foods into their diet.

Who Is a Vegetarian?

You haven't eaten red meat in years, but you still occasionally enjoy chicken and fish. Your training buddy drinks milk and eats cheese, but avoids eggs and meat of any type. So who's the vegetarian? Actually, vegetarianism means different things to different people. Vegetarian practices run the gamut from simply eliminating red meat to excluding all animal products, even foods derived from animal sources, such as honey and gelatin.

Athletes cite different reasons for reducing or eliminating animal products from their diet. You may want to improve your health, boost your performance, abide by spiritual guidelines, protect the environment, simply love animals, or have some other reason for following a vegetarian eating style.

The following terms describe the general categories of vegetarian diets:

- *Vegans* (or strict vegetarians) eat only plant foods, such as grains, beans, fruits, vegetables, nuts, and seeds, and consume no animal products (meat, fish, poultry, seafood, eggs and egg products, and dairy foods, such as milk and cheese).
- *Lacto-vegetarians* eat dairy and plant foods, but eliminate all meat, poultry, fish, seafood, and eggs.
- *Ovo-vegetarians* eat eggs and plant foods, but avoid meat, poultry, fish, seafood, and dairy foods.
- *Lacto-ovo vegetarians* include eggs, dairy, and plant foods in their diet, but exclude all meat, poultry, fish, and seafood.
- *Semi- or partial vegetarians* refuse red meat but occasionally eat chicken, fish, and seafood along with eggs and dairy foods.

Rewards and Risks of a Vegetarian Diet

With careful planning a vegetarian eating style can improve your health and your performance. Simply eliminating animal foods without finding appropriate substitutes, however, results in an unbalanced diet that does more harm than good.

Rewards

For the most part, opting for a vegetarian eating style is a healthy path to follow. Health experts continually urge us to eat more plant foods and less animal products, which lack fiber and tend to be high in fat and cholesterol. Think about the Food Guide Pyramid. Daily recommendations call for six to 11 servings of bread, cereal, rice, and pasta, three to five servings of vegetables, and two to four servings of fruit, accompanied by two to four servings of milk, yogurt, and cheese and two to three servings of meat, poultry, fish, dry beans, eggs, and nuts. Adding it all up, the pyramid prescribes at least 11 to 20 plant-food servings but only a few servings of animal foods. Planning meals around grains, beans, soy foods, vegetables, and fruit definitely supports optimal health. Several recent studies show that compared with the general public, vegetarians have lower rates of hypertension and certain cancers, as well as a much lower risk of developing heart disease and diabetes. Eating a plant-based diet can also make it easier to maintain a healthy weight.

A plant-based diet also supplies plenty of carbohydrates that help to replenish glycogen stores—a prerequisite if you work out daily, train more than once a day, or want to keep moving for hours on end. Endurance athletes need to consume approximately 60 percent of their daily calories from carbohydrate-rich foods. Foods from the Bread and Cereal group, Fruit and Vegetable groups, as well as beans, soy foods, milk, and yogurt fills the bill. If you're filling up on these foods, you're most likely already adopting a vegetarian or near-vegetarian diet. You should be able to obtain the rest of the nutrients you need, including enough high-quality protein, if you eat a variety of foods daily and make some savvy substitutions for the foods you eliminate.

Risks

Despite all the benefits associated with a vegetarian eating style, I find it difficult to comment specifically about endurance athletes performing better on meatless diets. Too many variations exist on the vegetarian theme. Many athletes eat healthy, well-balanced vegetarian diets, but others struggle with vegetarian meal plans that are too restrictive. The bottom line is that you shouldn't automatically assume that your health or performance will improve simply because you eliminate red meat or other animal products. A vegetarian lifestyle, in fact, has been linked to menstrual abnormalities, and in some athletic women, vegetarianism may even be a red flag signaling an eating disorder.

I've counseled a number of semi- or near vegetarians who make poor food choices and end up with diets low in protein, iron, zinc, and calcium. How does this happen? Try this diet on for size: no red meat, few, if any eggs, dairy, or soy foods, and limited amounts of fish, poultry, and beans. Survival depends on eating lots of bagels, salad, pasta, and desserts or snack items. You're likely to end up in this rut if you make little effort to shop and prepare snacks and meals, if you aren't keen on trying new foods, or if you live in a carnivorous (meat-eating) household and routinely eat only the starchy parts of family meals.

Consuming the nutrients and calories needed to partake in endurance endeavors becomes more difficult as you eliminate foods and food groups. Vegan diets pose the greatest challenge. Eliminating two food groups increases the risk for deficiencies, especially of some key nutrients such as vitamins B_2 and B_{12}, iron, zinc, and calcium. Endurance athletes often struggle to meet their high calorie needs on vegan diets as well.

Special Nutrient Concerns for Vegetarians

Vegetarians typically define themselves by the foods they *don't* eat. It's common to hear a vegetarian say, "I don't eat meat," but how often do you hear, "But I do eat bok choy, tofu, and garbanzo beans?" To reap the benefits of vegetarianism, you need to seek alternative sources of nutrients for the foods you choose to eliminate. The easiest way is to focus on including a variety of foods in your daily diet, such as whole grains, dark green leafy vegetables, and soy foods.

If you're curious about how your vegetarian eating style stacks up, ask yourself a couple of questions. Do you, or are you willing to, explore new foods to meet your nutrient needs? Do you, or are you willing to, plan meals and snacks to meet the high energy needs of being an endurance athlete? If you can answer yes to both questions, you're on your way to eating a healthy, well-balanced vegetarian diet.

Calories, Carbohydrates, and Fat

Vegetarian athletes typically have little problem eating enough carbohydrates. Breads, cereals, pasta, rice, fruits, vegetables, beans, lentils, soy foods, milk, and yogurt all supply carbohydrates. By their nature, vegetarian diets rank higher in complex carbohydrates and fiber and lower in saturated fat and cholesterol than diets containing meat. Eating enough whole grains, however, can be a challenge for some vegetarians. Developing a taste for barley, brown and wild rice, bulgur, couscous, kasha (buckwheat), millet, and quinoa is particularly important for vegetarian athletes. Besides complex carbohydrates these foods provide protein, iron, zinc, and other trace minerals. An easy first step: switch to eating whole-grain cereals and whole-wheat bread, crackers, and pasta.

Your daily fat requirement (at least 20 percent of total calories) doesn't change if you follow a vegetarian diet. In fact, many vegetarians assume that eliminating animal products ensures a low-fat diet. Don't count on it. You can easily rack up fat calories if you rely too heavily on nuts and seeds, cheese and other whole-milk dairy foods, and high-fat snack and convenience foods. If this is an area you need to work on, read food labels and choose low-fat alternatives whenever possible. If you rely on nuts and cheese for protein, consider leaner options, such as dried beans and peas, lentils, and soy foods. Don't forget that you can always cut back on how much or how often you eat a particular food.

Plant foods are bulkier and usually lower in calories than animal foods so some athletes end up feeling full before they consume enough calories. Vegan diets, in particular, are high in fiber and low in fat. If you're having trouble consuming enough calories, don't skip meals or snacks (plan to eat six or more times a day), and concentrate on including plenty of high-calorie, nutrient-dense foods such as nuts and seeds, nut butters, fruit juices, dried fruit, and dairy foods. Cooking with small amounts of fat or oil will also help boost your calorie intake. Desserts and snack foods supply loads of calories just be sure to eat more nutritious foods first.

Protein

Getting enough protein is a concern for many vegetarian athletes. Because endurance athletes have higher protein needs, sprinkling a few chickpeas on a salad or crumbling a little tofu into a vegetable stir-fry won't get the job done. Most female endurance athletes need 65 to 90 grams of protein a day; active males typically require 95 to 120 grams daily.

Keeping up with your protein needs requires a two-pronged approach: eat a variety of plant foods daily and consume enough calories to maintain your weight. Too few calories means protein gets used for energy rather than for building, repairing, and maintaining body tissues, including muscle. If you continue to eat poultry, fish, eggs, and milk products, getting enough protein shouldn't be a problem. Animal foods provide all the essential amino acids (the ones our bodies cannot make) that you need to make new proteins. Plant sources of protein, such as grains, dried beans and peas, nuts, seeds, and vegetables do not contain all the essential amino acids and are considered incomplete proteins. Soybeans are the exception. They contain certain amino acids in higher amounts than found in other beans, so ounce for ounce, soybean protein is equivalent in quality to animal protein.

In the old days, vegetarians were advised to combine specific plant foods within a meal (such as rice and beans) to form complete, or complementary, proteins. Today we know that combining plant foods at the same meal isn't necessary. The body makes its own complete proteins if a variety of plant foods (and enough calories) are eaten each day. Of course bean burritos, lentil soup with corn bread, and peanut butter sandwiches made with whole-wheat bread taste good, so you still have a valid reason for eating these combinations!

To boost your protein intake and avoid the carbohydrate-overload trap, consciously include a protein-rich food at all your meals and snacks (see table 7.1). Lacto-ovo vegetarians, for example, can add milk products (regular or soy) or eggs to any meal or snack. Eat hot or cold cereal with milk, dunk a bran muffin into yogurt, snack on a slice of cheese pizza, or prepare French toast for breakfast. Another good strategy: make sure you don't eat your grains plain. Smear nut butters, low-fat cottage cheese, or hummus on a bagel. Vary your pasta toppings such as canned spicy beans one night and a vegetable and tofu stir-fry another. Keep in mind that anything made for pasta can just as easily be spooned over brown rice or instant couscous or rolled in tortillas.

Vegetarians who eliminate animal foods without substituting traditional vegetarian staples have the most trouble meeting their protein needs. A good rule to follow is to eat legumes (dried beans and peas and lentils) and soy foods daily. Quick-fix beans (precooked canned varieties) and meat substitutes made from soybeans provide an easy and simple way to get the protein you need. Choose hearty soups and stews made with lentils, split peas, and

Table 7.1 Protein Content of Commonly Eaten Foods

Food	Typical Serving	Protein (grams)
meat (red meat, poultry, fish)	3 oz cooked	21-25 g
milk or yogurt	1 c.	8 g
cheese	1 ounce	7 g
egg	1 medium	6 g
beans	1 c. cooked	12 g
soy milk	1 c.	10 g
tofu	3 oz (1/5 block)	10 g
peanut butter	2 tbsp.	8 g
nuts or seeds	1 ounce	5 g
bread	1 slice	3 g
pasta or grain	1 c. cooked	6 g
potato	1 small	2 g
starchy vegetables (peas, corn, etc.)	1/2 c. cooked	2 g

beans. Try baked beans on your next baked potato. Or serve a quick "meal in a can" such as vegetarian chili. When it comes to soy foods, experiment with different forms. Serve meat substitutes (check the freezer section in natural food stores and the health food section of grocery stores) and use textured vegetable protein in dishes that traditionally call for meat, such as chili and tacos.

Keep in mind that animal foods provide a more concentrated dose of protein than plant foods. A typical small hamburger or chicken breast (three ounces or the size of a deck of cards) supplies 25 grams of protein. You'll have to eat a generous cup of cooked beans plus a cup of cooked grain or two cups of pasta topped with three ounces of tofu to match that. You can determine the amount of protein in the foods you typically eat by checking the nutrition facts label on food packages. Be certain to compare the serving size against the portion you actually eat.

TIPS FOR ADDING MORE SOY TO YOUR DIET

You've heard all about the wonders of soy, but how do you actually eat the stuff, or at least sneak some into your diet? This list contains some simple suggestions to get you started.

1. Drink soy milk (fortified with calcium and vitamin D) and use it in place of skim milk in recipes for soups, muffins, pancakes, waffles, and pudding.
2. Create smoothies by blending fresh fruit (bananas and strawberries work well) with vanilla-flavored soy milk.
3. Add diced firm tofu or chunks of tempeh to your favorite spaghetti sauce, chili, vegetable soup, stew, stir-fried dish, and casserole.
4. Combine soft tofu with cottage cheese or ricotta cheese in lasagna and stuffed shells or use it as a cheese substitute in pasta dishes.
5. Blend soft tofu into low-fat sour cream for a baked-potato topping or use it instead of sour cream or yogurt.
6. Crumble tofu into scrambled eggs during the last minute of cooking.
7. Snack on roasted soynuts (found in most supermarkets).
8. Prepare tempeh on the grill. Steam it first, marinate in barbecue sauce, and then grill until brown. Add cubes of firm or extra-firm tofu to shish kebab.
9. Add soy protein isolate (powder) to milk shakes, fruit smoothies, and fruit juices or sprinkle it on hot cereal for an added protein boost.
10. Try tofu dogs (soy hot dogs), veggie patties (soy-based burgers), and other meat alternatives; replace ground meat with textured vegetable protein in tacos, spaghetti sauce, and chili.

To estimate your daily protein requirement, multiply your weight in pounds by 0.55 to 0.75 grams protein per pound (1.2 to 1.7 grams per kilogram body weight). Athletes eating primarily vegetarian foods should select the higher end of the range, especially those participating in ultraendurance events.

See table 7.1 for the protein content of some commonly eaten foods. Use this list as a reference to keep track of your daily protein intake.

Iron and Zinc

Athletes eating a meatless diet run a greater risk of getting too little iron and zinc. Even marginal deficiencies can hamper your performance. With an iron-poor diet, you won't form enough hemoglobin and myoglobin, the oxygen-carrying molecules in the blood and muscles, which will leave you feeling weak and fatigued. Female athletes, in particular, are at a greater risk for low iron levels due to smaller reserves and greater losses through menstruation. Athletes need adequate zinc to fight off infections and help wounds and injuries heal.

Absorbability is a key issue when it comes to getting enough iron and zinc. About 20 to 30 percent of the iron in meat (heme iron) is absorbable, compared with only 2 to 8 percent in plants (non-heme iron). The zinc from animal sources is generally more absorbable too since fiber and compounds called phytates found in whole-grain foods can interfere with zinc absorption.

All types of meat contain the more-easily-absorbed heme iron, not just red meat. You'll benefit by including poultry (especially the dark meat), fish, and seafood in your diet. Don't rely on dairy foods or eggs to come through in this department as both are poor sources of iron. Some good plant sources of iron include fortified breakfast cereals, wheat germ, dried beans, peas, and lentils, leafy dark green vegetables like spinach, kale, and collard greens, tofu and textured vegetable protein, nuts and seeds, dried fruit, and prune juice.

Vitamin C enhances the absorption of iron, so serve vitamin C-rich foods with the iron-rich plant foods listed above. (Foods high in vitamin C include strawberries, kiwi, cantaloupe, citrus fruits, red and green peppers, broccoli, and tomatoes to name a few.) For example, drink a glass of orange juice with a bowl of iron-fortified cereal or cook beans in a tomato sauce. Cooking in a cast-iron pot or skillet will also raise the iron content substantially as the mineral leeches into the food. Meat contains a compound, the MFP factor, that promotes the absorption of nonheme iron too, so have your iron-rich vegetables and any meat you may eat together.

Animal foods (especially oysters) contain abundant amounts of zinc, while plant foods provide only moderate amounts. You need to make an effort to include several servings of zinc-rich foods in your diet every day. If you consume enough protein, you're most likely getting enough zinc.

Significant plant sources of zinc include lentils, beans, whole grains, whole-wheat bread, wheat germ, nuts, soy and dairy foods, and some fortified breakfast cereals.

Don't be too quick to reach for supplements that provide beyond 100% of the RDA for iron and zinc. Clearly, if iron-deficiency anemia is a problem, additional iron will help. You should start, though, by monitoring your iron levels through routine blood tests that look at your hemoglobin, hematocrit, and serum ferritin (storage form of iron) levels. Too much iron can interfere with the absorption of zinc and copper, and cause constipation. Oversupplementing with zinc may cause a relative deficiency in other minerals, such as copper, because they all compete for absorption. Eating plant foods rich in iron and zinc, however, won't cause any problems. Play it safe—make the effort to include good meatless sources of iron and zinc.

Calcium and Vitamin D

Besides building strong bones and teeth, calcium helps your muscles to contract and relax, your nerves to send messages, and your blood to clot properly. Vitamin D aids in the absorption of calcium and phosphorus, nutrients essential for healthy bone tissue. Your daily calcium needs vary depending on your gender, age, and (for women) your menstrual status. Shoot for at least 1,000 milligrams a day. If you eat dairy foods, you can get plenty of calcium from fat-free and low-fat milk, yogurt, and cheese. Plant foods that contain calcium include dark leafy greens (such as kale and mustard, collard, and turnip greens), bok choy, broccoli, beans, dried figs, soy nuts, sunflower seeds, and other calcium-fortified foods, such as orange juice, cereal, breakfast bars, tofu (processed with calcium sulfate), and fortified soy or rice beverages. If you occasionally eat animal foods, canned sardines and salmon (be sure to eat the bones) are a good source of calcium, too.

Check the nutrition facts label on your orange juice, soy and rice beverages, and tofu. If you're relying on these foods for calcium, select calcium-fortified varieties and tofu prepared with calcium sulfate or you'll miss out. Green leafy vegetables can provide adequate calcium, but you'll have to eat enough of them to make it count. For example, you need to eat three cups of broccoli or one and a half cups of kale to equal the calcium in one glass of milk or one cup of

Vegetarian Calcium Sources*

1 cup milk
1 cup fortified soy milk or rice milk
1 cup yogurt
1 1/2 oz cheese
1 cup tofu (made with calcium sulfate)
1 1/2 cups cooked dark leafy greens—kale, collard, turnip greens
2 cups cooked bok choy
3 cups cooked broccoli
1 1/2 cups canned baked beans
1/2 cup soy nuts
11 dried figs
3 tbsp sesame seeds
4 oz canned salmon or sardines (with bones)
1 cup fortified orange juice
fortified breakfast cereals (varies)

*Contains at least 300 milligrams per serving.

Quick Vegetarian Snacks and Meals

Whole-grain pancakes

Whole-grain muffins or cookies

Graham crackers, rice cakes, whole-grain crackers, tortillas

Instant macaroni and cheese, couscous with lentils, polenta, or mashed potatoes

Instant brown rice or other grains

Bagels or whole-grain bread with nut butter

Oatmeal or cold cereal with milk

Dried fruit—raisins, apricots, dates, figs, papayas, apples

Frozen juice bar

Bean taco, burrito, or enchilada

Lentil or split-pea soup

Fruit shakes or smoothies

Low-fat cottage cheese

Yogurt (dairy or soy)

Canned beans, vegetarian chili

Ethnic frozen meals—Mexican, Chinese, Thai, or others

Tofu hot dogs

Veggie burgers

Quick mixes of tabouli, humus, refried beans, black beans

Roasted soy nuts or other nuts

Vegetable pizza

yogurt. (Don't forget, at 300 milligrams a cup, you need the equivalent of at least three glasses of milk a day to reach your daily goal of 1,000 milligrams of calcium.) If you think calcium supplements are the answer, be aware that a diet low in calcium is also likely to be low in protein and vitamin D. Calcium supplements won't help with that. To increase absorption, take calcium supplements with meals, in doses of 500 milligrams or less at one time, and not along with an iron supplement.

Few foods are naturally high in vitamin D. Our bodies usually make enough when our skin is exposed to sunlight (at least 15 minutes several times a week.) Fortunately, athletes routinely spend a great deal of time outdoors wearing little clothing! Keep in mind that your skin becomes less efficient at making vitamin D as you age and sun exposure may not be adequate in northern climates during the winter months. Good food sources of vitamin D include fatty fish (like salmon), egg yolks, and fortified foods such as milk, butter, margarine, breakfast cereals, and soy beverages. Vegans should consider a vitamin D supplement (200 IU/day or 400 IU/day for athletes over 50 years of age.)

B Vitamins

If you eat a well-balanced vegetarian diet, full of whole grains, enriched grains, legumes, nuts, seeds, fruits and vegetables, and plenty of calories, you should have no trouble meeting your need for thiamin, riboflavin, niacin, vitamin B_6, and folic acid. Vitamin B_{12} is needed to maintain healthy red blood cells and nerve fibers. It's a unique vitamin, produced by bacteria in the soil and in animals. Unless you're in the habit of ingesting soil along with your greens (as animals do), most people meet their needs by eating animal foods, so you're covered if you consume eggs, dairy products, fish, or poultry. Deficiencies are rare, even in vegetarians, because our daily requirement is small (two micrograms a day), and the human body carefully hoards and guards its supply.

The only plant foods that are *reliable* B_{12} sources are fortified foods such as soy milk, soy burgers, and certain breakfast cereals (such as Total or Product 19). Nutritional yeast (Red Star brand T-6635), not regular baking yeast, is also a reliable source. Don't count on tempeh, spirulina, sprouted legumes, miso, sea vegetables, or umeboshi plums; these foods don't contain the active form of vitamin B_{12}. Vegans who don't routinely eat fortified products should take a supplement because subtle neurological damage can occur before you know you have a deficiency.

Profile of a Vegetarian Endurance Athlete

Laurie Brandt Hauptmann, former full-time NORBA national circuit mountain bike racer, is the four-time winner of the Leadville Trail 100 Mountain Bike Race, a mountain bike race featuring 10,000 feet of climbing, most of which is above 10,000 feet. Hauptmann holds the course record of 7:58:53 and is the only woman to break the nine-hour mark. Hauptmann is also a lacto-ovo vegetarian. In her diet she includes eggs, cheese, cottage cheese, and yogurt but abstains from eating meat and milk.

Hauptmann shares the following advice with vegetarian athletes participating in endurance activities:

- If your sport is a lifestyle, make your nutrition a lifestyle, too. Educate yourself by reading nutrition articles written by credible people involved in your sport, as well as gleaning information from food labels.

- Include protein at every meal. It will help you feel better and recover from workouts more quickly. If you have trouble meeting your protein needs by eating protein-rich foods, experiment with a powdered protein supplement. Stir supplemental protein powder into beverages and foods, such as oatmeal, cold cereal, pancakes, and other foods you prepare from scratch including bread, muffins, and cookies. Experiment with different flavored powders. Hauptmann's favorite use for powder is creating a smoothie by combining fresh fruit (banana, orange, or kiwi), a quarter cup of vanilla soy protein powder, wheat germ, and cottage cheese or yogurt. Add water to obtain the desired consistency.

- Pack a powdered protein supplement for use when traveling. Powders travel well and won't spoil. Supplemental protein is particularly important for international travel, as well as for traveling to and from day-long ventures, when it can be difficult to locate or store reliable food sources of protein.

- Take advantage of the high-quality protein delivered in eggs. Eat eggs in several easy and quick-to-prepare forms: scrambled, hard-boiled, omelets, and egg sandwiches.

- To incorporate more beans into your diet, try burritos or make multibean stews effortlessly by using an electric cooking pot or slow cooker. Serve bean stews over baked potatoes or rice or with whole-grain bread. If you haven't enjoyed beans in the past, try them again topped with cheese.

- Just because you're a vegetarian doesn't mean you'll automatically get the minimum five servings of fruits and vegetables you need daily. Get off to a good start by including a piece of fruit or a glass of fruit or vegetable juice at breakfast.

• Don't become stuck in a rut eating the same few foods. Incorporating vegetarian alternatives will increase the variety of food in your diet. Some foods to try: veggie burgers, imitation bacon in BLT sandwiches or crumpled on a salad, and grainburger (textured vegetable protein) tossed into tacos, stews, and casseroles. Check out new foods each time you shop and experiment with something new each week. Switch to a different staple (for example, from potatoes to rice), experiment with different toppings, or try a new way of preparing a food.

• Don't rigidly control your fat intake. Let go of the idea that being a successful endurance athlete depends on eating an exact number of fat grams. Concentrate on making wise food choices that optimize your intake of carbohydrate and protein. Let your fat intake fall where it does. Hauptmann regularly snacks on homemade oatmeal raisin cookies and chocolate, and enjoys an occasional bowl of ice cream. Eating a reasonable amount of fat allows you to train more vigorously, which translates into more muscle mass and more strength. Think of your body fat as a ready reserve that you can tap into during long races.

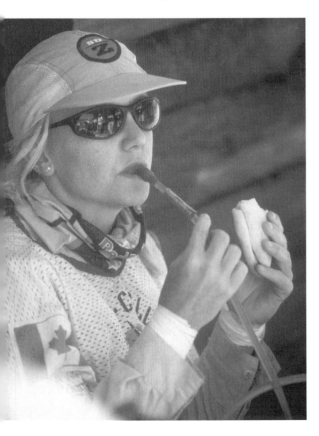

Special Health Concerns for Vegetarians

A meatless diet does not guarantee good health and better performances. Unless you stick to some basic guidelines and stay abreast of your calorie and nutrient needs, you may encounter some difficulties. Two particular problems that may slow vegetarian athletes down are amenorrhea (in women) and disordered eating habits.

Amenorrhea and Vegetarianism

Female athletes who adopt vegetarian diets may be at a higher risk for amenorrhea, a medical condition character-

A well-balanced vegetarian diet contains a reasonable amount of fat that promotes good health and vigorous training.

ized by low estrogen levels and the loss of menstrual periods. Women who follow a plant-based eating style typically have lower levels of hormones that affect menstruation, such as estrogen and prolactin, than do nonvegetarian women. These hormonal levels appear to be altered by some component characteristic of a vegetarian diet; possibilities include a high fiber intake, low-fat content, or the presence of weak plant hormones. Since amenorrhea is also linked with extreme or extensive exercise, it's not surprising to find the problem compounded among vegetarian athletes. High rates of amenorrhea have been reported in vegetarian athletes, particularly in runners. In one study, vegetarians made up 25 percent of the amenorrheic runners but only 11 percent of the runners who had regular menstrual periods.

If you develop amenorrhea, don't ignore it. You're three times more likely to develop a stress fracture, and low levels of estrogen at any age can cause premature bone loss. Look at your current eating habits. You often need only to gain a small amount of weight (2 to 3 percent of your body weight, or two to four pounds for a 120-pound woman) to restart your menstrual periods.

Because it's easy for an endurance athlete to burn off large amounts of calories through exercise, you may develop amenorrhea because of an energy imbalance. You simply don't consume enough calories to sustain your high energy expenditures. If you feel that your current vegetarian eating style doesn't keep up with your calorie needs, eat more fat (at least 20 percent of your total calories) and protein and cut back on fiber-rich foods that fill you up quickly. If possible, cut back on how intensely you exercise and reduce your training volume by 10 to 20 percent; even more if you're trying to conceive.

Be certain you consume adequate protein. The research suggests that amenorrheic athletes tend to have diets low in protein compared with regularly menstruating athletes. Some studies show that adding meat (red meat in particular) has a protective effect on menstrual periods, although it's

A Day in the Vegetarian Life

Here's a nutrition-packed, one-day vegetarian menu. Preparation time for each meal: under 10 minutes.

Breakfast

1 cup quick oatmeal, topped with 1 cup fat-free vanilla yogurt and 2 tbsp raisins

2 slices hearty grain bread with 1 tbsp peanut butter

8 oz orange juice

Lunch

1 garden burger on a whole-grain bun, with sliced tomato and onion

1/2 cup pasta and bean salad

Handful of baby carrots dipped in yogurt salad dressing

Snack

1 cup calcium-fortified soy milk

1 soft pretzel

Dinner

1 cup black bean chili, over top of 1 cup cooked Aztec rice and corn mix

Dark green salad with 1 tbsp low-fat dressing

1 cup frozen yogurt with 1/2 cup fresh or frozen strawberries

The day's tally:

Calories: 2,660 calories

Protein: 100 grams

Carbohydrate: 400 grams

Fat: 74 grams

unclear why. Obviously, it's a matter of personal choice whether you include or exclude meat in your diet. Depending on your long-term goals, you may want to reevaluate the effect that including small portions of meat several times a week could have on your health and performance.

Disordered Eating and Vegetarianism

Some vegetarian athletes, male and female, inadvertently consume too few calories to sustain their high energy output. Others, however, consciously restrict the foods they eat under the guise of vegetarianism. In other words, they choose (or choose to continue) a vegetarian eating style as a way to control their eating habits and cope with pressures to be thin. These individuals may feel better about themselves or superior to others when they eat differently, or they may feel "more perfect" when they don't eat certain foods.

Some hallmark behaviors to look for are vegetarians who narrow their protein choices to a few "acceptable" items, avoid fat by shunning nuts and seeds, nut butters, dairy products, and other high-fat items, and skip meals or elect not to eat in social settings rather than prepare or search out vegetarian fare. If you, or someone you train with or coach, pursue vegetarianism primarily as a politically correct means to lose weight or achieve a lean appearance, heed the warning signs. Such harmful and ineffective eating behaviors set you up for anemia, stress fractures, and possibly a full-blown eating disorder.

Parents and coaches of teenage athletes need to be particularly vigilant when it comes to young people and vegetarianism and the reasons teens give for renouncing foods and the effectiveness with which they replace these foods with healthy substitutes. Girls, in particular, may adopt vegetarianism as a socially acceptable way to mask their disordered eating habits.

Researchers at the University of Minnesota recently surveyed high school students across Minnesota and found that teenage vegetarian girls are twice as likely to diet, four times as likely to induce vomiting and eight times as likely to use laxatives as are their meat-eating peers. These findings support a reverse study of 116 patients suffering with anorexia nervosa (self-induced starvation): 54 percent avoided red meat, although only 4 percent had done so before the onset of their eating disorder.

One of my clients, a 13-year-old who adopted a vegetarian diet at the age of five, played soccer, swam, ran, and participated in gymnastics during a typical week. When a swim coach at a summer camp delivered the erroneous message that athletes should avoid eating fat, she began to count calories and fat grams, skip meals (saying she was not hungry or that the vegetables tasted terrible), and exercise twice a day. After she lost 10 pounds and her menstrual periods stopped, her parents took action.

Upon meeting her, I found that besides not eating meat, she didn't like fish, rarely drank milk, ate eggs only if they were prepared for her, and wrinkled her nose at the mention of beans or tofu. Obviously, she wasn't doing too well at covering her protein, iron, and calcium needs. She also wasn't consuming enough calories to balance those burned through exercise. Fortunately, a strong desire to continue at her sports activities motivated this teen to gain weight. She ate more of the foods she liked and after a few months began to eat some foods she had previously considered forbidden.

The bottom line is that a vegetarian diet can be a healthy way to eat or it can be a haphazard eating style that comes up short in many key nutrients. To reap the benefits of vegetarianism, you must be willing to do two things: stock your kitchen with some vegetarian staples (and know how to prepare them!) and invest some time and energy exploring new foods that will help you meet your nutrition needs.

Adapted, by permission, from S. Girard Eberle, 1997, "The vegetarian runner," *Marathon & Beyond* 1(5):69-77. © 42k(+) Press, Inc.

Hitting the Wall

"It wasn't until I got to the Olympic Training Center that I had any serious testing of my iron levels done. They couldn't believe how low my ferritin stores were for an endurance athlete. Training 25 to 40 hours a week at altitude pushes them even lower. I make a conscious effort to eat red meat several times a week and I take a liquid iron supplement twice a day, otherwise my levels drop right back down. It definitely helped me in Hawaii and I'm going to stay on top of it as I train for the Olympics. Taking too much iron can be dangerous, though, so my brother (a physician) monitors my blood once a month."

—Tim DeBoom, third-place,
1999 Hawaii Ironman

Just when you think you have everything under control, something pops up that snaps you back to reality. It could be a tree root, a flat tire, or a broken ski binding. It may also be one of the common nemeses discussed in earlier chapters that athletes face every time they head out the door to exercise such as dehydration, glycogen depletion, or bonking due to a low blood sugar. On the other hand, it may be something you're not as familiar with, such as anemia or recurring muscle cramps. A food allergy or intolerance may threaten to slow you down, too. On top of that, female endurance athletes face some particular challenges, such as feeling bogged down certain times of the month and dealing with the physical and emotional changes associ-ated with pregnancy. In any case, nutritional strategies exist to help you get back on track quickly.

Muscle Cramps

If you've ever suffered with a muscle cramp, you know that they always seem to strike just when you need to make your push toward the finish line. Unpredictable in nature, a cramp is a muscle contraction gone out of control, locking the muscle into a sustained and painful spasm. The exact cause of muscle cramps and how best to treat them remain unclear. Calf muscles seem to be most susceptible, but any muscle in the body can be done in by a cramp.

Overexertion, or working a muscle to the point of exhaustion, is the most likely culprit, but predisposing factors such as dehydration, an electrolyte imbalance, or a mineral deficiency may play a contributing role. Undoubt-edly, athletes tend to suffer muscle cramps more easily when dehydrated, so don't overlook an obvious solution. Start out well hydrated, drink as much as you can tolerate while exercising (ideally eight ounces every 15 to 20 minutes), and be sure to rehydrate afterward.

One way to monitor your fluid needs during exercise is by noting your ability to urinate. No hard and fast guidelines exist for how often you should urinate during prolonged exercise. If you find yourself not urinating for more than a few hours at a time or you can't urinate for several hours following exercise, you need to pay more attention to your fluid needs during exercise. Don't forget, it's possible to lose two quarts of sweat per hour during vigorous exercise in the heat. Avoid becoming progressively dehydrated day to day, especially when training in warm conditions, by checking your weight before and after you exercise. Assume that all the weight you lost is fluid that you need to replace that day. Rehydrate by drinking at least two cups of fluid for every pound of body weight lost.

Besides drinking enough fluid, be sure to get enough electrolytes, such as potassium and sodium, in your daily diet. Potassium and sodium help maintain water balance in the body, and the electrical charges they carry help trigger muscles to contract and relax. A potassium-sodium imbalance may lead to muscle cramps. Although you lose both potassium and sodium in sweat, you should have enough body stores of both to cover these losses.

Most sports drinks intended for use during exercise, as well as foods typically eaten during ultralong events, provide both sodium and potassium.

Your best defense against muscle cramps is to eat potassium-rich foods daily and use the salt shaker liberally, especially if you sweat profusely, train in a hot environment, or are involved in ultraendurance events. Potassium-rich foods, such as pinto and kidney beans, potatoes, tomatoes, spinach, cantaloupe, orange juice, bananas, dried fruit, milk, and yogurt make good choices. Potassium supplements shouldn't be necessary, and they can be harmful if you consume large doses over a short period of time.

If you're in good health and don't have a family history of hypertension (high blood pressure), don't let the popular guidelines calling for a restriction on dietary sodium trip you up. These guidelines target the general population, with the hope of reducing high blood pressure in sedentary and overweight individuals. As an endurance athlete, a self-imposed salt-restricted training diet may send you to the medical tent on race day. Muscle cramps, especially if accompanied by fatigue and lethargy, can be due to a sodium deficit that develops during prolonged exercise. In fact, many exercise physiologists and nutritionists feel that sodium depletion is the major predisposing factor behind cramping during athletic performances, especially in warm weather conditions.

Keep the salt shaker handy at the dinner table and answer salt cravings when they arise by consuming salty foods, such as pretzels, salsa and chips, pickles, soup, and canned foods. If you participate in ultraendurance events and suffer from recurring muscle cramps despite a daily liberal salt intake, consider experimenting with salt or electrolyte tablets. Keep in mind that you must take these tablets with ample fluid or you run the risk of causing gastrointestinal problems and dehydration.

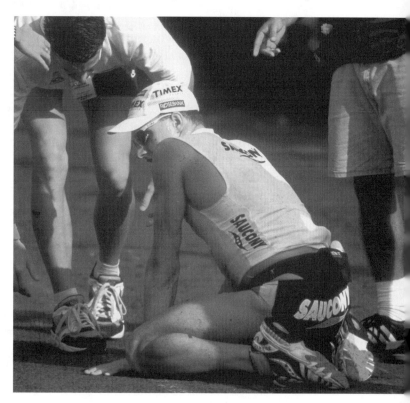

Ward off muscle cramps and heat exhaustion by drinking plenty of fluids and liberally salting your food prior to exercise.

A calcium deficiency in often blamed for muscle cramps, too. Calcium, the most abundant mineral in the body, plays an essential role in normal muscle function. It's unlikely that a calcium imbalance causes muscle cramps, because the body tightly regulates calcium levels in the blood. It does so by releasing calcium from the bones when enough dietary calcium isn't available, so sufficient calcium always remains available for normal nerve conduction and muscle contraction.

Nevertheless, some athletes may see their cramps disappear by boosting a calcium-poor diet with foods rich in calcium. To see if consuming more calcium makes a difference, consume at least two to three servings of calcium-rich foods daily. Dairy foods or other calcium-fortified foods, such as orange juice, soy milk, and tofu, make good choices. If you're unable to consume enough calcium through your food choices, round out your diet with a supplement. If nothing else, it will help protect your bones from becoming depleted.

In the end, if none of these nutritional strategies help in resolving muscle cramps, a physical therapist can help you explore potential biomechanical causes of muscle cramps, such as a leg-length discrepancy. A lack of flexibility or physical conditioning can also precipitate muscle cramps, so consult an athletic trainer or coach regarding proper stretching and training techniques.

Iron-Deficiency Anemia

Iron-deficiency anemia, characterized by a low blood-iron level, will slow even the fittest and best conditioned endurance athlete. Iron, although present in the body in relatively small amounts, plays a crucial role in the transport of oxygen. The body requires iron to form both hemoglobin and myoglobin. Hemoglobin, found in red blood cells, binds with oxygen in the lungs and then transports it (via the blood) throughout the body. Myoglobin, located in muscles, combines with oxygen and stores it until needed. If you suffer from anemia, your muscles receive less oxygen and, consequently, produce more lactic acid. As lactic acid builds up in your muscles, you fatigue prematurely when you exercise. Other possible signs and symptoms of iron deficiency anemia include muscle burning and shortness of breath during exercise, nausea, frequent infections, respiratory illnesses, and a pale, washed-out appearance.

The body's total iron content is small, averaging 2.9 grams in adult females and 3.5 grams in adult males. Most of the iron in the body is incorporated into hemoglobin (60 percent) and myoglobin (10 percent), with a small amount (2 percent) involved in other intracellular components and enzymes. About 30 percent (less in women) is stored as ferritin, primarily within the bone marrow, liver, and spleen. Outright low levels of iron in the blood indicate anemia, but low iron stores (nonanemic iron deficiency) can also be a problem for endurance athletes.

Iron Needs and Losses

Women have higher daily iron needs (15 milligrams) compared with teenage males (12 milligrams) and adult males (10 milligrams) because they lose iron through menstrual bleeding. If you suffer from recurring bouts of anemia, the first step is to take a closer look at your diet. A diet low in iron-rich foods is the primary cause of most iron deficiencies, particularly among active women. Even women who make smart food choices often have difficulty meeting their daily iron requirement. Female athletes who place a premium on having a lean physique by dieting or restricting calories will find it virtually impossible to consume enough iron. Vegetarian athletes, male or female, also have a higher risk of developing anemia. The iron in plant foods is not as efficiently absorbed as the iron in red meat, poultry, or fish.

Menstrual blood loss is the second biggest cause of low iron levels in women. Female athletes lose iron-rich hemoglobin each month if they menstruate regularly. This loss can vary substantially depending on the duration and heaviness of the menstrual flow.

Endurance athletes lose iron through various other avenues as well. Iron is lost through gastrointestinal (GI) bleeding that occurs with prolonged exercise, especially if diarrhea or cramping occurs during exercise. Less blood flows to the GI tract during exercise, especially during intense efforts, as more blood flows to active muscles. The lack of blood flow and nutrients in the lining of the GI tract causes cells to die and slough off. The result is occult, or hidden, blood in bowel movements. Some athletes suffer with bloody diarrhea occasionally, but in most cases you're probably not even aware of GI bleeding and this mode of iron loss. Dehydration, an inevitable consequence of participating in endurance events, exacerbates GI bleeding by further reducing the blood flow to the GI tract. Taking aspirin or nonsteroidal anti-inflammatory medications (Advil, Aleve, and so on) may also increase GI blood loss.

Iron losses through sweat and urine are usually negligible, but these losses can add up with prolonged exercise. For example, the physical jarring that the bladder endures during prolonged exercise, coupled with dehydration, can result in urinary blood losses. Daily exercise also appears to impair the absorption of iron from the GI tract. Normally, the body absorbs more iron in response to an iron deficiency. In athletes, this compensatory response appears to be blunted. One study, for example, found that iron-deficient runners absorbed only 16 percent of dietary iron as compared to nonathletes who absorbed 30 percent.

Iron depletion can also result simply from the slow loss of iron due to the chronic injury to red blood cells. The repetitive trauma of hard foot strikes in high-impact sports such as running, for example, destroys red blood cells. Athletes involved in swimming and other nonrunning sports, however, can have exercise-induced anemia, leading to the theory that muscle contractions, acidosis (a decrease in blood pH), or the increase in body temperature associated with exercise may also damage red blood cells. Your liver recycles released hemoglobin from damaged red blood cells up to a point. Beyond that, the hemoglobin is excreted into the urine, thereby compromising your iron status.

Monitoring Your Iron Status

An iron deficiency develops in three stages. In stages I and II, or nonanemic iron deficiency, the body's iron stores become depleted before the onset of anemia is clinically recognized. Stage I (iron depletion) is characterized by a serum ferritin level of less than 12 ng/mL, indicating complete depletion of iron stores. If this iron depletion continues for several months, stage II (iron-deficient erythropoiesis) can result, in which iron transport throughout the body and the production of red blood cells are affected. During both these stages, serum ferritin levels will be low, but hemoglobin and hematocrit (percentage of red blood cells in the total blood volume) values remain essentially normal. In stage III (iron-deficiency anemia), hemoglobin production falls and clinically recognized iron-deficiency anemia results, as evidenced by low hemoglobin and hematocrit levels.

The normal range for hemoglobin in teenage and adult females is 12 to 16 grams per deciliter. For hematocrit, the normal range is 37 to 48 percent. For teenage and adult males, normal values for hemoglobin range from 13 to 18 grams per deciliter. For hematocrit, the normal range is 45 to 52 percent. Athletes living and training at higher altitudes typically have more red blood cells, resulting in slightly higher hemoglobin and hematocrit values. Being dehydrated at the time you have your blood drawn can also produce elevated levels.

When it comes to interpreting serum ferritin values, it's generally accepted that levels below 12 ng/mL indicate completely depleted iron stores in the bone marrow, whereas values between 12 ng/mL and the lower limit of the normal range represent minimal iron stores. Diagnostic laboratories typically define normal, or adequate, iron stores as more than 20 ng/mL, whereas many exercise physiologists and exercise science researchers define serum ferritin levels of 35 ng/mL as the lower limit of normal for athletes.

You can easily monitor your iron status through specific blood tests that check your hemoglobin, hematocrit, and serum ferritin levels. Hemoglobin and hematocrit are typically included in routine blood work during a yearly physical. Unless you have a sports-savvy physician, though, you'll most likely have to request to have your iron stores, or serum ferritin, checked.

To get the most out of monitoring your iron status means you must first determine your baseline values. Anemia is defined by a hemoglobin or hematocrit value that falls below the normal range. Normal and abnormal values overlap significantly, though, and you should compare your test results only to your personal baseline range. For example, during my career

What If I Have Sports Anemia?

Incidentally, a low hemoglobin may not always represent a problem, as is the case in dilutional pseudoanemia. Commonly referred to as sports anemia, dilutional pseudoanemia is the natural dilution of hemoglobin that occurs when endurance exercise produces an increase in plasma volume. Your plasma volume, the watery portion of the blood, expands beyond its baseline in response to the exercise-induced release of various hormones. This increase in plasma volume artificially lowers hemoglobin and hematocrit readings.

Because the number of red blood cells remains normal and increases proportionately during exercise as water is lost from the blood in sweat, oxygen carrying-capacity is not compromised. Sports anemia doesn't usually last very long. It frequently occurs in athletes returning to training after inactivity or those who are increasing their training intensity. It doesn't respond to iron supplementation and can be distinguished from iron-deficiency anemia because your lab workup will reveal that the red blood cells do not appear pale or small as they do in true anemia.

as a competitive distance runner I kept copies of all my blood work and I've discovered over the years that I perform poorly when my hemoglobin dips into the 13's as my baseline runs closer to 14.5 grams per deciliter. A reading of 13 grams per deciliter, however, may not signal anemia for an athlete who has a lower baseline.

Unfortunately, most athletes typically have blood work performed only when they aren't feeling or performing well. This means it may take a series of blood tests over time, correlated with physical symptoms and your training and racing performances, to determine your ideal normal range. If you can swing it, have blood work performed when you're at the top of your game, too.

Treating Anemia

If you're diagnosed with iron-deficiency anemia, treatment usually consists of 50 to 100 milligrams of elemental iron, two to three times a day. To reduce possible side effects, such as nausea, diarrhea, or constipation, gradually increase the dosage from once a day to three times a day as your tolerance increases. Ferrous sulfate, available in a liquid form, is absorbed better than most other varieties. Slow-release products can help with reducing constipation.

To enhance the absorption of iron supplements, take them on an empty stomach with 500 milligrams of vitamin C or a glass of vitamin C rich juice. Allow at least four to six weeks before you have your blood work repeated to confirm that your hemoglobin concentration has improved. By eight weeks the anemia is usually corrected, although every athlete responds differently. You may need to continue with iron supplements for six to eight months to replenish your iron stores, as evidenced by normal ferritin levels. Be sure to do this under the care of a physician.

Treating Nonanemic Iron Deficiency

Athletes with low-normal or decreasing levels of serum ferritin, despite a hemoglobin reading in the normal range (nonanemic iron deficiency), should consider iron therapy, too. Anemia impairs athletic performance by reducing the delivery of oxygen to tissues, but a nonanemic iron deficiency can diminish your performance by a different mechanism. Iron-dependent metabolic processes at the cellular level, such as energy production in the mitochondria, may become impaired as your iron stores drop.

Studies of the effects of iron supplementation on performance in athletes with low iron stores have produced conflicting results. No improvements in $\dot{V}O_2$max have been shown, but other indicators of improved endurance, such as improvements in treadmill times and lower lactate levels during submaximal exercise, have been recorded. My personal experience and that of endurance athletes with whom I've trained suggests that low iron stores can hinder your performance well before you're diagnosed with anemia. As with hemoglobin, an individual threshold, or optimal level of iron storage, most likely exists for every endurance athlete. While living in Boulder, Colorado, my serum ferritin levels fell to 21, most likely due to training at altitude. Although considered "normal" by the physician, I began supplementing with iron. Another blood test three months later revealed that I had boosted my iron stores to almost twice that amount. More important, the chronic muscle soreness I had been experiencing cleared up in just a few weeks!

Whether it helps immediately, boosting low (less than 12 ng/mL) and borderline-low ferritin levels by controlled iron supplementation can prevent outright anemia from developing. The recommended treatment is 50 to 100 milligrams of elemental iron a day for three months, after which you should have your serum ferritin levels rechecked. Many times, the hemoglobin level will also increase, indicating that a mild anemia was already present although the initial hemoglobin level was technically in the normal range. Ideally, you want to maintain your iron stores as high as reasonably possible, as evidenced by serum ferritin readings of 50 ng/mL for women and 70 ng/mL for men. Your ferritin value can be elevated for 48 to 72 hours following a prolonged bout of exercise (for example, a marathon or triathlon) or if you're fighting an infection or inflammation. High-intensity training tends to decrease it gradually, so keep these variables in mind as you interpret your values.

Preventing Anemia and Iron Deficiency

Emphasizing iron-rich foods in your diet will help prevent an iron deficiency from turning into anemia. The iron in animal foods, particularly that contained in red meat, is more absorbable than the iron in supplements or plant foods (for a list of iron-rich foods see Iron Best Bets in chapter 1). Cooking in cast-iron skillets will also help you maximize your iron intake, as will eating a food rich in vitamin C (fruits, vegetables, or juices) along with iron-containing foods. Female athletes who don't eat meat should consider taking a multivitamin with iron or a low-dose iron supplement (15 milligrams per day).

Since iron deficiency is so common, especially among female athletes, screening for it at least once a year makes sense. Be sure to request a serum ferritin blood test along with the routine tests that look at hemoglobin and hematocrit levels. Keep a log of your blood test results and record other pertinent data, such as the type and amount of training you were doing, racing performances (if applicable), and comments on your general state of health.

Although it's tempting to diagnose and treat yourself when you feel rundown and tired, don't start taking appreciable amounts of iron without first seeing a physician. Certain individuals are susceptible to iron overload, or hemochromatosis, which can lead to serious and irreversible damage to internal organs. Besides, taking iron supplements when you don't have an iron deficiency won't boost your performance, and consuming too much iron can impede the absorption of other minerals, such as zinc.

Food Allergies and Intolerances

Athletes often let self-diagnosed food allergies get in the way of eating a well-balanced, healthy diet. After all, about 25 percent of American adults believe they

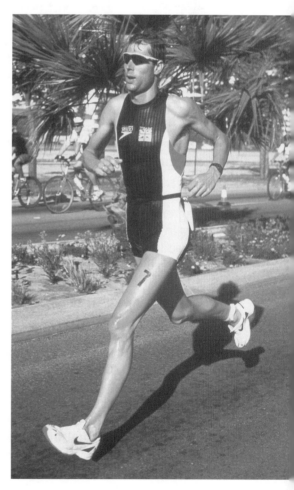

Triathletes and runners in particular need to eat an iron-rich diet to avoid iron-deficiency anemia.

have a food allergy, but only 1 to 2 percent actually do. A food intolerance, on the other hand, can affect nearly everyone at some point. This next section provides strategies for dealing with both.

Food Allergies

What's the difference between a food allergy and a food intolerance? A food allergy involves the immune system of the body. An allergen, usually a protein, in a food or ingredient causes an allergic person's immune system to overreact. Perceiving the allergen as being harmful, the body produces massive amounts of immunogloblin E (IgE), a type of antibody. IgE antibodies circulate in the blood and enter body tissues, stimulating other cells to release powerful substances, such as histamine. The reactions that occur, within minutes to an hour or two later, include tingling or swelling in the mouth and throat, stomach cramps, vomiting, diarrhea, skin rashes or hives, runny nose, sneezing, coughing, and wheezing. In highly allergic individuals, anaphylactic shock, a severe swelling of the throat, tongue, and airway that obstructs breathing, can occur.

Eight foods cause almost 90 percent of all severe food allergy reactions. In adults, shellfish (shrimp, crayfish, lobster, and crab), peanuts, tree nuts (almonds, cashews, pecans, and walnuts), fish, and eggs top the list. In children, eggs, milk, and peanuts are the main offenders. Soy and wheat round out the list. In general, if you're from a family in which allergies are common, such as hay fever, asthma, or hives, you're more likely to be predisposed to developing a food allergy. Although adults rarely lose their allergies, children will often outgrow their allergies, especially to milk, soy, and eggs.

Having a food allergy is a rare and serious condition that warrants a proper diagnosis by a board-certified allergist. Try to find one that specializes in food allergies. Keeping a food diary that details the allergic reactions caused by a specific food will provide valuable information, such as how much you can eat before experiencing a reaction and how quickly the reaction occurs after eating the suspected food. To narrow down the cause or help rule out a suspected food allergy, an allergist can perform various skin tests (PST, scratch or prick skin test) or blood tests (RAST, radioallergosorbent test). Be aware that a positive skin or blood test, by itself, doesn't make the diagnosis of a food allergy. You must have a positive test to a specific allergen and a history of reactions suggesting an allergy to the same food.

Self-diagnosing an allergy can get you into trouble. Avoiding foods unnecessarily deprives you of food choices and important nutrients. It can also be dangerous if you incorrectly identify the allergen. In a true food allergy, even minute amounts of the allergen will cause a reaction. Treatment focuses on avoiding the food after it is identified. Allergy shots, as well as injections of small quantities of extracts from foods you react to, are rarely effective in relieving food allergies.

Food Intolerances

If you have trouble tolerating a food, it's much more likely you have a food intolerance. You may suffer from many of the same symptoms as an allergy, but your immune system is not involved. Food intolerances tend to come and go in severity and are rarely life threatening. A prime example is lactose intolerance, which occurs when the body lacks enough lactase, an intestinal enzyme that breaks down the sugar in milk. Stomach cramps, gas, and diarrhea signal this problem.

Another important distinction from food allergies is that a food intolerance will often allow you to eat varying amounts of the offending food without experiencing any symptoms. Lactose-intolerance sufferers will often find they can tolerate milk in different forms, such as yogurt, cheese, and ice cream. Using Lactaid tablets, drinking milk with added lactase, or drinking small amounts of milk at meals, not on an empty stomach, can often alleviate the problem, too. The good news is that in many cases, your body can learn to adjust to the food as you build up a tolerance to it. For example, routinely drinking two to four ounces of milk at one meal can condition your body, over time, to handle larger amounts of lactose.

If you find your list of intolerable foods growing, other factors may be coming into play. Eating certain foods too close to exercise, when you're nervous, or when you're under stress may be causing a reaction. Milk, for example, is routinely blamed for causing cottonmouth—dryness in the mouth accompanied by thick, white saliva. The most likely culprit behind cottonmouth, however, is a combination of emotional stress and the loss of fluids during vigorous exercise and competition. Staying well hydrated before, during, and after exercise—rather than avoiding milk—is your best defense against cottonmouth.

A psychological trigger may be responsible for your food intolerance. It's common to have experienced an unpleasant event, often during childhood, tied to eating a particular food. Or you may be convinced that eating a certain food is associated with a poor performance in the past. Eating that food then becomes linked with a rush of unpleasant sensations that can resemble an allergic reaction to food.

Seeking a Solution

Eliminating a few foods from an otherwise healthy diet shouldn't cause a problem, especially if you eat a variety of foods most of the time. Athletes often temporarily avoid certain foods as they approach an important competition. You may be setting yourself up for nutrient deficiencies though, if you exclude entire food groups or regularly find yourself able to tolerate only a few foods. If this is the case, seek help from a registered dietitian or other qualified health professional to help you make food substitutions and plan a well-balanced diet. If your symptoms are linked to food additives, such as MSG or sulfites (common in asthmatics), it makes sense to avoid foods containing those substances. Check the ingredient lists on food labels and inquire how foods are prepared when dining away from home.

One way to investigate whether a specific food is the source behind your symptoms is to use an elimination diet. Keeping other factors the same, such as the amount and intensity of your training, eliminate one food at a time for several days. Monitor your symptoms for improvement. To confirm the connection, you need to eat the food again and see if the symptoms return. Obviously, you can't do this without medical supervision if you've been experiencing severe reactions that you believe are food related. In addition, elimination diets aren't that useful if the symptoms you experience occur infrequently.

Keep in mind that whenever you push your body to the limit, high levels of epinephrine (adrenaline) can interfere with the normal functioning of the GI tract. The rate at which food empties the stomach can be delayed, increasing the likelihood you'll experience nausea and indigestion. Mental and emotional stress can also slow the time it takes for food to leave the stomach. Eating smaller, more frequent meals, composed of low-fat, familiar foods, can help as you approach a competition or undergo periods of vigorous or stressful training. More often than not, modifying the timing of foods and fluids around exercise can make the difference.

No athlete wants to be slowed by bloating, flatulence, abdominal cramps, or diarrhea. Do your best to avoid abdominal discomfort before important events or races by staying well hydrated and avoiding gas-forming foods, such as carbonated beverages, beans, broccoli, cabbage, onions, and other problem foods you've identified during training. Establishing a consistent eating pattern and regular bowel habits are your best bet in preventing abdominal and intestinal problems.

Runner's Diarrhea

Any athlete may suffer from diarrhea and other intestinal problems during or after workouts or long races. Runners, however, appear to be affected by diarrhea and cramping more so than other athletes. Studies reveal that between 19 and 26 percent of marathon runners experience running-related diarrhea. Besides the lack of adequate blood flow to the GI tract during exercise and exercise-induced changes in GI hormones and the nervous system, runners suffer from another insult. The repetitive and jarring action of running may cause injury to the walls of your large intestine or colon, leading to diarrhea and GI blood loss.

While diet and medications can certainly be factors that cause runner's diarrhea, drinking plenty of fluids before and during exercise is your best defense against runner's diarrhea and other more serious GI problems, such as "athletic colitis." Experiencing bad diarrhea during exercise, but not at other times, might indicate that your colon becomes irritated due to the lack of adequate blood flow during exercise. During prolonged exercise, your body diverts blood away from the colon to active muscles and to the skin to disperse heat. Being dehydrated exasperates the situation as your reduced blood volume means that even less blood is available to the large intestine. The lack of blood flow can sometimes cause severe damage to the walls of the colon.

One elite female runner and two elite triathletes (one female and one male) have had parts of their colons surgically removed because of exercise-induced bowel problems. Concentrate on drinking fluids in the early stages of long races. As dehydration progresses, it becomes more and more difficult for your body to absorb the fluids that you do drink.

Take a look at your diet, too. Eating high-fiber foods, such as bran cereals and whole-grain products, too closely to the time you exercise (especially if you're nervous or anxious) can cause diarrhea, too. Insoluble fiber causes the colon to retain water and soften bowel movements, which can result in diarrhea during the stress of competition. Caffeine is known to have a laxative effect and artificial sweeteners, such as sorbitol and aspartame in candy and diet sodas can cause diarrhea, too. Develop and stick to a prerace diet of foods that you have tested and know you can tolerate. Check with your physician about the possibility of giardiasis (an infection of the small intestine caused by a parasite) or medications or herbal supplements causing diarrhea during exercise. Your health care provider can also advise you on the use of antidiarrheal medications during prolonged exercise.

Special Concerns for Female Athletes

Female athletes may face unique challenges including premenstrual syndrome, pregnancy, and breast-feeding. The following sections provide nutrition strategies that will help female athletes manage premenstrual syndrome, as well as advice on how to feel your best and remain fit and active while pregnant or breast-feeding.

Premenstrual Syndrome

If you feel that your ability or desire to train or perform suffers at certain times of the month because of your menstrual cycle, you're not alone. One likely cause is premenstrual syndrome (PMS), a condition that affects 90 percent of women to some degree, especially those in their 30s and 40s. Although exercise can help curb the symptoms of PMS, an athlete in touch with her body may be more aware or more sensitive to monthly hormonal fluctuations.

Women of all athletic abilities can suffer from PMS, a complex of emotional, behavioral, and physical symptoms that occurs in some women one to two weeks before the onset of menstruation. The symptoms vary widely among women but tend to fall into four categories: anxiety (mood swings, irritability, sense of being out of control), cravings (increased appetite, craving for sweets or salty foods, fatigue, headache, dizziness), edema (weight gain, breast swelling or tenderness, abdominal bloating), and depression (forgetfulness, crying, insomnia). With PMS, the symptoms resolve quickly (within four days) after the onset of menstrual bleeding. During the teenage years and early to mid-20s, symptoms may be minimal and barely noticeable. As you get older, the symptoms may gradually get worse from year to year or rapidly increase in intensity following the birth of a child.

The exact cause of PMS remains unclear. An imbalance in one of the two female hormones, estrogen and progesterone, or an imbalance of the ratio between these hormones, as well as alterations in brain chemicals, appears to play a role in susceptible women. Not all women suffer to the same degree with premenstrual symptoms. Athletic women may feel particularly hampered by physical symptoms, such as fluid retention, weight gain, and breast tenderness. Many also complain of feeling clumsy, less coordinated, and more susceptible to muscle or skeletal injuries. Mood swings, uncharacteristic fatigue, or the energy lows associated with PMS can also lead women to feel as if they can no longer complete their daily training routine.

Diet and Supplements

Although nutritional issues alone most likely don't cause and can't cure PMS, modifying your diet may help alleviate symptoms. No single treatment has proven effective for all women, so you may need to try different strategies to find relief. In some cases, it may take a few menstrual cycles to see any effects.

Eat small, frequent meals based on complex carbohydrates during the two weeks before your period is due. Going long periods without food causes your blood sugar to plummet, which accentuates many of the symptoms of PMS. Eating six small meals a day, about three hours apart, will help keep your blood-sugar level on a more even keel. Include plenty of complex carbohydrates, such as pasta, baked potatoes, cereal, crackers, bread, rice dishes, and vegetables. Choose whole-grain versions rather than sugary foods.

When blood-sugar levels get too low, adrenaline is released, which may interfere with the normal metabolism of progesterone. In addition, the extra adrenaline can make you feel more anxious, tense, or aggressive. Eating complex carbohydrates also increases the production of serotonin, a brain chemical that leaves you feeling satiated, as well as less depressed and less irritable.

• Limit your consumption of simple sweets. Resist the urge to self-regulate your mood or energy level with sugar. Simple sugars found in baked goods, soda, and candy can cause rapid swings in blood-sugar levels. You may feel better and temporarily have more energy only to find yourself in need of another sugar fix a short while later. Enjoy these foods in moderation at mealtimes, not on an empty stomach.

- Stay well hydrated. Dehydration can make PMS symptoms worse, especially feelings of fatigue. Limit or avoid alcoholic beverages.

- Avoid caffeinated beverages and other sources of caffeine. Try to eliminate, or at least cut way back, on the caffeine in your diet throughout the entire month. It's unclear why it may contribute to PMS, but as a stimulant, caffeine also induces the release of adrenaline. Many women find that eliminating caffeine is particularly helpful in alleviating breast tenderness or pain.

- Monitor your sodium intake. The traditional advice has been to cut back on sodium (10 days before your period) so that you retain less water, which may help some women alleviate the bloating, tender breasts, and headaches associated with PMS. Hormonal fluctuations, however, most likely induce the body to retain water (whether or not you eat salty foods) and even cause some women to lose sodium before their period. Increase your sodium intake slightly to see if it makes a difference, particularly if you typically crave salty foods.

- Boost your calcium intake. During certain phases of the menstrual cycle, fluctuations in calcium-sensitive hormones that regulate calcium levels may set off a host of PMS symptoms by interfering with the brain chemical serotonin. If you don't get 1,200 milligrams of calcium a day by eating calcium-rich foods (see Best Bets: Calcium in chapter 1), boost your intake to the recommended level with a daily calcium supplement (in divided doses of 500 to 600 milligrams at a time). Daily calcium supplementation has shown promise in reducing symptoms of mild to moderate PMS, including generalized aches and pains, food cravings, water retention, depression, and mood swings. It may take two to three menstrual cycles to see positive effects.

- Boost your magnesium intake. Magnesium also plays a role in the synthesis of brain chemicals, so make sure you regularly eat plenty of magnesium-rich foods. Good sources include legumes, whole grains, dark green leafy vegetables, nuts and seeds, tofu, and seafood. Supplemental doses (200 milligrams) may help some women with mild symptoms of PMS, such as bloating.

Here's some advice on other popular treatments for PMS:

- Use caution with vitamin B_6 supplements. Vitamin B_6 is involved in the synthesis of brain chemicals, such as dopamine and serotonin, and in the way the body metabolizes hormones. Some women report relief of PMS symptoms with supplementation, although most studies do not find it superior to a placebo or sugar pill. Doses as low as 200 milligrams a day, taken for an extended time, may cause irreversible nerve damage, including tingling or numbness of the hands or feet and difficulty walking.

To derive the possible benefits, eat foods rich in vitamin B$_6$, including whole grains, soybeans, soy milk, potatoes, salmon, poultry, spinach, broccoli, bananas, and cantaloupe. If you choose to take a supplement, take an entire vitamin B complex containing no more than 50 milligrams of vitamin B$_6$. Take doses over 100 milligrams a day only under the supervision of a physician.

• Many women find relief from female problems by turning to herbal remedies. Black cohosh and chaste berry tree are purported to reduce PMS by balancing hormone levels, St. John's Wort by acting as a natural antidepressant, and valerian root by serving as a mild tranquilizer and sleep aid. To reduce possible side effects, try one herbal remedy at a time. Check with your physician first, especially if you take any medications, including oral contraceptives, estrogen, or antidepressants.

Managing Your PMS Symptoms

When it comes to PMS, your best bet is to establish healthy eating patterns, modify your training and racing schedules as needed, and seek healthy ways to manage daily stress. Avoid remedies that promise to cure PMS if you abstain from eating long lists of "offender" foods, such as refined white sugar, white flour, and so on. Such an extreme diet is not proven to be effective, is difficult to follow, and can create more anxiety than it's worth.

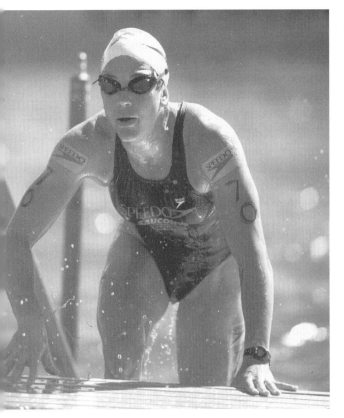

Keeping a daily chart of your three to five most severe symptoms will help you recognize the effects of PMS on your appetite and athletic performance. Record the absence or presence of your symptoms, their severity, and the day of your menstrual cycle (day 1 starts with menstrual bleeding.) Ovulation (approximately days 12 to 14 of a normal menstrual cycle), for example, boosts a woman's daily energy needs by 100 to 200 calories. You'll be less anxious, less irritable, and less prone to food cravings if you're aware that an increase in appetite is natural and normal at this time.

Eating regular meals, reducing stress, and modifying your training shedule can help you manage premenstrual syndrome.

If self-help techniques, such as healthy nutrition habits, dietary supplements, and a stress management program, prove to be ineffective, explore other treatment options with your physician. Oral contraceptives, natural progesterone, or antidepressants may also be indicated to help alleviate the emotional and physical symptoms associated with PMS.

Nutrition and Pregnancy

Even when you plan to become pregnant, your game plan may not include sitting around for nine months waiting for the baby to arrive. Many female athletes desire, and are able to retain, a high degree of fitness during pregnancy. Returning quickly to competition following the birth of a child is also a powerful motivator for many female endurance athletes. Listening to your body and maintaining healthy eating habits before, during, and after your pregnancy is key to ensuring a healthy baby and a healthy, fit mom.

Prepregnancy Diet Concerns

Paying attention to your diet *before* you plan to conceive can reduce your risk of having a baby born with a birth defect affecting the brain or spinal cord (neural tube defects), such as spina bifida or anencephaly. The first eight weeks after conception are the most crucial time in your baby's development. By the eighth week, the developing fetus has a complete nervous system, a beating heart, a fully formed digestive system, and the beginnings of facial features. Neural tube defects occur during the first month of pregnancy when the neural tube is forming. As many as half of all pregnancies are unplanned, so many women, including female athletes, don't realize they are pregnant at this time. Weight gain can be minimal during these first few weeks, and a woman may attribute a late or missed menstrual period to hard training efforts or the stress associated with competitions.

Consuming 400 micrograms a day of the B vitamin folate or folic acid will help your developing baby form and develop new and normal body tissues. (Folate is used when the vitamin is found naturally in foods; folic acid is used when it is found in supplements.) Natural sources of folate include legumes, such as lentils and dried beans, leafy green vegetables (especially spinach and broccoli), whole grains, orange juice, and some fortified breakfast cereals. Grain products, such as breads, pasta, rice, cornmeal, and enriched flours, are now being fortified with small amounts of folic acid, too. Nevertheless, most women do not consume adequate amounts of folate in their diet.

If you're contemplating pregnancy, see your doctor before you try to conceive and begin taking a prenatal vitamin-mineral supplement as directed to obtain the folic acid you need. Because so many pregnancies are unplanned, the March of Dimes recommends that all women of childbearing age, whether planning to become pregnant or not, take a multivitamin with 400 micrograms of folic acid daily and eat folate-rich foods. (Excessive levels of vitamin A can be toxic to a developing baby. Avoid taking a daily multivitamin containing more than 5,000 international units of vitamin A.)

Abstaining from alcohol makes sense, too. No safe level of alcohol consumption has been determined for pregnant women. Consuming limited amounts of alcohol after conception, before becoming aware you're pregnant, shouldn't cause you distress. Regularly consuming alcoholic beverages, however, does affect the developing fetus. Having one to two drinks a day can result in a smaller baby. Drinking greater amounts can lead to birth defects associated with fetal alcohol syndrome. The earlier you eliminate alcohol, the better.

Dealing With Morning Sickness

Weight gain, food cravings, fatigue, and morning sickness are issues all pregnant women have to deal with. Most female athletes are prepared to slow down as they gain weight throughout their pregnancy. You may even be looking forward to satisfying a craving or two. You may not be prepared, however, for the slowdown caused by morning sickness and fatigue during the first few months of your pregnancy.

Morning sickness, characterized by nausea with or without vomiting and fatigue, affects 50 to 90 percent of pregnant women to some degree. Despite being studied for at least four thousand years, the exact cause remains a mystery. Fluctuating hormonal levels, dehydration, and a trigger of some sort most likely combine to produce the next round of nausea. It's usually worse in the morning upon rising, although it can occur anytime throughout the day. Morning sickness usually resolves itself by the end of the first trimester (week 13), but don't worry if you still experience it into the fourth or fifth month.

Because every pregnancy is different, what triggers morning sickness will also vary from woman to woman. You'll have to experiment to find what works for you in reducing or alleviating the symptoms of morning sickness. Some age-old remedies that have stood the test of time include keeping soda crackers near your bed to nibble on before you get up and not brushing your teeth right after eating. You may find that eating a snack before go to bed or when you awaken during the night may ward off nausea in the morning. A heightened sense of smell is typical during pregnancy, and smells or odors may play a large role in triggering bouts of morning sickness. Try to sleep with the window open. Avoid cooking odors, perfume, aftershave, and cigarette smoke. If the smell of some foods make you sick, avoid them.

Be prepared to eat small meals every two to three hours to keep your blood sugar from getting too low, which may induce nausea. Don't worry about craving or only being able to tolerate junk food during bad periods of morning sickness. The goal is to find foods you can eat and keep down. Your favorite workout food, the one you can stomach during a hard effort or in the middle of a race, might just do the trick. Concentrate on eating nutritious foods once the nausea and vomiting pass. Eating typically causes you to drink more, which will help you to avoid becoming dehydrated. Drink beverages slowly and in between meals to further combat nausea. Of course, you'll want to pay particular attention to drinking enough fluids before, during, and after exercise.

Weight Gain and Energy Needs

You may be surprised that eating for two requires only an extra 300 calories a day, primarily during the second and third trimesters. That's not much—in fact, three glasses of lowfat milk will do the trick. As you reduce your training, you may not even need to eat any extra food to meet your energy needs. Let your rate of weight gain be your guide. You'll want to gain at least 25 to 35 pounds during your pregnancy to reduce the chance of complications, such as having a baby that weighs too little or is born prematurely. Pay particular attention to eating two to three hours before you exercise, as well as immediately afterward, to minimize exercise-induced falls in blood sugar. Keep supplemental carbohydrates (for example, sports drinks, energy gels, and energy bars) on hand to ingest during exercise as needed, even during short sessions when you typically wouldn't need anything.

Gaining less than five pounds in the entire first three months is perfectly normal. Typical gains are about a pound per week after that. Athletic women may easily gain more than the recommended range, particularly if you're lean and enter your pregnancy with a low body-fat level. If that's the case, don't worry about what the scale says. If you're eating healthy foods and continuing with your exercise routine (with modifications as necessary), your baby will profit from the extra weight you gain.

Nutrient Needs and Food Cravings

During pregnancy, you need more of certain nutrients. Besides folic acid, active women need to pay particular attention to getting enough calcium, iron, and protein. Your calcium needs jump to 1,200 milligrams a day, or the equivalent of four servings of dairy foods (see Best Bets: Calcium in chapter 1). As your baby's bones calcify, calcium moves out of your bones and across the placenta. Without adequate calcium stores, you run the risk of weakening your bones. This increases your risk of developing a stress fracture when you return to training, and for developing osteoporosis earlier in life.

Pregnancy doubles your iron requirement to 30 milligrams a day, because you need to make hemoglobin for extra red blood cells for yourself and the developing fetus. Along with the inevitable loss of iron that occurs with blood loss at birth, your iron stores will also be used to create your baby's iron stores. Since many woman athletes, particularly those involved in endurance sports, have low iron stores, you should have your iron status checked early in your pregnancy and at regular intervals thereafter. Although it's

Competing After Pregnancy

Julie Moss, former competitive triathlete (1982-1990), was bitten by the Ironman bug again following the birth of her son Mats in 1993. She returned to complete two Ironman competitions at age 39—the 1997 Australian Ironman (seventh overall, first in age group) and the 1997 Hawaii Ironman (second in age group).

"It takes nine months to make a baby (first trimester), nine months to recover (second trimester), and then another nine months (that's the third trimester) to pick and prepare for an athletic goal and find your competitive self again."

common to experience fatigue, especially during the first trimester, developing iron-deficiency anemia only makes matters worse.

You also need an extra 10 grams of protein every day—the amount supplied by one glass of low-fat milk and a piece of whole-grain bread. Although most female athletes can easily meet their increased protein needs through food alone, supplementing with calcium and iron makes sense. Incidentally, individual food cravings do not typically reflect any particular nutrient deficiency. Go ahead and appease your cravings within reason. Food aversions and cravings probably arise during pregnancy due to changes in your sensitivity to tastes and smells.

Foods to Avoid While Pregnant

Food safety during pregnancy is simple. Just be careful about ingesting anything you wouldn't serve your baby. Besides alcohol, watch out for caffeine, artificial sweeteners, contaminants from pollution or bacteria, and herbal supplements. Restrict your daily intake of caffeine (considered a necessary substance by many athletes!) to 300 milligrams or less, about the amount in two cups of brewed coffee. Some studies suggest that drinking more than that may increase your risk of giving birth to an underweight baby. Although artificial sweeteners appear to be safe for pregnant women to consume, relying on natural sweeteners, like sugar, honey, or molasses, is a safer route to follow.

Skip soft cheeses such as feta, blue cheese, Brie, Camembert, and Mexican-style cheeses during your pregnancy. These items, as well as hotdogs, luncheon meats, and cold cuts, can be contaminated with a bacteria called listeria, which causes a flulike illness. Transmitted across the placenta, listeriosis food poisoning can lead to premature delivery, miscarriage, stillbirth, or serious health problems for your newborn child. Because of the risk of bacterial contamination, you should also stay away from raw or undercooked meat, poultry and shellfish, sushi, unpasteurized milk or juice, and raw eggs found in homemade ice cream, eggnog, and raw cookie dough.

Because of their potential mercury content, restrict your intake of tuna and swordfish to twice a week.

As for herbal supplements, few if any of these products have been tested for safety during pregnancy or lactation. If you're considering taking herbal supplements during your pregnancy (or while breast-feeding), consult with your physician first.

Breast-Feeding

Breast-feeding, not pregnancy, is the time more aptly referred to as eating for two. Your body requires an additional 600 or more calories a day to produce enough milk. Studies have shown that most breast-feeding women who exercise seem to increase their daily food intake spontaneously by 400 to 500 calories to cover their increased energy needs. The rest of the energy comes from fat stores accumulated during pregnancy for that purpose.

Dieting or excessively restricting your calories to speed up the process of returning to your prepregnancy weight doesn't make sense. You'll end up irritable and low on energy just when you need it the most during the first few months when you're fighting off the effects of sleep deprivation and adjusting to a new schedule. Don't try to lose more than one to two pounds per week. It took nine months or more to gain the weight, so it will most likely take at least nine months to lose it, although regular exercise can speed up the timetable.

To keep up with your baby's demand for milk, you'll need to consume enough calories, adequate carbohydrates, and plenty of fluid. Plan to have a minimeal each time you nurse, such as a piece of fruit or half a sandwich, plus at least eight ounces of fluid, such as water, milk, or juice. A poor diet is more likely to decrease the quantity, not the quality, of the milk produced. If you're having trouble producing enough milk, reevaluate your food choices and boost your calorie intake. (A baby that gains a quarter to a half pound per week is getting enough milk and gaining weight appropriately.) Your calcium needs remain high (1,200 milligrams per day) during lactation, and you should continue to monitor your iron stores (serum ferritin) and supplement with iron as needed. Women often find it helpful to continue taking a prenatal vitamin-mineral supplement while breast-feeding.

Dehydration can be a problem until you recognize how much your fluid needs have increased. Drink enough so you feel you have to urinate every time you feed your baby. The clearer your urine, the better hydrated you are. Don't plan to exercise strenuously if your urine isn't clear. Dark, concentrated urine indicates that you're already in a dehydrated state.

Substances such as alcohol and caffeine enter breast milk, and large amounts consumed in a short period can affect your nursing infant. Intense exercise efforts also affect the composition of breast milk by decreasing immunoglobulin A, a substance important for a healthy immune system, and by increasing the amount of lactic acid that appears in breast milk. The increase in lactic acid causes a sour taste that your baby may find unpleasant. Within 60 to 90 minutes after exercise, however, breast milk returns to normal, so these changes don't appear to be significant. If your infant appears to react to your breast milk following exercise, try breast-feeding your baby before you head out to train.

part II

Endurance Nutrition Programs

9

Marathon Running

"It's a good thing I don't look like what I eat (when training for a marathon) otherwise I'd be Tony the Tiger or Captain Crunch."

—Keith Brantly,
1998 United States Men's
Marathon Champion

Keith Brantly
Event: 1998 United States Men's Marathon Championship
Pittsburgh Marathon
First place, 2:12:31, U.S. course record

Prerace Nutrition

Carbohydrate loading: Minidepletion of muscle glycogen stores by avoiding carbohydrates after 6 P.M. Thursday, followed by a brisk four- to five-mile run on Friday morning. Following the run, replenished glycogen stores by grazing on five to six light carbohydrate-rich meals throughout the day for the next two days. Did not use a carbohydrate-loading beverage.

> *KB:* "I've had to experiment a lot with carbohydrate-loading and the last thing I want to do is be depressed (a possible side effect during the carbohydrate depletion phase) heading into a major race, so I limit the depletion phase to 12 hours followed by a run."

Hydration: Relied on water and a sports drink (no particular brand, looks for one that contains maltodextrins).

> *KB:* "I know I'm doing a good job drinking when I have to pee at what seems like every 15 minutes."

Prerace Meals (Race Start: 8 A.M.)

Night before: Ate dinner between 8:00 and 8:30 P.M., ordered soup and pizza from room service. No steadfast prerace meal. He chose foods he enjoys, had access to, and are filling enough to help induce sleeping through the night. Consciously continued to drink water.

> *KB:* "I cut my odds of getting food poisoning by not eating with a group. I know I can't always get the same foods, so why worry about it? The race is difficult enough! I have a window of OK foods that I can eat. I've actually had steak the night before a race and haven't felt any different. Besides, the prerace meal is only one factor that goes into preparing for a marathon."

Morning of race: Breakfast for elite athletes in the hospitality suite, approximately 5:30 A.M.: one and a half bagels (no condiments), orange juice, banana, coffee (two cups), water.

Continued to nibble on a bagel in his hotel room and drank a mixture of sports drink, water, and glycerol up to an hour before the race, then switched to drinking plain water.

KB: "My goal is to eat and drink as much as possible right up to the start of the race. I've hit the wall a couple of times while running a marathon and it's the most depressing feeling, as you can't do anything about it. I can gain up to four or five pounds before the race from carbohydrate loading and holding on to water. I know I'm filled with fuel. In fact, the more sluggish I feel is a sign that I'm going to run really well. Since I feel so full, I'm never really that famished, so I have to force myself to eat the morning of the race."

Supplements: Used glycerol, 1.7 ounces per 32 ounces of fluid (as directed based on body weight). Drank approximately 32 ounces of Gatorade-water-glycerol mixture up to one hour before the start to hyperhydrate and added the same solution to race bottles in varying dilutions.

KB: "I think glycerol really works, but I don't use it unless it's really warm and humid. I haven't had any negative experiences yet."

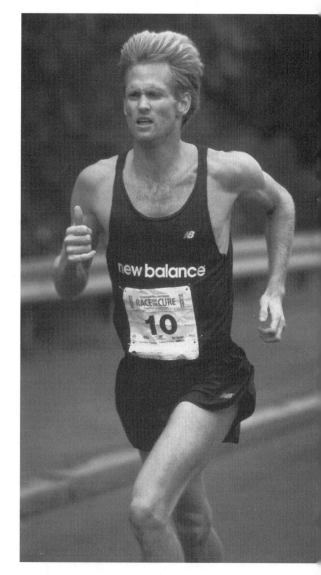

1996 Olympian Keith Brantly views the marathon as a race to the finish before his energy reserves run out.

During the Event

Aid stations: Drank a mixture of Gatorade, water, and glycerol throughout the race. Brantly premixed his drinks the day before and prepared his water bottles by adding foot-tall U-shaped handles (made from postal strapping tape) to make them easy to spot and grab. Race officials placed them on elite-athlete tables at eight predesignated aid stations. He has never used energy gels in a marathon race.

Early miles:	up to 15K (9 miles)	75% Gatorade, 25% water
	around 20K (12 miles)	60% Gatorade, 40% water
	around 25K (15 miles)	50% Gatorade, 50% water
	around 30K (19 miles)	40% Gatorade, 60% water
	from 35K (22 miles)	100% water

> *KB:* "The plan is always to hit every aid station, especially the early ones, and I spend the extra time and effort to do it. The marathon is not a race against others; it's a race against physiology. You just hope to get to the finish line before your body shuts down. I want to get sugar and electrolytes in early on during the race. I've experienced problems in the past with dehydration, especially in hot weather marathons. I can tell because I don't want what's in my bottle to taste too sweet. I know I'm in trouble, and I immediately try to rehydrate with water only. Water is my lifeblood in a marathon. I know I need to drink early and often."

Postrace Recovery

Immediately: Drank plenty of sports drinks, nibbled on bananas and bagels, enjoyed a beer or two. Grazed on light meals (e.g., soup) and eventually dined on rewarding foods.

Following week: Consciously drank a lot of water and ate whatever he wanted! One of Brantly's favorites: PopTarts (toasted, of course).

> *KB:* "My eyes are bigger than my stomach after a marathon. I basically just want to sleep. My recovery includes stretching, hot baths, massage, light jogs, swimming, and sailing. One of the perks of training (100-mile weeks) and racing marathons is that I should be able to eat anything I want!"

Tips for All Marathoners

1. Start the race well hydrated and well fueled. Start pushing fluids at least 24 hours before you toe the line. Keep a water bottle close at hand all day. If you've trained properly and eat a normal diet the few days prior to the race, you can expect to store roughly 2,000 calories of glycogen to use as fuel during the race. Since every mile you run burns approximately 100 calories, it makes sense to boost your glycogen stores by carbohydrate loading in order to reduce your chances of "hitting the wall" at about the twenty-mile mark of the marathon.

Keep in mind that carbo loading does not require you eat enormous quantities of food, nor does it mean loading up on high-fat foods. To enter the race feeling fresh and well rested, you'll want to taper your training as race day approaches. You'll be expending less energy (calories), so it's not necessary to eat hundreds of extra calories in order to boost your carbohydrate intake. Instead, concentrate on increasing the percentage of your calories that come from carbohydrate-rich foods. As long as you fill up on carbohydrates and not fat, don't be alarmed if you feel bloated or gain a couple of pounds in the days leading up to the race. Your body stores a considerable amount of water as it stows away carbohydrate as muscle glycogen. This extra water will help delay dehydration during the race. Experiment with carbohydrate loading before long training runs to find a routine that works for you.

2. Plan to eat a high-carbohydrate breakfast a few hours before the start of the race, especially if the race features a late morning or midday starting time. Eating breakfast can help settle your stomach and ward off hunger pangs as you wait for the race to begin. More importantly, eating breakfast refills your liver glycogen stores, which are critical for maintaining a stable blood sugar level during exercise. If you're simply too nervous to eat the morning of the race, try drinking your breakfast in the form of a breakfast shake or meal replacement product. Or try eating a substantial late-night snack before going to bed. Experiment before long training runs or shorter races leading up to the marathon with the types and quantity of food you can tolerate eating for breakfast.

3. If the race involves travel and meals eaten away from home, be sure to take with you any special or favorite food items that you can't do without. Consider using a high-carbohydrate beverage or meal-replacement product to supplement your carbohydrate needs if time-zone changes or your travel schedule will interfere with your regular eating habits. As much as you can control it, don't try new foods or experiment or change your diet in the week leading up to the race.

4. Save your glycogen stores and extend the distance you are able to run by eating during the marathon. Without a doubt, drinking your calories via sports drinks remains the easiest way to meet energy (and carbohydrate) needs in a marathon. Pudding-like energy gels, however, provide another option. Easy to ingest while running, energy gels need to be taken with four to six ounces of water (not a sports drink) to reduce the risk of stomach upset. Plan ahead and ingest a packet right before an aid station where water is available. Waiting too long into the race, when you're more likely to be dehydrated, also increases the risk you may suffer gastrointestinal problems. (Of course, don't wait until the race to experiment with energy gels, try them out during training runs first.)

Most gels supply 80 to 100 calories per packet. If you plan on carrying more than one energy gel packet with you, use one of the convenient palm-sized flasks that clip to the waistband of your running shorts. These refillable flasks can carry and dispense up to five servings (packets) of gel as you desire it. Runners who plan to take longer than four to five hours to complete the marathon course may consider wearing a waist pack instead, to tote energy gels or other well-tolerated solid foods, such as energy bars. Consuming at least 30 grams of carbohydrate every half hour (check labels of your favorite race foods beforehand) will boost your spirits and help you keep moving all the way to the finish line.

5. Experiment with glycerol during long training runs in the heat before trying it on race day. You need to see if you can consume and tolerate the large volume of fluid (generally a quart or more) recommended for hyperhydration. Most athletes prefer a combination of water and a sports drink to plain water for the mixture. Keep notes on how long it takes you to drink the mixture comfortably, how long it takes to clear your gastrointestinal tract, and if you feel bloated, how long the feeling lasts. Be aware that you will still need to replace your fluid losses as much as possible by drinking water and fluid replacement drinks throughout the race.

6. Beware the bonk. A marathoner "hitting the wall" has essentially depleted his or her muscle glycogen stores. Your legs have gone on strike, even though you may have been consuming adequate fluids and calories. (Your training, or lack thereof, improper pacing and general fatigue can contribute to this phenomenon). Runners are often able to continue and finish the race, albeit not with the desired performance. Bonking, when the body completely shuts down due to a severe drop in blood sugar, is a much more serious situation. The glycogen stored in your muscles and liver is gone and you have no fuel for your muscles or more importantly, your brain. If left untreated, you may become increasingly irritable, confused and disoriented, may find yourself sitting or lying down, and you could possibly even lapse into a coma. Stop walking or running and boost your blood sugar by consuming readily absorbable carbohydrates, such as sports drinks, or energy gels, soda, fruit juice, or glucose tablets, if available. Seek or ask for medical attention if necessary.

Libbie Hickman, who recorded a 2:28:34 personal record in only her third marathon, and Brantly share the following tips on meeting your fluid and energy needs during the marathon:

- Brantly compares the water stations in marathons to the pit stations in autoracing. He advises fellow marathoners to not even think about bypassing them, especially the early stations. Your running pace will determine which water stops to really key on, as you need to drink water and/or a sports drink every 15 to 20 minutes (aim for four to eight ounces). Don't wait until you feel thirsty—once you're dehydrated, you won't catch up. Drinking a sports drink is the easiest way to replace water and carbohydrates while you're running. If you have a particularly sensitive stomach, find out beforehand which sports drink will be used during the race and practice drinking it during your long runs.

- Drinking while running is an art and a science. Simply grabbing a cup or two isn't good enough; it's about getting the fluid down. Hickman, a marathon neophyte is still "learning the game." She recommends using shorter races to practice the following favored technique: grab a cup, pinch or crush it lightly it to form a funnel and take one or two gulps at a time. Keep in mind that even if you have to slow to a walk to drink enough fluid, it's better than dropping out of the race due to being dehydrated or glycogen depleted.

- If you're fast enough to warrant picking up water bottles at aid stations designated for elite marathoners, use your imagination and decorate your bottles. You want them to be easy to spot and easy to grab. Brantly and Hickman caution athletes not to panic if a bottle is not where you planned it to be. Slow down slightly to try and spot it, but don't waste too much time. Remind yourself that you can get plenty of water or sports drinks along the course. Start grabbing cups of fluid immediately and slow down if necessary to be sure you consume enough.

- Drink the water offered along the course, don't pour it over your head. While it may temporarily cool you off, it doesn't make sense to pour water over your head instead of drinking it. Brantly compares it to driving a car that's over heating to the gas station, pulling up to the water hose, opening the hood of the car and then spraying the water all over the over-heated engine.

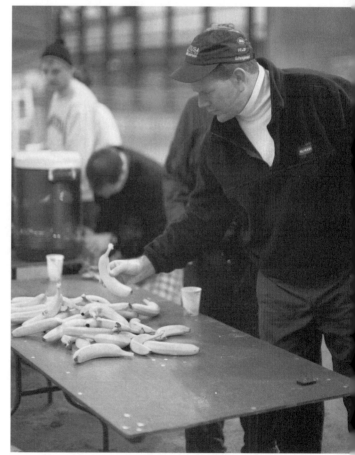

Enjoy a speedier recovery by consuming carbohydrate-rich foods as soon as possible following the marathon.

7. Be aware of the possibility of hyponatremia (low blood-sodium level) when competing in marathon races. To prevent hyponatremia, maintain or increase your intake of salt leading up to the race, particularly if you'll be competing in hot weather or if the conditions will be warmer than you normally train in. Add table salt to foods and/or eat your favorite salty foods. During the marathon, keep up with your fluid losses by rehydrating with a sports drink. Don't be afraid to drink plain water, just don't rely solely on it throughout the entire race. Female marathoners, racers taking three hours or more to complete the marathon, as well as marathoners not acclimated to the heat are at particular risk. If you've had problems with hyponatremia or dealing with the heat in the past, see your physician before taking salt (or electrolyte) tablets while exercising in the heat.

8. Shorten your recovery time by replenishing your glycogen stores as soon as possible following the race. You'll experience less muscle damage and soreness if you take advantage of the first 30 minutes (the carbohydrate "window") after crossing the finish line. Be prepared: anticipate that you won't feel hungry following a marathon race. Begin by drinking carbohydrate-rich beverages, such as sports drinks, fruit juice, milk shakes or smoothies, lemonade, soda, or high-carbohydrate or meal-replacement beverages. Ease in carbohydrate-rich foods as soon as you can. Include a quality source of protein at your next meal (ideally within an hour or two) to further enhance the glycogen rebuilding process.

9. Drinking alcohol following a marathon may impede your recovery by hampering your efforts to rehydrate (as a diuretic, alcohol causes your body to lose fluid) and by interfering with your body's ability to replenish its glycogen stores. Your best bet: make rehydrating with nonalcoholic beverages your first priority. Beyond that, realize that following a strenuous effort such as running a marathon, your body may not be able to tolerate or process alcohol as well as it normally does, so indulge in moderation.

10. Counter losing weight from heavy training demands with a recovery period. Many marathoners lose a substantial amount of body fat while meeting the high energy demands of marathon training. Give your body a full chance to recuperate, including gaining a modest amount of weight (if necessary), before jumping back into your full training regimen. Both Hickman and Brantly's recovery plans include indulging themselves with high-fat foods for up to several weeks following a marathon race. To avoid becoming run down or susceptible to injuries, Hickman, for example, consciously regains the five pounds she routinely loses while training for a marathon. Treating herself to Captain Crunch cereal, Cheetos, and McDonald's Big Macs, Hickman gets a much needed "mental recovery" as well, which allows her to return to her ambitious training schedule and healthy eating habits with renewed motivation.

Triathlon

10

"You can keep getting better as you age as long as you take care of yourself. I do constant body check-ups, focusing on good nutrition and not overtraining. In the long run I know I will perform better by consistently training year after year. Shortcuts like overtraining or starving yourself to get thinner may allow you to race well for six months, but you'll never reach your true potential."

—Karen Smyers,
1995 winner of the International Triathlon Union World Championship and the Hawaii Ironman

Karen Smyers
Event: 1995 Hawaii Ironman Triathlon*
First place, 9:16:46

*2.4-mile swim, 112-mile bike, 26.2-mile run

Prerace Nutrition

Carbohydrate loading: Goal was to be mentally fresh and enter the race in top physical shape. Continued to eat normal diet that emphasized carbohydrates and protein, without being too restrictive regarding fat. Consciously consumed carbohydrates by drinking Shaklee Performance (fluid-replacement drink) on bike rides and Champion Nutrition Metabolol II (recovery drink) following workouts.

> *KS:* "I don't aim to eat a perfect diet. I try to eat semibalanced meals with some protein, mostly carbohydrates, and I certainly don't restrict my fat intake. I don't want to lose any weight the last few days before the race, so I make sure I'm not missing meals. You can easily get depleted in the heat, so I only go to Hawaii about one week in advance, and I especially make sure I get carbohydrates in right after my workouts that week."

Hydration: Relied on water and sports drinks.

> *KS:* "Being in Hawaii, I'm conscious of my fluid needs and I drink plenty of water in the days leading up to the race. I had a beer two nights before but not the night before. I have too much respect for how important hydration is and every little bit helps."

Prerace Meals (Race Start: 7 A.M.)

Night before: Prepared and ate dinner at the condo, approximately 8 P.M.—pasta with red sauce (included chicken or meat in sauce), white bread, and cooked vegetables.

> *KS:* "I make my own dinner so I have control over when and what I eat. I like a simple, light, carbohydrate-based meal—some type of pasta with red sauce and vegetables, but I stay away from salad. Salad takes longer to digest. I want whatever I eat to be in and out quickly before a race."

Morning of race: Breakfast at the condo, 4:30 to 5:00 A.M.—oatmeal with banana, one cup of coffee, water.

> *KS:* "I don't really feel like eating—I need my sleep—but oatmeal sits well and will carry me through the swim until I can refuel again on the bike. I drink one cup of coffee the morning of a race because it's a 'mover' and clears out my system. After that I just drink water [about 20 ounces] all the way from breakfast to the race start."

Supplements: Did not use salt tablets or glycerol. Took two Advil tablets during the race toward the end of the bike segment.

> *KS:* "I've never used salt tablets during a triathlon. I get salt through my food beforehand. I listen to what my body tells me [in training]. If I'm craving salt, I eat salty foods such as chips or I salt my meat and potatoes, and I get it through canned foods too. I seem to do OK during the race with just my electrolyte-replacement drink, although some athletes

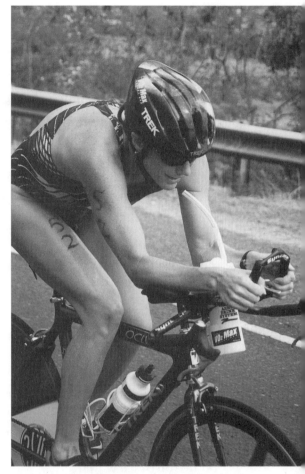

Professional triathlete Karen Smyers knows that success in the Ironman depends on making the right nutritional choices on race day.

definitely do use salt tablets to try to prevent cramping. It's tricky trying to figure out what your body needs."

During the Event

Swim and first transition: Drank water up to the start of race. Prepared bike beforehand by loading a handlebar carrier with Gatorade Relode energy gel packets. Also taped a few to the top of the bike's top tube (total of 10 energy packets.) Mounted three standard water bottles on bike; one full of water, two full of Shaklee Performance fluid-replacement drink (one at double strength). Used a seat-mounted water bottle carrier, as well as one bottle mounted on the down tube.

Bike: Planned for approximately five hours on the bike. Goal was to ingest 350 to 400 calories per hour. Consumed approximately one energy gel packet (80 calories) every 45 minutes and one bottle of sports drink (200 calories) every hour, plus water from aid stations as often as needed to ingest energy gels or dilute the double-strength sports drink. Feed bag at turnaround contained two more bottles of Shaklee Performance drink. Due to missing her pick-up at the turnaround, switched to drinking Gatorade the second half of the ride.

> *KS:* "Solid food works OK in training, but I learned I just couldn't eat in the heat. I had no saliva, plus it's hard to chew and breathe hard at the same time. My goal was to drink one bottle an hour and eat two gels for a total of 350 to 400 calories. I actually got down one energy packet about every 45 to 50 minutes, for a total of six while on the course. I have to let my stomach calm down a little, so I start drinking about 10 minutes out on the bike and take the first energy gel within 20 minutes of starting the bike.
>
> In two years of trying, I've never gotten my bag at the turnaround. I wasn't willing to stop because it's your first chance to see your competitors and you try to put an extra bit of distance on them. I knew I could switch to another drink [Gatorade available at aid stations along course]. I trained with Gatorade so I knew I would be OK."

Second transition: Drank water and fluid replacement drink leaving transition area.

Run: Planned for three hours of running. At every aid station (every mile) grabbed at least one cup of Coke and one cup of water, as well as a water bottle full of ice water.

> *KS:* "In the run I go from aid station to aid station. I drink the Coke and the water and pour the ice over my head or into my hat. That lasts for about a half mile and then you just hang on until the next oasis [aid station] appears. I probably end up drinking close to 13 cups of Coke during the race—a half cup per aid station! You want to keep it coming; otherwise, you'll get a sugar low.
>
> "In my first Ironman (second place, 1994 Hawaii Ironman) I figured it was easier to drink on the bike than on the run, so I tried to fuel up as much as possible on the bike. I only drank water the first eight miles of the run, but then I fell apart the next two to three miles. I went from running my regular 7:30 to 8:00 miles to 10:30 to 11:00 miles. I knew I was bonking and needed carbohydrate, and Coke gave me an instant energy shot. That's when I learned the importance of keeping the carbos coming the whole race."

Postrace Recovery

Immediately: Drank plenty of cold water. Eventually able to eat solid foods.

Following week: Daily multivitamin, consumed Champion Nutrition Metabolol II recovery drink after any training efforts.

> *KS:* "It's hard to eat right after. I finally had some pizza. I may have been able to squeeze one beer down later, but celebrating mostly comes the next day. I'm hungry for several days after! The next day I just play around on the beach. Swimming and easy bike rides are added back first. I don't run for about a week, then go for an easy run. I always take a multivitamin, and after any training I drink a protein drink (Metabolol II) for insurance purposes. I know I've broken down a lot of muscle tissue, so I eat more meat and chicken, too."

Tips for All Triathletes

An Ironman is a swimming, biking, running, eating, and drinking contest. No matter how much training you've put in or how accomplished you are in the first three, the last two can just as likely determine your success on race day. Smyers contends that her 1995 victory was half due to accomplishing the right training and half due to making the right nutritional decisions on race day. In the same vein, even though her training indicated she was in better physical condition in 1996 as she prepared to defend her title, Smyers was fortunate to rally and finish third after making one error in her drinking regimen during the bike segment.

Obviously, you can't complete an Ironman triathlon without doing the proper training. You can't just show up and drink and eat your way to the finish. Nutrition, however, is often the area that triathletes can improve the most. Balance your nutritional awareness and knowledge against your training. Ignorance, laziness, or becoming too focused on your training will doom you on race day. Eating and drinking during the race provides the fuel you need to get the job done. It's simple—you're not going to finish if you don't give the nutritional aspect of the triathlon the respect it deserves.

1. Start the race well hydrated and well fueled and keep on top of your needs during the race. Start pushing fluids at least 24 hours before you toe the line. Keep a water bottle close at hand all day. Ironman competitors expend 8,000 to 10,000 calories or more during the race so it makes sense to top off your glycogen stores by eating breakfast the morning of the race. Experiment with carbohydrate loading and prerace meals to find a routine that works for you.

2. During the race, aim to replace at least 30 to 50 percent of the calories you expend, which translates into approximately 2,500 to 5,000 calories or more for most triathletes (less for triathlons shorter than four or five hours). To maintain hydration and a stable blood-sugar level, most triathletes need roughly 250 to 400 calories per hour. Most of these calories (70 to 75 percent) should come from carbohydrates—sports drinks, energy gels and bars, and other solid foods that are well tolerated. Consuming a small amount of protein and fat will also help you over the long haul.

3. Practice your race strategies at every opportunity in training and shorter races. American Tim DeBoom, winner of the 1999 Ironman New Zealand, his first Ironman win in seven attempts, offers the following additional race-day tips.

- **Swim:** Because urinating isn't a problem on this segment, hydrate right up to the start of the race. In ocean swims, you'll inevitably swallow some salt water, so be prepared for a burning sensation in your throat. Swallow enough salt water and your tongue will swell, and you may begin the bike ride feeling sick to your stomach. Some triathletes even suffer from seasickness during choppy open-water swims. The best plan of attack is to wear earplugs to combat nausea and know how to breathe bilaterally to minimize the effects of a choppy sea.

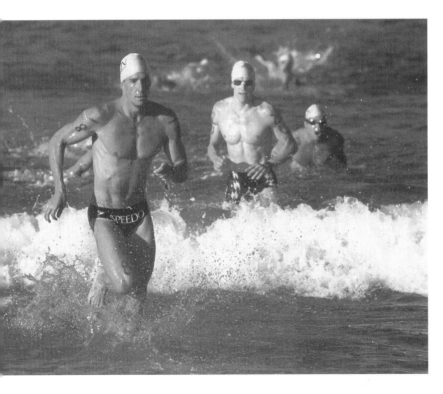

Take time between race legs to rehydrate and refuel.

- **Bike:** Become one with your bike. Triathletes spend the most time in a race cycling, so you need to become proficient at eating and drinking on your bike. During training rides, be sure to practice your drinking and eating techniques at your intended race pace. During a race, control or slow your pace slightly when it's time to rehydrate and refuel. Keeping a sleek aerodynamic bike on the road can be challenging as you juggle food and water bottles, especially in windy conditions.

- **Run:** Gastrointestinal distress, such as nausea and bloating, can be common during the running segment. The jostling nature of running and the progressive dehydration associated with several hours of continuous exercise slow the absorption of fluid and nutrients from the stomach. Get used to the feeling of fluid sloshing around in your stomach during training efforts and shorter races. Recognize that an inability to urinate during the running segment is a red flag indicating that you've become too dehydrated. Slow or stop when you approach aid stations to ensure that you consume some fluid and aren't just pouring it on yourself or the ground.

  If vomiting ensues during the run, think of it as wiping the slate clean. Slow or stop, regroup, and start over with your rehydrating and refueling efforts. It's definitely a setback, but you can rebound once you actually start absorbing the fluid and calories you need. Remind yourself that the only way to finish is by replacing, mile by mile, the fluid, calories, and carbohydrates you need. Sometimes chewing solid food, such as an energy bar or a banana, can help settle a queasy stomach and provide a much-needed mental lift. Some athletes find that chewing on a Tums tablet helps also.

- **Transitions:** Relax and take your time, as you transition both onto the bike and into the run. Set up your transition area in a logical, organized manner so you can't possibly exit the transition area without your essentials. For example, if you're wearing a bike jersey or fanny pack to carry food while on the bike, put it on top of your unbuckled helmet or across your bike seat. Obviously, you should pack fanny packs and bike jerseys beforehand, and tape any food items you desire to the bike. (In shorter races, you can tuck a packet or two of energy gel into a swimsuit or the waistband of bike or running shorts.)

  Always keep an extra water bottle handy in the transition area to drink from as you head out on the run. DeBoom, for instance, takes advantage of his slower pace as he transitions into running by using it as an opportunity to refuel. You may feel better by getting fuel in at the start of the run (for example, by drinking a sports drink) than by cramming food down during the latter stages of the bike portion.

Finally, to simulate race conditions, practice your transitions by racing against a friend during training.

4. Experiment with and choose a carrying system that works best for you, such as wearing a fanny pack, a bike jersey with pockets, or taping food items to bike stems. Several hydration strategies exist, such as traditional mounted water bottles (on the down tube and seat tube), aerobar-mounted drinking systems, seat-mounted bottle carriers, and bladder hydration systems. If you go with a bladder, choose an aerodynamic model made specifically for cyclists. Insulated water bottles that help keep liquids cold may also help you consume more fluid while on the bike.

5. Most people tolerate drinking and eating better on the bike than while running. You can get in trouble, however, by drinking or eating too much, too soon during the bike leg. Blood redirected to the stomach for digestion can interfere with reestablishing blood flow to hardworking leg muscles. Concentrate initially on sipping drinks and hold off on eating anything for the first 20 to 30 minutes. Solid foods can be well tolerated if you can get them down. For example, if you carry energy bars with you, remove wrappers and cut them in half or into bite-size pieces. Don't plan to eat anything that doesn't hold up well in the heat, such as chocolate. If the race features individual feed bags at the turnaround and it contains something essential to your race plan, be prepared to stop for it. DeBoom packs his turnaround bag full of many different foods, hoping that at least one item will seem appealing at that point in the race. Try including a treat that you can't get at aid stations on the course.

6. Drinking the majority of your calories is a safer bet. Figure out in training, ideally under conditions similar to those expected in the race, the minimum amount of fluid you'll need to drink per hour to stay reasonably hydrated. Twenty ounces, or one standard water bottle, is the minimum that most triathletes will need. Along with your sports drink, figure out what you need to eat to consume at least 60 grams of carbohydrate every hour. Remember, try to take energy gels with six to eight ounces of water, not a sports drink. Monitor your hydration efforts by keeping tabs on your ability to urinate at least once or twice during the bike and running portions of the race.

7. If you choose to drink soda (for example, Coca-Cola), consume water with it. You'll dilute the carbohydrate concentration of the soda into a more optimal range that favors absorption. Keep in mind that soft drinks also contain minimal amounts of sodium compared with a typical sports drink, which may increase the risk of hyponatremia in susceptible individuals. Although Smyers typically drinks Coke from the outset in Ironman-length triathlons, DeBoom prefers to hold off as long as he can. Reaching for Coke can provide an almost immediate psychological boost, but realize that in most cases it's only a temporary lift. Be prepared to continue with Coke once you've started drinking it.

8. To improve your odds of being successful in the future, record your thoughts and observations about your nutritional strategies as soon as possible following races. Smyers could recount the details of her 1995 race four years later simply by looking it up in the training logbook she always keeps.

9. Be sensitive to blood-sugar lows. Dips in your blood-sugar level can leave you feeling overwhelmed and questioning your ability to continue. Before you make any drastic decisions, consume readily absorbable carbohydrates, such as sports drinks, energy gels, soda, candy, or fruit, and give the necessary carbohydrates a chance to be absorbed.

When you hit a tough patch, rely on strategies that have worked in the past but be willing to try new things too. Successfully finishing an Ironman hinges on your ability to solve problems and keep yourself in the race. Trust your training and give it a chance to come through. When you least feel like eating or drinking is when you most likely need to do so.

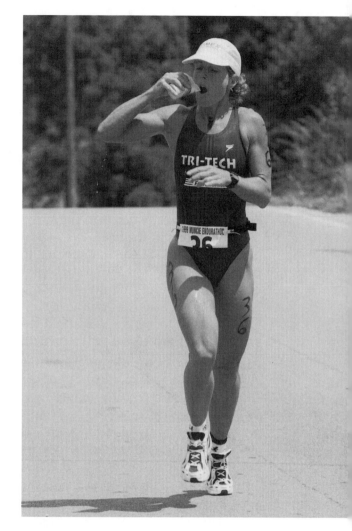

Drink a sports drink at regular intervals during the race.

10. Be aware of the increased risk of hyponatremia (low blood-sodium level) associated with ultraraces conducted in the heat, such as most Ironman triathlons. Female triathletes, triathletes coming from cooler environments who didn't have time to acclimatize properly, and slower triathletes are at increased risk.

The best way to prevent this imbalance is not to restrict your fluid intake during the race, but to increase your salt intake. Acclimatize as much as possible by training in similar hot weather conditions as those you expect to compete in (you'll train your body to lose less sodium via your sweat) and increase your salt intake for several days leading up to a long race by eating salty foods and drinking fluid replacement drinks. During the race, drink a properly formulated sports drink and consume solid foods, as tolerated. Don't drink only water and cola as these beverages supply fluid but very little sodium, thereby increasing your risk of hyponatremia.

If you've had muscle cramps or other problems dealing with the heat in the past, experiment in training with the use of salt or electrolyte tablets. No clear-cut guidelines exist, so you simply have to experiment before race day and determine what your needs are. Don't overdo it. Salt tablets can irritate the lining of the stomach and induce vomiting so take them with at least six to eight ounces of water. If you have a health problem, check with your doctor about the use of salt tablets and your ability to exercise in the heat.

11. Glycerol may be of benefit during an Ironman because it can help the body store more water than normal. Experiment with it first during long training efforts in the heat. The incidence of gastrointestinal complaints is high among triathletes competing in Ironman triathlons. The potential bloating, nausea, and abdominal distress associated with glycerol use may only further complicate the situation. If you choose to hyperhydrate with glycerol before a race, it doesn't mean you can take shortcuts during the race. You still need to replace your fluid losses as much as you can by ingesting water and a fluid-replacement drink throughout the race.

12. The use of nonsteroidal anti-inflammatory drugs (NSAIDs such as Advil, Nuprin, Aleve, Actron, and so on) is not recommended before or during exercise, especially for ultraendurance events like Ironman triathlons. NSAIDs may cause stomach irritation and bleeding, contribute to the development of hyponatremia, and, combined with dehydration, increase the risk of kidney problems. Pay particular attention to your fluid intake before and during the race if you choose to take NSAIDs.

13. Enhance your recovery by making smart nutritional choices following the race. Granted, you'll be sore and tired following an Ironman no matter what you eat or drink after the race. But you can lessen somewhat your discomfort and the extent of muscle damage. Rehydrate with something other than plain water or alcohol. Sports drinks are still the beverage of choice because they contain sodium that will help you retain the fluid you drink. Eating salty foods, if tolerated, will also help.

Ease solid foods in as tolerated. Aim to include adequate amounts of protein, in combination with carbohydrate-rich foods, at every meal to help with glycogen resynthesis, as well as to help repair damaged skeletal muscle. Of course, don't ignore your cravings—you've earned the right to celebrate. DeBoom, for instance, often finds that fried onion rings really help him get back on track!

Cycling

11

"Eat right or eat muscle."

—Kieran "Kerry" Ryan,
member of the winning team
in the 1998 Race Across America,
Team Division

Kieran "Kerry" Ryan
Event: 1998 Race Across America, Team Division*
First place, Team Division: 5 days, 11 hours, 2 minutes

*Represented Team Action Sports (including Pat Tafoya, Mike Wracher, and Tim La Frombaise). Race Across America is a nonstop transcontinental bicycle race. Racers compete as solo riders, tandems, or relay teams.

Prerace Nutrition

Days before the race: Because the 1998 course was considered to be flatter than usual, prerace body weight was not as much of an issue. Riders, therefore, did not restrict their fat or calorie intake going into the race. Spizerinctum (Spiz), a liquid food-replacement product (500 calories and 97 grams of carbohydrate per serving) used during the race, was routinely consumed before rides and afterward to speed recovery.

KR: "Without a doubt, most of the guys ate a controlled diet while training. We would definitely put the right type of fuels in the body, but I was not afraid to have a dessert. It's a mental reward if nothing else. Your body is so well trained, and we weren't worried about our body weight because we wouldn't be in the mountains for a couple of days. We were probably putting in more protein and more fat than a normal diet—not quite as heavy as the 40-30-30 but more like 60 percent carbohydrate, 25 percent protein, and 15 percent fat.

Our percentage of body fat needs to average no less than 7 percent before we get into this race. When you don't put enough calories in and you go through a form of voluntary starvation like we do during the race, the end effect is myoglobinuria—it's where you digest muscle. I was at 151 [pounds]; in years previous with hillier courses I would start the race at 147.

You always keep Spiz in your system so you're used to it and your stomach tolerates it. You're not just going to put something new into your diet. We've trained on it—we've used it before rides and for recovery after rides, as well as a meal when we get busy."

Prerace Meals (Race Start: 9 A.M.)

Day and night before: Primarily liquid food (Spiz) the day before, dinner meal at 8:30 P.M., eaten as a team. Goal was to enter the race with a "clean" digestive tract.

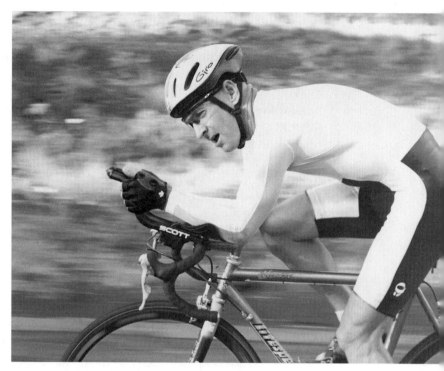

Bicycle shop owner Kerry Ryan enjoys coaching other cyclists to eat, drink, and ride around the clock.

KR: "We do a lot of liquid foods the day before the event, so our digestive tracts are really clean. This translates into fewer bowel movements and less discomfort in that direction.

　　We are not superstitious in what we put in our stomach, and basically we know this is really the last time we're going to get real food for about five days. It's like the Last Supper, with all our crew members, the Disciples, hanging out. We're all laughing because this is going to be the last time we're not at odds with somebody. We practice good hydration, of course, and maybe some liquid food before bed."

Morning of race: Approximately 6 to 7 A.M. consumed serving of Spiz (full strength). Teammates had pancakes also.

KR: "We start drinking as soon as we get up, since dehydration is such a factor in the race. Mostly Spiz, although some of the guys did meet for pancakes this time. Usually, I like to keep my tract really clean."

Supplements: No extra regular vitamins taken; relied on a fortified liquid-food product (Spizerinctum). Did not use electrolyte tablets or glycerol during the race.

KR: "Liquid food, in my opinion, gives you a balance in your system that you can't get eat at the table—all the major nutrients plus vitamins and minerals. This is the year I basically went with no vitamins and no supplements. I just worked on establishing a really good base and always having the correct nutrition and correct hydration level before every ride. They do Olympic drug testing on us at the end. I don't want to subject anything to controversy. My philosophy is I don't want anything and don't give anything to me.

We've never taken electrolyte or salt tablets, even before we started using IVs. One year we mixed sodium straight into our electrolyte drink. Up to a half tablespoon into a 20-ounce bottle—it tasted salty, based on the rider's tolerance."

During the Event

Hydration/Fuel: The race covered 2,900 miles from California to the East Coast, 24 hours a day of continuous riding, each rider cycling for 20 to 25 minutes at a time followed by approximately one hour of rest. Relied primarily on Spiz, sports drinks, and energy gels. Supplemented with favorite foods. Received proactive saline IVs approximately every second hour throughout the race.

KR: "This is all anaerobic-level time trialing. Every time you get on the bike you ride to your max potential at that time of day and depending on how well your body has recovered. You need to constantly reevaluate nutritional needs—the right amount of fuel to the body, plus the type of fuel your stomach can tolerate. You become intensely sensitive as you spend more and more time in the saddle. After you ride a few rides really, really hard, you have no desire to eat. You don't even feel like chewing. We use liquid foods and try to drink our calories. Most of the guys started at 153 or 154 [pounds], and we need on average 11,000 calories per rider per day.

In 1996, here's what we would typically do. You ride for 20 to 25 minutes. You get off the bike and within two or three minutes try to down an entire bottle of Spiz so it gets ingested. I could tolerate on average two and a half scoops (in 22 ounces). From there, I would chase it by sipping on water. If I'm feeling a little bit flat, I'll go ahead and do an energy drink with a sugar base—Cytomax, PowerAde, Gatorade, etc. Right before your next ride, you would slam one or two energy gels—GU or Power Gel—around the clock for five days.

On occasion, somebody would stop for a cheeseburger or a Subway sandwich. It had to be at the right time at the right gap. You or your partner couldn't be on the bike because you have to be following him in the van. In 1996, I remember going to a minimart. In training, I would typically have a tuna sandwich at lunchtime, so I got a tuna sandwich for the first time in two days and I had the best race of my life. That taught me something for future races.

We knew in 1996 that we always felt flat in the head. You always felt a weird sense that you just didn't recover and your head just couldn't motivate yourself to get on the bike. What I realized from the tuna sandwich, and pizza I had somewhere else, was that I needed more of what I trained on—either for the mental stimulation or for what it did for me. Fun carbohydrates, fun fat. I couldn't wait to ride.

In 1998, we took peanut butter and jelly, deli turkey, tuna sandwiches. I told everybody we were going to try to get almost half our calories from regular foods, to get away from that flat feeling and the mental boredom. One night, somebody gave us 20 hotdogs at midnight as they were about to close. We weren't afraid to eat anything. You've got to throw superstition out the window in those types of races. You need the calories.

We also did proactive IVs. We took an ambulance, an EMT vehicle, and six medical people—three EMTs, two paramedics, and a doctor—with us. We had never done it in the past. Other teams had done it before, usually using the IVs as a last-ditch chance to save someone. The average temperature the first three days (passing through Texas) was 110. In 1998 we did Spiz, GU packets, and more real food. But if you're eating food, you're not drinking the calories. So for hydration, every second hour we were taking 1,000 milliliters, or one liter, of a saline IV, plus a potassium injection sometimes, too. We never had a single cramp in any of our riders. We never got behind in our calories because we felt good enough to eat regular food. At night we would only take the IV bag once because we were able to drink better and our core body temperature was lower.

Everyone on the team was very intelligent with their training and their thinking. The focus is so intense you tell yourself you can't fail your team. It's one thing if you're on your own—you're just screwing yourself if you don't eat. But if you have a team, you just force it down. Voluntary starvation definitely happens during this race to all of us, by hour 40. You do not want to eat. You've already made incredible rides and you're competing against other teams in the beginning, so you just keep going faster and faster.

It's really more about hydration than the calories, in my opinion. With the IVs, we had regular bowel movements, regular diets, frequent urination. We were able to eat solid foods, able to tolerate anything. We were a lot more friendly, and we weren't dead headed, no blood-sugar problems."

Postrace Recovery

KR: "You have 24 people who have slaved for you and they want to celebrate. You don't want to let them down so you party for two days. The real recovery comes in just sleeping. I've always driven back [in two days]. Now I'm eating everything in sight—a whole-on binge.

Two to three candy bars at every rest stop. I have a voracious appetite for weeks. I lost seven pounds this year. I'm eating everything in sight—every sweet, every dessert.

The day afterward, we get a massage and go for a small spinout of some sort. After the drive back, we'll get on the bike the next day and spin our legs out. Spiz is out of the question now. You have no tolerance for GU, Spiz, or anything else that reminds you of RAAM."

Tips for All Road Cyclists

1. Keep your thinking cap on. As a cyclist, you walk a finer line than most endurance athletes do when it comes to staying on top of your nutritional needs during exercise. Your fluid and energy needs are some of the highest due to the distance and duration of endurance cycling events. Despite knowing that, cyclists often find themselves caught off guard when trouble sets in. Bonking, the depletion of muscle glycogen stores that causes you to slow your pace dramatically, is a prime example.

Keep in mind that rapid evaporation of sweat can give you the false sense that you're losing only minimal amounts of fluid. The windchill factor that occurs during cycling may prevent you from feeling warm or overheated, which can delay or mask the feeling that you need to drink. On top of that, your body weight is supported while cycling, so you don't receive any feedback from ankles or legs being traumatized by pounding. Drafting and coasting allow you to "cheat" while you continue to perform. In other words, it's easy to ignore or underestimate your nutritional needs because you don't feel that poorly until it's too late. Anticipate your needs and adhere to a plan.

2. Fuel up before you go. Stockpiling calories and topping off your glycogen stores by eating carbohydrate-rich foods is essential before heading out for a long ride or race. Experiment with carbo loading and preevent meals, including high-carbohydrate or liquid-meal products, to find a routine that works well for you.

Eating breakfast will help ensure that you don't dig yourself into a hole early, especially in competitive events lasting less than one and one-half to two hours. In events of that duration, you may choose not to eat while on the bike because your preride glycogen stores should be enough to meet your energy needs. Starting off with a stable blood sugar extends your muscle glycogen stores, eliminates hunger pains, and keeps your head in the game. Eat early enough (two to four hours before getting on the bike works for most athletes) so you don't feel bloated or as if your diaphragm is being crushed.

3. Hydrate before, during, and after the ride or race. First, start paying attention to your fluid intake the day before, not the morning of, your ride. You know you're starting out well hydrated if you're urinating frequently and it's pale in color. Second, train yourself to start drinking on the bike

immediately, before you feel thirsty. Set your watch or look at your computer as a reminder if necessary. Aim for approximately four to five ounces every 15 to 20 minutes, or a minimum of one regular water bottle (16 ounces) per hour, under normal conditions. (Remember that weighing yourself before and after training rides can help you determine your personal fluid needs while cycling. A drop of a pound or two is generally acceptable. Larger weight losses indicate that you need to reassess your hydration habits.

Riding in extreme conditions, such as heat and wind or high humidity, further increases your fluid needs. Your stomach should cooperate and be able to tolerate up to a quart (32 ounces) an hour, so aim for two small or one and a half large bottles per hour in extreme conditions. If drinking colder liquids doesn't make you nauseous (because of delayed emptying from the stomach), it can help cool you down and provide a needed boost on a ride in extreme conditions. Add ice to bottles or freeze half a bottle of water or sports drink the night before and top it off immediately before you get on the bike. On extended or self-supported rides,

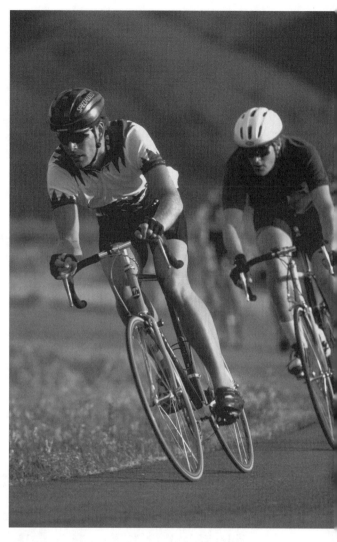

Sweat evaporation and windchill during a ride can mask feelings of dehydration so drink before you're thirsty.

wearing a bladder system allows you to carry large volumes of fluid without worrying about the need to stop and possibly lose your group. Be sure to choose a model designed specifically for cyclists.

When it comes to consuming sports drinks, don't assume you need to drink less just because they contain electrolytes and carbohydrates. If you find that the sweet taste deters you from drinking enough on extended rides, carry an extra bottle of plain water and drink alternately from it. Competitive cyclists who plan to drink cola drinks or apple juice during races should experiment first during vigorous workouts to determine how well their stomachs will tolerate these drinks.

4. Keep up with your energy needs while on the bike. Replenish the carbohydrates you burn as you burn them. By topping off liver and muscle glycogen stores and eating breakfast, most riders can perform well for the first one and a half to two hours of cycling (for example, the first 30 miles of a century ride), relying only on an electrolyte-replacement drink. If you expect to cycle longer than two hours, plan to refuel while on the bike. Begin to eat as soon as the event or race starts to extend your glycogen stores. Don't wait until you bonk or your blood sugar bottoms out to try to remedy the situation.

Your calorie needs will vary tremendously depending on a multitude of variables, such as road surface, terrain, weather, wind resistance, speed or intensity, and your fitness level. Figure on 30 calories per mile as a rule. Keep in mind that your estimated calorie needs increase dramatically as your speed increases (see table 11.1).

Your speed is your "air speed," so add a headwind to the ground speed indicated by your computer and subtract a tailwind.

Kerry Ryan and Cindy Staiger, a two-time solo finisher of RAAM, offer the following pointers for road cyclists:

- The less fit you are, the fewer shortcuts you can take. Knowing what you can survive on and still perform well comes with experience. Being less fit or having a less efficient riding style (that is, being a novice rider) means you can't take any shortcuts. Set your watch or computer and train yourself to drink (every 15 to 20 minutes) and snack (every 30 minutes) on a regular schedule to replace the estimated calories you burn per hour. Practice this in training so it becomes automatic on race day. Eating on the bike becomes even

Table 11.1   Calorie Burn Rate*

	Miles Per Hour						
Rider Weight	**12**	**14**	**15**	**16**	**17**	**18**	**19**
110	293	348	404	448	509	586	662
120	315	375	437	484	550	634	718
130	338	402	469	521	592	683	773
140	360	430	502	557	633	731	828
150	383	457	534	593	675	779	883
160	405	485	567	629	717	828	938
170	427	512	599	666	758	876	993
180	450	540	632	702	800	925	1048
190	472	567	664	738	841	973	1104
200	495	595	697	774	883	1021	1159

* Assuming an upright position on flat terrain with no wind.

more of a necessity if you are a slower rider because of the longer time
you spend on the bike.

- The best way to avoid bonking is to create a calorie buffer. Ryan
  and Staiger both favor liquid calories in the form of electrolyte-
  replacement drinks and high-energy liquid products because they
  tend to be well tolerated and require less effort to get down than
  solid foods. Experiment with flavors and brands until you find
  palatable varieties.

- You might want to try Ryan's "no-failure nutrition system" for a
  cyclist (150 to 160 pounds) attempting a hilly century ride (approximately five hours). Start off with a Camelbak full of water, one bottle
  of electrolyte-replacement drink, and one bottle of a high-calorie
  drink, like Spiz (500 calories in 16 to 20 ounces). Carry Baggies
  containing premeasured powder and refill your bottles at every rest
  stop or along the way as needed. Consume 500 calories or one bottle
  of your high-energy drink per hour religiously right from the start!

- Consider how your body processes foods. Rely on simple carbohydrates during high-intensity (closer to your VO_2max) rides when
  your gastrointestinal tract is less efficient, or when you need a rapid
  energy boost. Choose electrolyte-replacement drinks, energy gels
  (take with water), glucose tablets, and if tolerated, soda or juice. On
  longer rides of moderate intensity, add solid foods and high-calorie
  liquid drinks to boost your calorie intake and your spirits. Snack
  frequently rather than eating a large quantity at any one time, which
  diverts blood away from your muscles.

- Use your common sense when eating on a bike. Concentrate on the
  road, look ahead for hazards, and slow down if necessary. When
  riding one-handed as you reach for food or a water bottle, keep your
  bike from veering by gripping the center of the handlebar next to the
  stem. Always empty your down-tube bottle first, then switch it with
  your full seat-tube bottle.

- Stay with foods you are used to eating as much as possible. Eat after
  cresting a hill, not shortly before a substantial climb or while climbing. Eat when you're at the end of a pace line, not in the middle or
  while pulling.

- Always carry something with you, such as prepackaged powdered
  drink mix and a snack (for example, energy bars or a peanut butter
  sandwich), in case you don't like what's offered at rest stops or need
  to refuel before or after a scheduled rest stop. What you take with you
  will determine how you carry it—jersey pocket, fanny pack, or taped
  to your bike.

- Recreational riders may choose to stop and eat at organized rest stops
  provided during century rides and daylong or multiday events.

Foods typically provided include fruit, such as apples, oranges, and bananas, energy bars, energy gels, granola bars, bagels, peanut butter sandwiches, cookies, mini candy bars, and sometimes even sandwich fixings. Stopping to enjoy a real lunch break can provide a psychological boost; just don't gorge yourself. Save your big meal for the end of the ride.

5.   Speed up your recovery time by refueling after long rides or races. You may be off your bike, but you still have work to do, especially if you're participating in a multiday ride or bike tour. Consciously plan to replace fluids and carbohydrates as quickly as possible. Anticipate having a suppressed appetite following long hours of cycling by keeping a high-carbohydrate sports drink or a liquid-meal product handy. Drink it within the first 10 to 15 minutes and follow up with a high-carbohydrate meal within one to two hours.

6.   Beware of hyponatremia (low blood-sodium concentration), particularly in events or races lasting beyond four to five hours. Often caused by consuming large volumes of sodium-free fluid, such as water (which dilutes the blood-sodium concentration), hyponatremia can cause fatigue, nausea, confusion, and even seizures. Be realistic about your fluid losses (urine and sweat) and your fluid intake while on the bike. Ingesting 16 to 20 ounces of fluid per hour during prolonged exercise is reasonable for most cyclists under normal conditions. (Remember that high-intensity rides and extreme conditions boost your fluid needs.) Substitute an electrolyte-replacement drink for plain water on rides or races lasting longer than 60 minutes and increase your intake of salty foods before riding or racing in hot and humid conditions.

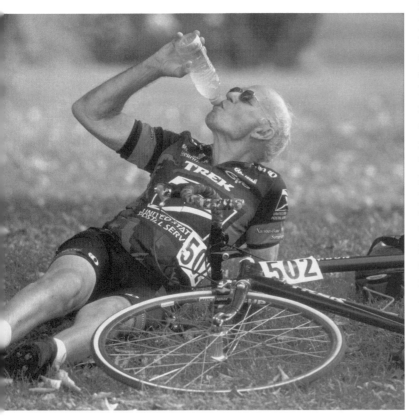

Avoid hyponatremia during prolonged exercise by drinking a fluid replacement drink containing sodium.

Generally, the sodium in sports drinks and the food you ingest before and during your ride or race should provide adequate sodium. Some individuals, however, may need to supplement with electrolyte or salt tablets when riding in extreme conditions. No clear-cut guidelines exist, so experiment on training rides first. Be sure to take electrolyte or salt tablets with six to eight ounces of water and don't overdo it. If you have a health problem, check with your physician about the use of salt and your ability to exercise in the heat.

Riders particularly at risk for developing hyponatremia include slower riders (more opportunity to "overhydrate"), undertrained riders (more sodium loss by sweating), and riders competing in hot and humid conditions.

7. Try glycerol on training rides first. The "hyperhydration" effects of glycerol may minimize the negative impact of dehydration in endurance cycling events. Your performance won't improve, however, if potential side effects, such as bloating and abdominal distress, slow you down. Experiment with dosages and timing in training situations before using it before an important ride or race.

8. Be aware of the risks of using nonsteroidal anti-inflammatory drugs (NSAIDs, for example, Advil, Aleve, Actron) during endurance cycling races or events. Combined with dehydration, taking NSAIDs during prolonged exercise can increase your risk of kidney problems, as well as predispose you to hyponatremia. Pay particular attention to your fluid intake before and during the ride or race if you choose to take NSAIDs.

TIPS FOR CREW-SUPPORTED RACES

Ryan and Staiger, a highly sought after RAAM crew chief who now works as an official for the race, offer their expertise on crew-supported cycling races.

For the rider:

1. Be selective about who makes your crew team. Choose at least one person you respect more than yourself. Otherwise, you won't have anyone to answer to when the going gets tough. In multiday races, in which you increasingly rely on your crew as time passes, be certain that at least one crew person has considerable nutrition knowledge.

2. Be aware of your needs—your typical eating and drinking habits on the bike, what usually works well, what doesn't work—and share this information freely with your crew.

3. Be mentally prepared to drink and eat the calories you need. If you can't successfully meet your estimated calorie needs in shorter events (for example, a century ride), don't fool yourself into thinking you can do it for a daylong relay race or a multiday race. Establish good habits in shorter rides or races before stepping up to more challenging events.

4. Eat before you get hungry. Devise an hourly refueling schedule and stick to it, whether you feel hungry or not. A stable blood sugar allows you to think better and stay awake longer. Consume liquid calories and small snacks on the bike. Solid foods tend to promote sleepiness, so supplement with solid foods only when you're not riding. Avoid eating large quantities of food at any one time unless you have a substantial rest break or are going to sleep.

5. Drink plenty of water. Stay on top of your hydration status by monitoring your urine output. If you have difficulty urinating or it's dark yellow, you're dehydrated. Urine that is too clear (like water) indicates that you're overhydrated. Staiger figures solo riders need to drink at least one full bottle (12 to 16 ounces) of plain water per hour, besides the liquid high-energy beverages they are consuming. A rule of thumb is that a rider should be able to urinate a minimum of once every four to six hours.

6. Don't rely on supplements or drugs to improve your performance. The keys to success are training, pacing, eating, and drinking.

7. Go easy on caffeine. Caffeine provides a mental boost and helps you stay awake, but don't underestimate its dehydrating effects. Limit your intake on long rides, especially during hot weather.

8. To avoid mouth sores, which can make eating unbearable, routinely rinse your mouth with a dilute, tepid solution of one tablespoon of Listerine stirred into eight ounces of water.

9. Settle an upset stomach by consuming saltine crackers or drinking a can of ginger ale, bottled seltzer water, or plain water with a small amount of baking soda stirred in.

For the crew team:

1. Keep a detailed log. A little planning can go a long way, especially if you're in charge of more than one rider. Make extensive notes on each rider as the race unfolds—weather and terrain, speed and mileage, estimates of calories required and consumed hourly or per leg, fluids and sodium needed and consumed, pit stops, presence or absence of gastrointestinal distress, muscle cramps, cravings, low blood sugar, and any other information you find useful. Keeping a log helps you anticipate and ward off problems before they become insurmountable.

2. Monitor your rider's calorie intake closely. Aim for your rider to stay ahead of, or at least match, estimated calorie needs; otherwise, the body begins to break down its muscles to use as fuel. Individual needs vary, but Staiger figures that riders generally need at least 400 to 600 calories per hour. Don't focus on overloading your rider with protein. Consuming enough overall calories (from whatever source) is what counts.

3. Think of endurance cycling as essentially cycling with scheduled breaks. Plan breaks carefully to incorporate as much as possible into each stop, especially when crewing for solo endurance cyclists. Establish from the start that the rider is required to eat whenever possible, including while standing up during a rest break.

4. Baby-sit your rider or riders. A rider's success depends on his or her crew taking care of the smallest details. For example, keep fluids cold to encourage consumption, be certain riders start each leg with clean water bottles, and keep plenty of salty foods and electrolyte-replacement beverages on hand during hot-weather rides. In multiday events, recognize that it may take two to three days of around-the-clock cycling before a rider gives up total decision-making control to his or her crew. When the time comes, be prepared to do everything but push the pedals for your rider.

5. Keep your rider or riders happy about their food. Solid "normal" food helps riders stay properly fueled and mentally satisfied. Expect the unexpected. As the day or days progress, riders will crave weird foods. Be prepared to try to get them a small amount of it or a close substitute. If the food they desire goes against your better judgement, convince them to wait until a slightly better time (for example, before going to sleep).

6. Recognize the symptoms of bonking and intervene immediately. Warning signs include lethargy, decreased pedaling cadence or speed, inconsistent thought patterns, shakiness, glazed eyes, and acting spaced out. Treat a low blood sugar immediately with liquid foods, such as juice, soda, and energy gels (taken with water). In severe cases, it may take 60 minutes or more for a rider to revive sufficiently. Monitor your rider's calorie intake more closely after a bonk.

7. Feed yourself. Your rider's safety and success hinge on your ability to carry out your duties. You may not be able to do anything about getting more sleep, but frequent snacking will help you stay awake and be more alert.

Tips for Off-Road Cyclists

Laurie Brandt Hauptmann, four-time winner of the Leadville Trail 100 Mountain Bike Race and a former Colorado cyclo-cross champion, shares her tips for mountain bikers and cyclo-cross competitors.

1. Set up a drinking schedule and stick to it. Keep it simple. Drink one standard bottle (16 ounces) of your favorite sports drink one hour before you get on the bike, one bottle per hour while riding, and one bottle when you finish. Because it's easy to lose track of time when you're undertaking a

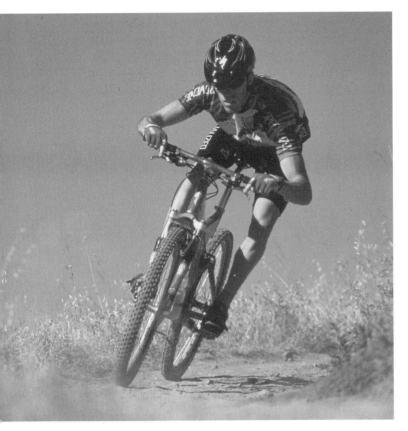

Drink and eat on a regular schedule to minimize spills and "endos" during mountain bike adventures.

serious personal effort, especially when it involves clearing terrain and negotiating descents, set your watch to remind yourself to try to drink every 15 minutes. Take advantage of any opportunity you have to down a few sips. For example, drink during easy ascents, when you tend to sit more upright and can more easily steady the bike with one hand.

Depending on the length of the ride or race, carry extra sports drink powder with you in premeasured amounts. Spend the time to stop and mix up more as needed. Establish good habits in shorter races or events before you venture into longer rides. For example, develop a feel for where your water bottle is on your bike so you don't have to take your eyes off the trail each time you reach for it.

2. Keep your hands free by using a bladder hydration system. From a safety standpoint, a bladder system is superior because your hand will be off the handlebars for only a split second while you grab the drinking tube. Clean your bladder system promptly if you put a drink containing carbohydrate into it. These drinks promote the growth of bacteria and mold, especially in hot weather. To avoid time-consuming cleanups, put only water in the bladder and make the sports drink in your bottles two or three times more concentrated. Then alternate drinking between the two.

3. Fuel up on "real" food. Over the long haul, real food is more fulfilling than energy bars and gels. In shorter mountain bike races (two to three hours), supplement the calories in your electrolyte-replacement drink by eating easy-to-carry finger foods (toss in your jersey pocket) that go down easily, such as raisins, grapes, small baked potatoes (eaten cold), and fig bars. Stick with foods that have worked for you on training rides. In longer races, in which you rely primarily on liquid calories from concentrated drinks, snack on real food for a psychological boost.

4. In 24-hour mountain bike racing, make food an important part of the experience. Get together with your teammates, figure out what everyone wants, and then shop for it together. On the bike, rely on a sports drink and water. Off the bike, refuel with real food. The key to a strong finish is to drink a recovery beverage (for example, a high-carbohydrate or meal-replacement product) immediately upon completing each leg to restock your glycogen stores. Follow up with a small meal within an hour.

5. Drink up during cyclo-cross races. Don't be fooled by the relatively short duration, 45 to 60 minutes, of cyclo-cross races. Intensely anaerobic, these races place huge energy demands on your body. Grab a bottle containing your favorite sports drink each time you pass through the feed zone. If you don't have a coach, recruit a friend or family member to help you. If you're completely solo or no feed zone is offered, wear a small (20-ounce), form-fitting bladder hydration system.

6. Capitalize on the carbohydrate "window" following rides or races. Traveling home from your favorite off-road ride or race often entails a long car ride. Don't wait until you reach home or your appetite returns to begin replenishing your glycogen stores. Get in the habit of packing a recovery drink (powder to mix with water or a canned supplemental beverage) and drink it within 15 to 30 minutes of getting off your bike. Plan to follow up with a well-balanced meal within two hours. You'll benefit by feeling more energetic the rest of the day, and your quadriceps muscles will be less sore in the following days.

Ultrarunning

12

"The hardest part about an ultrarun isn't the running. It's getting my stomach to cooperate."

—Ann Trason,
*winner of the 1998 Western
States 100-Mile Endurance Run*

Ann Trason

Events: 1998 Western States 100-Mile Endurance Run, first place, 18:46

1998 Vermont Trail 100, first place, 17:11, course record

1998 Leadville Trail 100, first place, 20:58

1998 Wasatch Front 100, first place, 22:27, course record

1998 Arkansas Trail 100, first place, 18:02

Prerace Nutrition

Carbohydrate loading: No depletion phase, supplemented normal high-carbohydrate, moderate-protein, low-fat diet with extra carbohydrate-rich foods (rice, baked potatoes, and pasta) for three days leading up to the race. Also included protein-rich food (usually chicken) at lunch each day in anticipation of muscle breakdown during the race. Main goal was to prevent gastrointestinal problems. Consumed one eight-ounce serving (two the day before the race) of Cytomax Metabolol Endurance drink (sports drink providing carbohydrates and protein).

> *AT:* "At this point I'm most worried about eating something that will get me sick, so I stick to bland, boring foods. I don't eat anything that could potentially upset my system, such as Mexican food. I use the Metabolol Endurance drink because it goes down so easy. I just try to eat normally, and I would never do a depletion phase. The last time I ran Comrades [54-mile race in South Africa], I stayed with a gentleman who turned into a major lunatic when not eating carbohydrates. On top of that, he couldn't run three miles four days before the race! He actually went on to race very well, but there's some things I just won't do."

Hydration: Water, sports drink.

> *AT:* "I know what I need to do—drink, drink, drink, and I rely mostly on plain water."

Prerace Meals
(Races Started Early, 4:00 to 5:00 A.M.)

Night before: Two large baked potatoes with butter and salt.

Breakfast (one to one and one-half hours before race): Energy bar (280 calories), one eight-ounce serving of Cytomax Metabolol Endurance (200 calories), and a cup of coffee.

> *AT:* "I like to eat my largest meal at lunchtime (chicken and rice), plus I eat and drink a lot throughout the day, including the Cytomax energy drink. I don't have any magical prerace meal the night before. It's always changing, as is my breakfast too. I used to drink Ensure until it began to make me sick during the first part of the race. I could never imagine starting an ultra without a good cup of coffee; the race starts too early."

Supplements: Two Imodium anti-diarrheal tablets the night before, two more the morning of the race. One electrolyte tablet (340 milligrams sodium, 20 milligrams potassium) the day before and one the morning of the race, taken at mealtimes with water.

> *AT:* "Another ultrarunner suggested the Imodium to me, and it's really helped since I've had a lot of problems with diarrhea in the past. The salt tablets are a very individual thing. My husband, Carl, also an ultrarunner, has to take a lot more than I do."

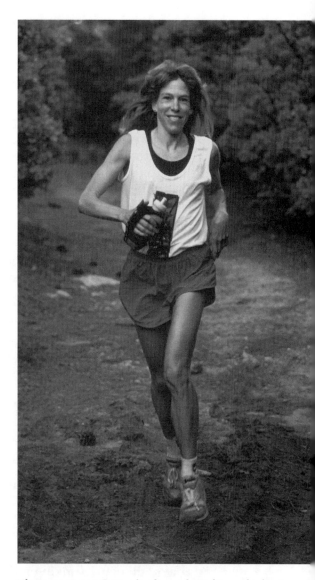

Ultrarunner Ann Trason is often referred to as the best ultrarunner in the world—male or female.

During the Event

Hydration and fuel: Cytomax Exercise and Recovery Drink (electrolytes and carbohydrate) mixed half and half with Metabolol Endurance for the first 25 miles, then just Cytomax Exercise and Recovery Drink, energy gels, and pretzels, boiled potatoes, hard candy, and M&Ms as backup foods, although rarely eaten. Began with Cytomax mixture. Bottles prepared beforehand, packed in ice, typically 10 ice chests set out at predetermined drops or aid stations as race permitted. Carried two insulated water bottles (20 ounces) one filled with water, one filled with sports drinks as well as GU packets (number depended on distance between aid stations). GU packets: one every 30 minutes.

> *AT:* "I drink the Cytomax mixture as long as possible, but by the end it's whatever I can take, which is usually water. I would drink defizzed Coke mixed with water before I'd drink another sports drink. I like to carry my bottles (by hand carries) because I remember to drink more. I know the minimum I need to drink is one bottle an hour. Ideally, I try to drink two. When it comes to food, simple is better. I eat two GU packets an hour (plain flavor). I set my alarm on my watch to beep every 30 minutes and I know it's feeding time. Pretzels help settle my stomach and sucking or chewing on ice cubes [she fills her water bottle with them] near the end of the race helps too."

Electrolyte tablets: As needed, at least one every four hours, and as often as every 90 minutes depending on the weather.

> *AT:* "I'm thinking all the time when I'm running. I don't follow a strict regimen. You have to get to know your body."

Postrace Recovery

Immediately and following week: Water, vanilla milk shake the following morning, food eased in as tolerated.

> *AT:* "Right after the race I can't eat, drink, or sleep, so I just lie on the couch wondering why I did this! I'm waiting for my stomach to settle, so I sip water, but basically, nothing is appealing. I really don't want any more liquid. I always have a vanilla shake the morning following a 100-miler but have to force myself to eat anything the following few days, although drinking milk seems to help. I'll also drink Cytomax ProScore 100 (whey protein) mixed into milk and try to get my carbohydrates from solid foods. I usually take the day off following the race but will be back running at least five miles two days later. Sitting in the hot tub and massage (at least 72 hours after the race) is part of the plan too."

Tips for All Ultrarunners

1. A 100-mile race is a running, drinking, and eating contest. Don't leave your nutrition game plan up to chance. Trason has hers detailed on a computer spreadsheet. Know the location and timing of aid stations and drop points so you can prepare accordingly what to have available and what

to carry. Write down or record your thoughts in some manner following training runs and shorter races and compile a database of what works for you and what doesn't. Experiment with food, supplements, hydration strategies, carbo loading and prerace meals, and gear as much as you can before the actual race. Establish good habits in shorter races before attempting a 100-mile race.

2. Tim Tweitmeyer, five-time winner of the Western States 100, helped compile these pointers on how to avoid three classic mistakes that ultrarunners make:

- Not drinking enough early in the race. Don't just tote fluid around with you, concentrate on drinking it. Most runners carry two sources of fluid—plain water as well as a rehydrating sports drink (contains carbohydrates and electrolytes). Most bottles hold 20 ounces, the minimum amount of fluid needed per hour. If you arrive at aid stations with your bottles still full, consider adding handles to your bottles and carrying them as a reminder to drink more often. (Don't forget to experiment on training runs first.) You should be urinating frequently, and it should be light in color.

- Not taking in enough calories early. The crucial time to pay attention to your nutritional needs is the first 70 percent of the race. You must make smart decisions about your fuel needs (as well as fluid and sodium) during the first 70 miles, or you won't be around to finish the last 30. It's easy to forget when things are going well or seem under control early. If you dig yourself into a hole, though, its not likely that you will recover enough to continue even if you desperately attempt to shovel in calories during the latter stages of the race. All your training will be for naught if you don't make smart decisions concerning your nutritional needs early in the race.

- Not paying enough attention to the need for salt. To avoid hyponatremia (low blood-sodium level), you may have to supplement your sodium intake (from sports drinks and food) with electrolyte or salt tablets. There are no clear-cut guidelines or recommendations because the need for sodium varies due to individual sweat rates and the weather. In hot and humid conditions, some runners may need as much as 800 to 1,000 milligrams of sodium an hour.

Before the race, check the labels of products you intend to use (energy gels, drinks, and so on) to determine how much sodium they provide (in the amounts you intend to consume). During the race, choose at aid stations salty foods such as soup or broth, pretzels, chips, boiled potatoes sprinkled with salt, and so forth. You'll have to experiment with salt (electrolyte) tablets to determine what works best for you. If you plan to carry them with you, keep in mind that they disintegrate quickly if they contact moisture (for example, sweat) so place them in small plastic bags. Take salt tablets with six to eight ounces of water and don't overdo it. Salty foods tend to stimulate thirst, but salt tablets don't, so it is possible to ingest too much. If you have a health problem, check with your doctor about the use of salt tablets and your ability to exercise in the heat.

3. Learn to drink your calories. Not all ultrarunners can go the distance on energy gels alone. Although gels supply quick energy that goes down easily, they provide only 80 to 100 calories per packet. Aim to consume roughly 250 to 500 calories per hour. The easiest way to get in substantial calories is by drinking more-concentrated energy drinks and using liquid meal-replacement products. Find one you can tolerate since it definitely requires a lot less energy to drink your calories than it does to try and eat them. No single product works for every runner, so experiment on your long runs. You want to be sure you can continue to drink the beverage over a long period of time without it causing nausea. Save caffeinated beverages such as cola and Mountain Dew for when you really need a quick pick-me-up such as in the later stages of the race.

4. Supplement with solid foods as tolerated. Realize that nothing will taste good or sound appealing as time passes, so nibble on a variety of foods as you pass through aid stations or meet up with your crew. Aid stations typically provide fruit, bagels, cookies, candy, pretzels, soda crackers, boiled potatoes, and soup. Have your crew stock other foods that you've experimented with on training runs.

5. Time your eating and drinking so the majority of it occurs when you're walking. In ultraruns, this typically means when you're heading uphill. In the same vein, if your crew is meeting you somewhere other than an established aid station, have them meet you at the foot of a hill or mountain rather than waiting for you at the top.

6. Be sensitive to blood-sugar lows. When you're convinced you aren't making any forward progress or you're just about ready to drop out, keep eating and drinking as much as you can tolerate. You're most likely suffering from low blood sugar by consuming readily absorbable carbohydrates such as energy gels, soda, juice, glucose tablets, or candy. Slow your pace or walk and give your blood sugar a chance to stabilize (usually within 15 minutes unless you're severely depleted). Heed this as a warning sign that you need to do a better job at keeping up with your energy needs.

Your blood sugar can also bottom out if you exceed your stomach's capacity to absorb fluids. This may be the case if you feel uncomfortably full or bloated in your lower abdomen (as if you have "two stomachs") or the fluids you've been ingesting seem to just sit in your belly and slosh around. In extreme cases, veteran ultrarunners report relief by vomiting or "wiping the slate clean and starting over." If you opt to try this remedy, immediately begin your recovery by sipping on a properly formulated sports drink, not plain water. Remember, you will need fluid, carbohydrates, and sodium to keep going.

7. Weigh-ins during the race are a common practice at most 100-mile races. Be prepared to be detained (to drink and eat) or pulled from the race if you can't maintain your weight within an acceptable range (generally within 3 to 5 percent of your starting weight). As you attempt to rehydrate, consume sodium-containing sports drinks, soup or broth, and salty foods. The sodium in these items will help you retain the fluid you consume.

8. Do your best to speed your recovery by eating nutritious foods as soon as possible after the race. Again, drinking the nutrients and calories you need, (e.g., by meal-replacement products) may be the easiest way. Be sure to include high-quality protein sources at all meals. Try dairy foods. Both Trason and Tweitmeyer find that they tolerate milk and ice cream well in the few days following an ultrarun.

9. If you choose to use nonsteroidal anti-inflammatory drugs (NSAIDs, for example, Advil, Nuprin, Aleve, and Actron) during an ultrarun, be aware of the risks. Although acute kidney failure among ultrarunners is rare, be ex-

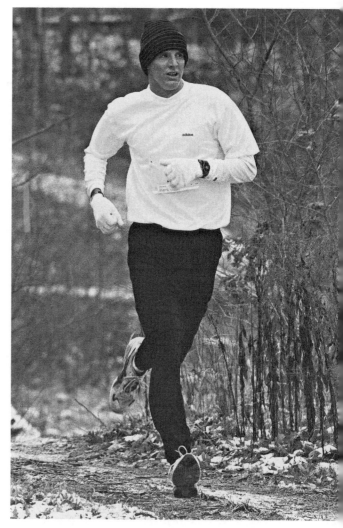

Be prepared to run, drink, and eat your way to the finish line of an ultrarun.

tremely cautious when using NSAIDs while running in the heat. Taking NSAIDs during prolonged exercise combined with severe heat stress or dehydration magnifies the potential for kidney problems and may contribute to the development of hyponatremia. Pay particular attention to your fluid needs before and during the race to minimize these risks. Taking NSAIDs may also upset your stomach.

10. Plan ahead when you travel to races, especially international races. Trason has traveled for the last 10 years with her rice cooker, as well as other standbys like energy bars and replacement drinks. Figure out what you can't do without and take it with you.

11. Learn from more experienced ultrarunners. Read about ultraendurance running and talk to other ultrarunners. That's how Trason started 14 years ago while training with a local running group. You'll never be able to simulate the last third of a 100-mile race in training, though. In the end, you just have to jump in and try it. Experience plays a large role in being successful at 100-mile races.

TIPS FOR SUPPORT CREWS

When they're not racing, there's a good chance that Ann Trason and Tim Tweitmeyer are crewing for another ultrarunner. Here's some advice they share for when it's your turn to crew at an ultrarun. I put all these tips to good use when I crewed for my husband at the Leadville Trail 100 race in Colorado.

1. As a support-crew member, make sure you have your own food and drinks. It's usually an extremely long day, and you don't want to become hungry. You are the brains behind the operation, so you need to be alert. You want to have fun, too, and it's a lot easier to do that when you have plenty on hand to eat and drink.

2. Have the runner write down a plan for you. If the runner won't do this, at least talk to him or her about the race as much as you can before the event. Do this a few days before the event, not the day before. A good ultrarunner will want to make your life easy. For example, you need to know what the runner might need and what he or she must absolutely carry with them when leaving the various aid stations.

3. Don't bombard your runner with questions as he or she arrives at an aid station. Before the race, have the runner give you a short list of questions that you should always ask. Trason, for example, has her crew ask if she wants more ice in her bottles and if she thinks she is getting enough salt. Make sure your runner is eating and drinking. For example, make sure you check the runner's bottles when he or she arrives at the aid station.

   Because your runner might not even remember his or her name after 70 miles, Tweitmeyer suggests asking a basic set of questions to draw out important information that the runner might otherwise forget. As a support-crew member, take care of the details as well as the big things. Even simple stuff can bog down a runner late in the race.

4. Have available as much information as you can about the various drops and aid stations. Write it down so there is no confusion. Most important is knowing what time to expect your runner to arrive so you can be there! Be ready to share information with your runner, such as how far the person has run and the distance to the next aid station. Split times from previous years can be useful to have on hand. If you keep split times of other runners, you can share how the race is going.

5. Expect your runner to go through emotional difficulties. Stay positive, flexible, and work at solving problems as they arise. Always think of yourself as the brain behind the operation. It's OK to play games with your runner to keep him or her going. If the runner wants to drop out, for example, tell him or her that dropping is not an option at this point. Reassure the runner that if he or she makes it to the next scheduled place and still wants to drop, you will talk about it then.

13

Open-Water Swimming

"Rhythm and consistency is as important to nutrition as it is to your stroke technique and race strategy. No matter what may be going on during the race, never miss a scheduled feeding."

—Tobie Smith, 1998 Open-Water World Champion 25K

Tobie Smith
Event: 1998 Open-Water World Championship 25K
Perth, Australia
First place, 5:31:20.1

Prerace Nutrition

Carbohydrate loading: No depletion phase. Boosted carbohydrate intake by supplementing with GatorLode (high-carbohydrate beverage with 50 grams of carbohydrate and 200 calories per eight ounces.)

> *TS:* "I've learned from other more experienced swimmers to really load up on carbohydrates before a 25K race. I typically eat three meals and snacks while doing heavy training. Less than a week before, I start supplementing every couple of hours with GatorLode. I probably have up to three or four two-liter water bottles of GatorLode a day. I don't really have any negative experiences, except that when having that much of one thing I start forcing it down at some point. In open-water swimming, you don't think about weight changes. Every pound doesn't count like it does in a pool swim."

Hydration: GatorLode and water.

> *TS:* "I'm drinking plenty of water along with the GatorLode. I'm definitely peeing all day long."

Prerace Meals (Race Start: 8 A.M.)

Night before: Ate a pasta dinner at an Italian restaurant at approximately 7P.M. GatorLode and a snack before bedtime.

> *TS:* "I eat something that goes down easy and settles well. I wouldn't eat steak or a hamburger, nothing greasy or spicy. Just bland food. I don't have anything magical that I eat. I did have some ice cream as comfort food. I certainly wouldn't go to bed hungry before a long race."

Morning of race: One and one-half hours before race—toast, half of a PowerBar, GatorLode, and water.

> *TS:* "I was really nervous that morning. I could only eat some toast and I forced down a half of a PowerBar with water. I drank more GatorLode because I could hardly eat anything. I drank water up to the start of

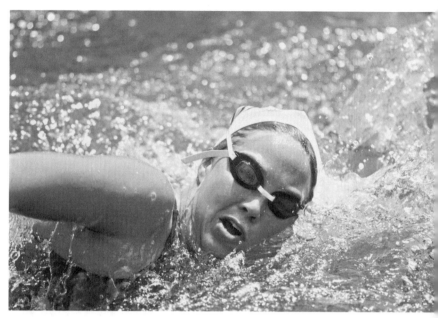

Open-water swimmer Tobie Smith swam the English Channel as her last race before retiring to attend medical school.

the race, especially since we were sitting on the beach after our warm-up and it was getting warm."

Supplements: Advil (two tablets) before the race, double dose of children's liquid painkiller at the halfway point of the race. Supplemented with iron in the weeks preceding the race.

> *TS:* "The liquid painkiller is easy to add to a feed and really helps cut down on the pain. I wasn't anemic but my ferritin was low at one point, so I was being really good before this race about taking my daily dose of iron."

During the Event

Feeds: Premixed several two-liter bottles (hold eight cups) the night before using powdered Gatorade and bottled water. Slightly stronger concentration than standard formula of 1 scoop per eight ounces (10 to 12 scoops per eight cups). Feeds administered from crew boat approximately every 20 minutes initially through halfway point, then every 15 minutes. Feeding pattern was Gatorade, Gatorade, water. PowerBar cut up into pieces as backup and carried on boat.

> *TS:* "About 20 minutes into the race was the first time I could get to the boat. My coach was adamant about not allowing me to miss any feeds. I make my drinks stronger so that I can taste them. A flavored drink is

really refreshing since your mouth and tongue start to swell and your throat burns from the salt water. The drinks are kept slightly chilled on the boat but not freezing cold.

You know when to start looking for the boat. Every 20 minutes is about a mile. I don't like the feeding stick, so my coach puts out a cup. I grab it, roll on my back, and take a big drink in about five seconds. Ideally, you drink the whole 8 to 12 ounces. I bet I get most of it. I don't like the taste of energy gels. They're too sweet. I did have a PowerBar as a backup, but I didn't eat any of it. It's just easiest to drink the calories.

I feed by how I feel. Usually it's every 20 minutes in the early part of the race. In the middle I had to regroup and slow down my intensity, so the feeds were dropped to every 15 minutes. In some races by the end you're feeding every 5 to 10 minutes, but that didn't happen in this race. I know what a low blood sugar feels like. I feel really weak and lose power. If my coach hasn't caught on, I yell 'feed' if I want quicker feeds."

Postrace Recovery

Immediately: Drank water, Gatorade, and soda. Snacked a few hours later after returning to hotel room. Ate Chinese food for dinner.

Following week: Resumed eating a normal diet.

> *TS:* "After the race, I drink a lot of anything I feel like drinking. Since I was being drug tested and needed to provide a urine sample, I even drank soda that was available. I snacked a few hours later on whatever we had in the room. I didn't have a race the following weekend, so I didn't care about getting carbohydrates back in. I eventually ate dinner because I definitely had to eat something before bed. You're so tired, but you can't sleep that night, and you ache all over, especially your neck and upper back. For the next three days you feel like you're overtrained. It's not comfortable. Since I decided I was retiring, I ate a regular person's diet, you know, hamburgers and beer."

Tips for Open-Water Swimmers

With help from competitive open-water swimmer Karen Burton, 1996–97 U.S. Marathon Swim champion and former national open-water team coordinator, I put together these pointers:

1. Start the race well hydrated and well fueled. Increase your glycogen stores by preloading with carbohydrate-rich foods and supplemental high-carbohydrate drinks (50 to 70 grams per eight ounces) for at least three days before the race. You may experience some lethargy and feel sleepier, so you may need to nap more than usual. Drink plenty of water leading up to the race. Plan to eat the morning of the race, too.

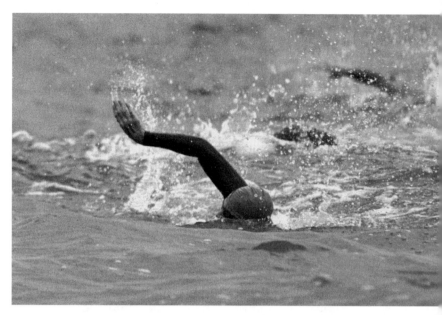

Work out a feeding plan with your support team before getting in the water.

2.   Feed on a regular, consistent schedule during the race. The standard feeding schedule is eight ounces of an electrolyte and fluid-recovery drink every 15 minutes. Aim for 20 grams of carbohydrate per feed, or 70 to 80 grams per hour. Avoid drinking only water if you will be swimming for more than 90 minutes, because you need the carbohydrates and electrolytes provided by a sports drink. In five seconds or less you should be able to grab a cup held out on a feeding stick or by hand, roll on your back, drink, dump the cup, and return to swimming.

Don't skip feeds, especially if you're feeling good and everything is going to plan. Be sure to experiment in training with the drink you plan to use during the race. Plan to drink the majority of calories that you need. Urinating every 30 minutes or so is a good sign that you're drinking enough. This does vary depending on the water temperature. You may urinate more frequently when swimming in cold water, and you will likely urinate less frequently while swimming in warm-water races.

3.   Bring solid foods as backup energy. Cookies, energy bars (precut into small pieces), canned fruit, bananas, and candy are some options. You need something on the boat to give yourself a lift during low points in the middle of the race. The calories these foods supply should supplement the calories provided by your drink. Be sure to drop your feeds to every 10 to 12 minutes, or even less, if you are feeling poorly.

4.   Replenish glycogen stores soon after the race. Speed your recovery time by immediately drinking 32 ounces of a high-carbohydrate beverage. Eat a meal within two hours of completing the race. The race isn't over when you stop swimming. During the open-water swimming season, it's common to swim three or four weekends in a row, so recovery is paramount. Expect your appetite to increase during the few days following a race. You may get

hungry quickly so eat often and be prepared by keeping essential foods on hand.

5.   Be sensitive to air and water temperatures. Open-water swims can take place in 60-degree water with 50-degree air temperatures all the way up to 83-degree water with 90-degree air temperatures.

In general, you'll need extra fluids and feeds for both extremes. In hot-weather races especially, you run the risk of dehydration. In cold-water races, you burn fuel much more quickly trying to keep up your core body temperature. In warm-weather races, increase your feeds to as often as every six to eight minutes or double your feeds by drinking one cup of water along with a cup of a fluid and electrolyte-replacement drink. Pack a cooler of ice to keep drinks cool during warm-weather races. For cold-water races, bring hot water to make feeds.

6.   Be aware of the symptoms of hypothermia, which can occur in warm water as well as cold water. Remember, if you've been swimming in a pool with water temperatures in the 80s, competing in 70-degree water can feel cold. Becoming dehydrated also predisposes you to hypothermia. Early signs include feeling cold (especially along the back), being unable to hold your fingers together while swimming, and shivering.

The trainer or coach on the boat makes the call of when to pull a swimmer from the water. Don't leave this decision up to the swimmer. A swimmer in trouble will be unable to swim in a straight line, appear blue, have difficulty speaking, and may be disoriented. If in doubt, ask the swimmer some thought-provoking questions, such as the name of a family member, or ask the swimmer to count backward from 20.

7.   Feed the crew. Be sure to bring extra food and beverages for the boat crew. It can be a long day on the water, and you depend on your crew always to be alert.

8.   Develop a healthy relationship about your body weight and body-fat percentage. A couple of extra pounds and a higher body-fat percentage can be advantageous for open-water swimmers, providing buoyancy and improving tolerance for cold water. Follow a sensible diet, mostly carbohydrates and adequate protein and fat, and let your weight fall where it will.

9.   Be prepared for the challenges associated with international races. Take any drink mixes or foods you plan to use during the race. Prepare your own bottles using powdered mixes and bottled water. Because you may be without your usual support crew, be sure to discuss your feeding schedule with whoever will be in charge on your boat. If necessary, set a watch alarm to beep every 15 minutes to remind yourself of your feeds.

To avoid becoming sick before the race, follow the standard precautions for eating and drinking in a foreign country. If you have concerns about the quality of the water you'll be swimming in, don't wait until you arrive and are ready to dive in. Contact your physician or local health department and obtain a gamma globulin injection, as well as a tetanus booster if necessary (once every 10 years), before you depart.

Marathon Skiing

"When I'm getting ready for a ski marathon, the most important thing is to eat a lot of everything."

—Carl Swenson, second place in 1999 American Birkebeiner

Carl Swenson

Events: Worldloppet circuit, third overall:

- American Birkebeiner,* Wisconsin, second place, 2:06:33.4

  *A 51-kilometer (31.6 mile) cross-country ski race—the largest Nordic ski race in North America.

- Austrian Dolomitenlauf (65K), fourth place
- Italian Marcialonga (70K), fifth place

Prerace Nutrition

Carbohydrate loading: No deliberate depletion of glycogen stores. Goal was to consume as many calories as possible the day before and enter the race well fueled.

> *CS:* "I don't know if it's superstition or tradition, but I like to have a high-protein meal two nights before, such as steak, because I really like it. Or I may have salmon or swordfish. The day before, I just try to eat as much as possible. I'll have cereal with 2 percent milk, bacon, and eggs for breakfast, and I'll snack on yogurt, muesli, and fruit throughout the day."

Hydration: Relied primarily on plain water, as well as a sports drink.

> *CS:* "I always have a water bottle with me."

Prerace Meals (Race Start: 9:00 A.M.)

Night before: Ate a high-carbohydrate meal between 6 and 7 P.M. Late P.M. snack of yogurt and muesli.

> *CS:* "I can eat a lot. I always outeat everyone around me. The more the better. I had pasta with meat sauce and bread. I eat less salad and vegetables than I normally would because they fill me up with less calories. I had just about everything, including some rice and potatoes, too. I don't have any special foods. There's nothing that I can't do without. In Spain [before a mountain bike race], I filled up on tortillas."

Morning of race: Ate breakfast provided by race directors from approximately 5:00 to 5:30 A.M. Consciously hydrated by drinking plenty of water up to the start of the race.

CS: "My breakfast used to be three hours before, but I've moved it back to four hours because I was feeling my stomach in races. It would feel full or blocked. I had cereal with milk, French toast, and a small amount of juice. I don't have a problem with dairy. I have it every morning, so I stick with that. I also have a little bit of protein, such as oatmeal or an egg. I have trouble eating and drinking during the race, so I try to eat as much as possible before."

Supplements: No supplements, including no vitamins. Does not use any type of protein powders or supplemental high-carbohydrate beverages. Uses energy bars as backup snacks.

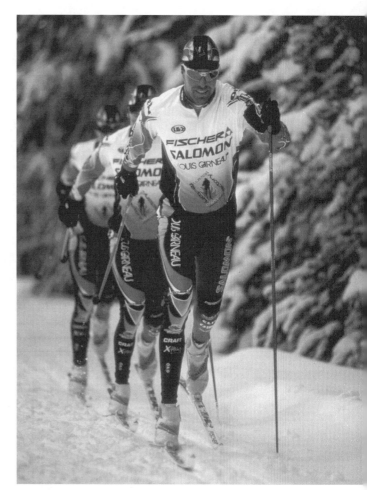

In 1998, marathon skier Carl Swenson became the only American to win the Birkie since it began in 1973.

CS: "I don't find that stuff that enjoyable to eat or that helpful. I don't feel I really need any supplements because there's nothing I don't like to eat. I would burn out if I lived on energy bars, although I always carry them with me, especially when I travel in Europe. They make good backup for my usual snacks."

During the Event

Feeds: Prefilled seven 16-ounce water bottles with a weak solution of Internutria Race Day sports drink (diluted with water to half strength or less). Picked up from predesignated feed stations throughout the race. Did not use energy gels.

CS: "There's great support at this race with seven feeds, spaced pretty evenly throughout the race, every 20 minutes or so. The feed stations are usually situated on a gradual downhill, so you can glide for a few seconds and drink. If I get down eight ounces that would be good. I missed one and skipped another, but I knew missing a couple would be OK. Four feeds are more than enough for me.

I keep my drink at half strength, even weaker in the summer [mountain bike races]. Otherwise my stomach feels full, as if the feed isn't absorbed by the time I go to put the next one in. I've gotten cramps in the past. Sometimes in Europe I'll drink defizzed Coke over the last 2K. I go with all liquid calories, but a lot of the other skiers tape GU or another energy gel to their bottle."

Postrace Recovery

Immediately: Replenished with water and supplemental foods. Ate a regular meal approximately three to four hours later.

CS: "Just plain water tastes good right after, and I'll drink a lot of it. It's hard to eat the next three to four hours. I tend to use more supplemental food after a race than before, such as Jogmate [puddinglike protein supplement in a tube] and energy bars. I just get back to eating regular meals, including some red meat, chicken, or fish at each meal. I'm tired the next day, but in two days I'm ready to go again."

Tips for All Winter Athletes

1. Start out well fueled. Cross-country skiing, in particular, uses the entire muscle mass of the body, so your energy needs are extremely high. Experiment with carbohydrate loading and prerace meals to find a routine that works well for you. Including fat and protein-rich foods will provide staying power and may help you tolerate the cold better, but don't let these foods squeeze out carbohydrate-rich foods. You need adequate carbohydrate reserves to power hardworking muscles and to fuel your brain so you can make wise decisions while racing. You may be able to compete in other sports on an empty stomach, but don't try it in a ski marathon venture. Plan to eat an adequate breakfast.

2. Pay attention to your fluid needs. You may not feel as thirsty while competing in cold weather or you may want to avoid making pit stops, but your hydration needs remain a priority. Swenson drinks similar amounts of fluid whether he's heading out on his skis or on his mountain bike. He jokes that he makes frequent pit stops no matter which competitive season he's involved in, cross-country skiing or mountain biking.

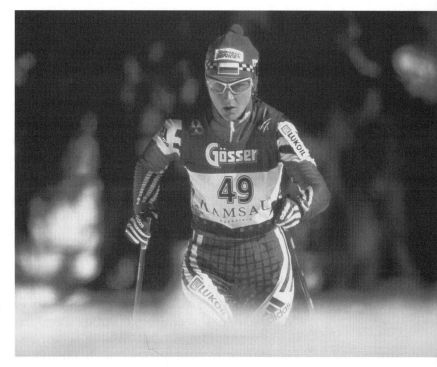

Plan for the cold. Skiers need to follow the same guidelines for drinking and refueling during competition as other athletes.

To keep your hands free, experiment with a bladder system. Choose one that is insulated, lightweight (Ultimate Direction has one designed for skiers), and nonrestrictive. Advances in technology have produced tubes and valves that are less likely to freeze up in cold temperatures, but these fluid-delivery systems aren't foolproof. If you've experienced problems before or expect extreme temperatures, wear a water-bottle carrier (with an insulated 16-ounce water bottle or larger) strapped around your waist instead.

3. Laura McCabe, two-time Olympian and the women's winner of the 1999 American Birkebeiner, offers the following nutrition tips for racers:

- Drink early in ski marathon races—ideally within the first 15 minutes. Choose an electrolyte-replacement drink to meet your fluid and carbohydrate needs.

- Practice drinking while on the move. McCabe suggests the following technique: on a slight downhill (a flat section can work, too, if you can keep moving without using your arms), whip your bottle carrier around to the front, pull the bottle out, and tuck the pole on that side under your arm. The idea is to remain aerodynamic by drinking in a tucked position. Take advantage of your position in a racing pack. If you're in front, gliding and drinking helps prevent people from passing. Drinking while drafting off others in a pack helps block the wind and keeps you from slowing.

- Refuel at every feed station. You can generally expect a feed every 10 to 15K in most ski marathon races. Be prepared to slow down to obtain a cup of fluid because volunteers may not be trained to deliver feeds by running alongside you. Save the sports drink you are toting for in-between feeds and during rough patches when you need an energy boost. Slower skiers may need to stop and refill their bottles at feed stations or wear a bladder system that allows for a larger fluid-carrying capacity. Foods typically available at feeding stations are sports drinks (water, too), hot chocolate, soup, orange slices, energy bars and gels, cookies, and brownies.

- Carry energy gels as backup fuel. Store energy gels in a water bottle carrier that has small pockets or tape a packet to the front of your jersey or to the inside of your arm (on top of your jersey). Choose a convenient place on your body that you can easily reach. You should consume energy gels with water, so time your intake with a feeding station.

- Be aware of the symptoms of bonking. You may feel unusually cold and experience shivering, or you may simply run out of energy. Two telltale warning signs that trouble is just around the corner are experiencing hunger pangs and having overwhelming negative thoughts. Recognize that your brain needs fuel immediately. Consume carbohydrate-rich drinks and foods as soon as possible and pay attention to your hydration and fuel needs for the rest of the race. Two situations that may boost your normal energy needs are hilly courses and extreme weather.

- Speed your recovery by refueling after races. It's easy to get lazy after the race. Concentrate on quickly replacing fluids and carbohydrates, especially if you have another race in a few days or the following weekend.

4. Make smart food choices on travel days leading up to race day. Traveling all day and eating poorly is a double whammy that can wipe out the fittest athlete. Be prepared by bringing foods that travel well and by stocking up on energy bars and powdered meal-replacement products. Swenson's philosophy is to stay flexible and eat as many different foods as he can (which for him meant trying a dish made with squid ink).

Adventure Racing

"In endurance sports such as the Eco-Challenge, good nutrition is the backbone and foundation to moving along and thinking clearly day after day. To fuel your body properly and to have it run as efficiently as possible, knowing what to eat and when to eat is the difference between winning and losing."

—Sara Ballantyne,
representing Team Vail, winners of the
1998 EcoChallenge Adventure Race

Sara Ballantyne
Event: 1998 EcoChallenge*, Morocco
First place, 6 days, 22 hours, and 15 minutes

*Represented Team Vail (including Mike Kloser, Andreas Boesel, and Billy Mattison). The race consisted of a 300(+) mile, nonstop, team adventure race combining segments of camel racing (9 miles), coasteering (3 miles), sea kayaking (50 miles), trekking and canyoneering (68 miles), horseback riding (30 miles), mountaineering (39 miles including a summit of North Africa's second highest peak at over 13,000 feet), and mountain biking (118 miles).

Prerace Nutrition

Six days before the event through the morning of the race: Prepackaged foods brought from the United States, bottled water, powdered sports drinks. A glass of wine or beer with dinner (another prepackaged meal) the night before. Instant oatmeal for breakfast. Avoided all ethnic Moroccan cuisine. Planned to buy butane gas for camping stove in Morocco (butane gas not allowed on airplane) but were able to purchase a hot burner plate to heat water.

> *SB:* "It was the guys' idea to bring all our own food, and it was also highly recommended by race officials. I always want to try the ethnic foods of the different countries I travel to. It turned out to be one of the keys to our success as many other teams were affected by the different bacteria and came down with traveler's diarrhea. You simply can't afford to start out stressed in an event of this nature. We don't have any particular good-luck meal, but I knew the next week would be total deprivation, so I wanted a glass of wine!"

During the Event

There is no such thing as a typical day because participants tackle various disciplines. Essentially, an EcoChallenge team is a self-sufficient team of four members who receive little outside assistance—including the offering of fluids and energy snacks—once the race begins. No support crews are allowed. The race features various mandatory checkpoints. This year's event included only one "oasis" where hot food was available, located at the midpoint of the race.

Hydration: Water and powdered sports drinks mixed with water. Team Vail relied on Camelbak hydration systems, carrying an average of 100 ounces (about three quarts) each. Bottled water was available at checkpoints and the oasis, but teams were advised not to rely on it. All teams were required to carry purification tablets to treat water found along the course.

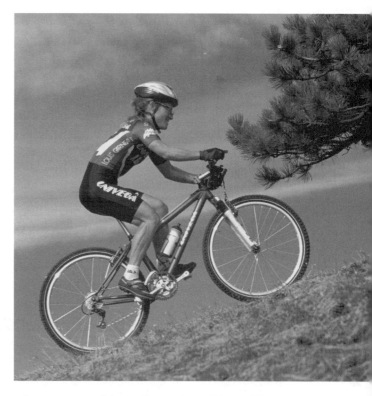

Adventure racer Sara Ballatyne honed her skills by winning the World Mountain Bike championships twice.

SB: "I couldn't imagine not using a Camelbak. I usually carry about 100 ounces, and we all carry our own unless we know that a water source is nearby. Then we'll share to lighten our loads. We've run out of water before while training in Utah and it's no fun. The first couple of days we were carrying 36 pounds of water between us (approximately four and a half quarts each) until water was so readily available along the course that we cut back. I probably drink about 200 ounces (six quarts) a day."

Food: Prepackaged foods included soup (eaten cold), jerky, powdered sports drinks (Champion Nutrition Metabolol), energy bars, gorp, chocolate, and so on. Ballantyne favored turkey jerky and Clif bars (especially all the chocolate flavors). Team Vail prepared no hot water or hot meals (including no morning coffee) once the race began. Oasis stop (midpoint of race) served hot ethnic Moroccan fare.

SB: "Everyone on our team carries their own food stash. I bring Clif bars because they're predictable and I like the taste. We all take responsibility for fueling and hydrating ourselves, and we sometimes assign a person to remind the rest of the group to keep eating and drinking. We also carry premade packets of team food that everyone picks through individually to supplement their own. We were very careful of what we ate at the oasis—only steaming hot rice and vegetables (we could see the steam rising off them), no poultry or cream-based dishes.

You can't just duplicate someone else's [teammate's] plan. You need to bring foods that you enjoy eating, whether it's sweets or salty foods. Lacking an appetite is part of the game; you won't eat it if you dread it. Losing weight is inevitable (I probably ate 3,000 calories a day), as it's impossible to keep up with the caloric intake needed to do something of this length."

Supplements: Multivitamin (daily), vitamin C (daily), over-the-counter anti-inflammatory drugs and aspirin (used as needed). Teams were required to carry salt tablets, but Team Vail never used them.

SB: "Most energy drinks have sodium and potassium in them, so I seem to get enough. The key is to never allow yourself to get too depleted of anything. It's a continual ongoing process of monitoring your body. Once you go too low, you can't get back. I try to avoid taking ibuprofen since I think it's responsible for some of the terrible edema you see some racers suffering with at the end of the race."

Postrace Recovery

Team Vail threw caution to the wind at this point, ate local fare, and paid the price!

SB: "The best thing to do is to try and do nothing at all. Just old-fashioned r and r (reading books by the pool) if you can, and drink plenty of fluids. You've stressed your body to the max and it needs downtime. Massage really helps. Recovery is a very individual process. I was riding such a high from winning that I was only home for two days and then went on a bike trip to Bolivia."

Tips for All Adventure Racers

1. Know where your next drink is coming from. Whether it's a one-day "sprint" or a week of classic adventure racing, an adequate fluid intake is paramount for survival and success. Experiment with different hydration systems while training. Try bladders, waist belts, or water bottle holsters that attach to the daisy chains on the front of a pack's shoulder strap. Keep in mind how rugged the terrain might be. A bladder system won't be of much use if it becomes punctured. In single-day races, determine how frequently you will pass through staging areas, which, in turn, will determine how much fluid you need to carry with you on each leg. Figure on a minimum of one water bottle (20 ounces) per person per hour, depending on the activity and the weather. In longer races, always use iodine tablets to purify water found along the course.

Because you're going to be on the move longer than an hour, drink a sports drink in addition to plain water. The electrolytes these drinks contain will help prevent muscle cramps and hyponatremia (low blood sodium) and will stimulate you to keep drinking. The carbohydrate provided by sports drinks will fuel your brain as well as your muscles. This is a definite advantage when the race hinges on navigation skills or your ability to decipher mysterious "special tests" throughout the race.

Don't wait until you feel thirsty to drink. Watch for the telltale signs of dehydration: headache, nausea, loss of appetite, personality change (stops bantering or answering questions), infrequent urination (dark color), clumsiness, lack of energy, and inability to tolerate hot or cold temperatures. Dehydration increases your risk for heat exhaustion, heat stroke, and hypothermia, all of which can prevent you (and your team) from finishing, especially during longer races. Stop before you allow dehydration to progress too far. In severe cases, stop, seek shade, and try to rehydrate by sipping on small amounts of water or other fluids as tolerated.

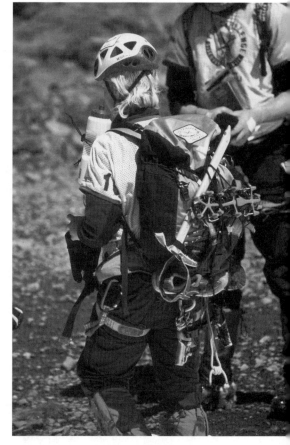

Don't leave home without a sports drink—it does triple duty supplying fluid, electrolytes, and energy.

2. Have a plan for refueling. A lack of appetite is the norm during adventure races, especially those stretching past a day or two. Just because you're hot, sweaty, dehydrated, fatigued, sleep-deprived, covered with mud, possibly well off course, and don't feel the least bit hungry, you still must replenish your limited glycogen stores. In single-day races, sports drinks, energy gels and bars, and any other carbohydrate-rich food you find appealing (bananas, fig bars, and so on) and have access to should do the trick.

3. If your adventure race takes you outside the United States, prepare by researching local resources. Take any foodstuffs you can't do without. If gastrointestinal risks are associated with eating the local cuisine or drinking the water, be cautious. Drink only bottled water, pasteurized juice, and soda (without ice), and take extra supplies for the days before the race. Powdered meal-replacement products and dehydrated camping fare come in handy before, as well as during, longer races. All of these items can be easily

prepared with bottled or purified water. Beware of "flavor fatigue," especially in longer races. Take many different flavors of energy bars, gels, and other staples because your favorite may not be so appealing by the third day.

Protein-rich foods are particularly challenging to locate in some countries. Be creative and try jerky, poptop cans of tuna or chicken, string cheese, individually wrapped rounds of hard cheese, peanut butter, and nuts. It's virtually impossible to carry all the calories an adventure racer needs in a long race. These foods provide substantial calories and are appealing complements to the array of sweet-tasting foods that you will typically be eating.

4. Keep an eye on your teammates. In adventure races, the first team to cross the finish line together wins. Teams that lose a member due to illness, fatigue, injury, or a team disagreement are disqualified. Obviously, you need to be responsible for staying on top of your personal fluid and fuel needs, but at the same time you must monitor your teammates. Be sure they are also eating and drinking. Share fluids and food as needed. Dehydration, depletion of muscle glycogen stores, or a low blood-sugar level makes the race seem even harder than it is. Be particularly sensitive to mood swings; a teammate in trouble may become extremely quiet or irritable and argumentative.

5. If you want to be a serious adventure racer, learn to travel light and fast. Cathy Sassin is an American who races with the French-based Spie Batignolles team in the Raid Gauloises. Her team placed second in the 1998 race held in Ecuador, finishing just two hours behind the winners in 8 days, 9 hours, and 46 minutes. The race included 58 miles (97 kilometers) of hiking, 22 miles (36 kilometers) of horseback riding and running, a 14-mile (24-kilometer) trek over the 19,000-foot summit of the Cotopaxi Volcano, 36 miles (60 kilometers) of Indian biking, another 55 miles (92 kilometers) of hiking, and a 155-mile (259-kilometer) water section completed by raft, canoe, and sea kayak. Sassin offers the following tips:

- Determine the food preferences of your teammates beforehand (as well as any food allergies), so you don't end up carrying food someone doesn't like or can't eat.
- Keep food and fluids near at hand. Easy access is the name of the game. Wear a bladder system or attach water bottles to the outside of your pack for easy access to fluids. Carry your own small stash of quick energy (Sassin favors fruit-to-go strips), such as dried fruit, energy bars and gels, trail mix, hard candy, or chocolate, in clothing pockets or in the outer pocket of one of your teammate's packs. Don't waste time taking your own pack on and off and repacking its contents every time you need to eat.
- Coordinate your refueling efforts with the inevitable stops you'll be making. Serious adventure racing requires a considerable amount of stopping for navigational purposes, so plan to access more substan-

tial preassembled team food (packaged in large zip-lock bags) at this time (as well as make adjustments in clothing and attend to foot problems). Keep it simple. Place the food in one person's backpack so it doesn't require a lot of effort or thought when you're in a hurry or feeling the effects of sleep deprivation. If one person needs to eat to continue, then everybody on the team should refuel.

- Learn to eat on the run. Sassin typically combines cold water and dehydrated fare in a resealable container (no time is wasted heating the water) and throws it back into her pack. After 20 minutes it's ready to eat. She and her teammates take turns passing the container around and squeezing the contents out of one corner—all while on the move, of course!

6.   Use salt and electrolyte tablets and glycerol wisely. Increase your salt intake by adding salt to the foods you eat and consuming salty foods in the few days before a warm-weather race. That and consuming a properly formulated sports drink during the race should be sufficient for most one-day adventure races. If you perspire heavily or will be competing for several hours or days in a warmer environment than you trained in, you may need additional sodium. Take salt or electrolyte tablets with plenty of water (six to eight ounces), otherwise you may find yourself slowed by nausea, vomiting, and diarrhea. Adventure racers competing in weeklong races are required to carry electrolyte tablets because the possibility of consuming only plain water for long periods increases the risk of hyponatremia. If you have a health problem, check with your physician about the use of salt tablets and your ability to exercise in the heat.

In longer races held in hot weather, "hyperhydrating" with glycerol could be beneficial as long as the possible side effects of bloating and abdominal distress don't slow your progress. Little is known about the day-to-day use of glycerol, so you'll need to experiment in training to determine your tolerance level and any potential benefits.

7.   Try to avoid using nonsteroidal anti-inflammatory drugs (NSAIDs) before or during adventure races. NSAIDs may irritate your stomach, contribute to the development of hyponatremia, and, combined with dehydration, increase your risk for kidney problems. Pay particular attention to your fluid needs before and during the race if you choose to take NSAIDs.

Facts About Vitamins and Minerals

Vitamins	DRI	Best sources	Functions
Water-soluble	**female/male** **(31-50 year olds)**		
Thiamin	1.1/1.2 mg	Wheat germ, whole grains breads and cereals, organ meats, lean meats, legumes, fortified grains	Release of energy from carbohydrates; maintenance of healthy nervous system
Riboflavin	1.1/1.3 mg	Milk and dairy products, green leafy vegetables, lean meats, beans, fortified grains	Release of energy from protein, fat, and carbohydrate; promotes healthy skin
Niacin	14/16 mg	Lean meats, fish, poultry, legumes, whole grains, fortified grains	Release of energy from protein, fat, and carbohydrate; synthesis of protein, fat, and DNA; promotes healthy skin and nervous system
Vitamin B_6	1.3 mg	Liver, lean meats, fish, poultry, legumes, whole grains	Protein metabolism; formation of hemoglobin and red blood cells; synthesis of essential fatty acids
Vitamin B_{12}	2.4 µg	Lean meats, poultry, dairy products, eggs, fish	Metabolism of carbohydrate, protein, fat; produces red blood cells; maintains nerve cells
Folic acid	400 µg	Green leafy vegetables, legumes	New cell growth; red blood cell formation
Biotin	30 µg	Meats, legumes, milk, egg, yolk, whole grains	Aids in metabolism of carbohydrates, fat, protein
Pantothenic acid	5 mg	Found in wide array of foods	Aids in metabolism of carbohydrates, fat, protein
Vitamin C	75/90 mg	Citrus fruits, green leafy vegetables, broccoli, peppers, potatoes, berries, kiwi	Maintenance of normal connective tissue; enhances iron absorption; antioxidant; helps heal wounds
Fat-soluble			
Vitamin A	4,000/5,000 IU	Liver, milk, cheese, fortified margarine, carotenoids in plant foods (orange, red, deep green in color)	Maintains healthy skin, mucous membranes, vision, and immune system; antioxidant
Vitamin D	200 IU	Vitamin D fortified milk and margarine, fish oil, sunlight	Promotes normal bone growth; aids in calcium absorption
Vitamin E	22 IU	Vegetable oils, margarine, green leafy vegetables, wheat germ, eggs, whole grains	Antioxidant; forms red blood cells
Vitamin K	65/80 µg	Liver, eggs, cauliflower, green leafy vegetables	Normal blood clotting

(continued)

Facts About Vitamins and Minerals *(continued)*

Vitamins Minerals	DRI female/male (31-50 yr olds)	Best sources	Functions
Calcium	1,000 mg	Milk, cheese, yogurt, ice cream, legumes, dark green leafy vegetables	Formation of bones and teeth; role in muscle contractions, nerve impulse transmission, and blood clotting
Phosphorus	700 mg	Meat, poultry, fish, eggs, milk, cheese, legumes, whole grains	Metabolism of protein, carbohydrate and fat; repairs and maintains cells; helps in formation of teeth and bones
Magnesium	320/420 mg	Milk, yogurt, legumes, nuts, whole grains, tofu, green vegetables	Metabolism of carbohydrate and protein; aids in neuro-muscular contractions
Iron	15/10 mg	Organ meats, lean meats, poultry, shellfish, oysters, whole grains, legumes	Aids in formation of hemo-globin and transportation of oxygen in red blood cells
Zinc	12/15 mg	Lean meats, fish, poultry, shellfish, oysters, whole grains, legumes	Energy metabolism; protein synthesis; aids in normal immune function and wound healing
Copper	1.5-3.0 mg	Lean meats, poultry, shellfish, fish, eggs, nuts, beans, whole grains	Necessary for iron absorption, manufacture of collagen; heals wounds
Fluoride	3/4 mg	Milk, egg yolks, water, seafood	Helps form teeth and bones
Selenium	55 µg	Meat, fish, poultry, organ meats, seafood, whole grains and nuts from selenium-rich soil	Component of antioxidant enzymes
Chromium	50-200 µg	Organ meats, meats, oysters, cheese, whole grains, beer	Regulates blood sugar; normal fat metabolism
Iodine	150 µg	Iodized salt, seafood, water	Component of thyroid hormone that helps regulate growth and development rate
Manganese	2-5 mg	Green leafy vegetables, whole grains, nuts, legumes, egg yolks	Aids in synthesis of hemoglobin
Molybdenum	75-250 µg	Legumes, cereal grains, dark green leafy vegetables	Involved in carbohydrate and fat metabolism
Sodium	2,400 mg or more	Table salt, found in virtually all foods	Acid-base balance, fluid balance; nerve impulses; muscle action
Potassium	3,500 mg	Fruits, and vegetables, (bananas, orange juice, potatoes, tomatoes), milk, yogurt, legumes	Fluid balance; acid-base balance; nerve impulses; muscle action; protein and glycogen synthesis

High-Carbohydrate Foods

Food group	Calories	Carbohydrates (grams)
Dairy		
Low-fat (2%) milk (1 cup)	121	12
Skim milk (1 cup)	86	12
Chocolate milk (1 cup)	208	26
Pudding, any flavor (1/2 cup)	161	30
Frozen yogurt, low-fat (1 cup)	220	34
Fruit-flavored low-fat yogurt (1 cup)	225	42
Beans		
Blackeye peas (1/2 cup)	134	22
Pinto beans (1 cup)	235	44
Navy beans (1 cup)	259	48
Refried beans (1/2 cup)	142	26
Garbanzo beans (chickpeas) (1 cup)	269	45
White beans (1 cup)	249	45
Fruit and vegetables		
Fruits		
Apple (1 medium)	81	21
Apple juice (1 cup)	111	28
Applesauce (1 cup)	194	51
Banana (1)	105	27
Canteloupe (1 cup)	57	14
Dates, dried (10)	228	61
Fruit roll-ups (1 roll)	50	12
Grapes (1 cup)	114	28
Grape juice (1 cup)	96	23
Orange (1)	65	16
Orange juice (1 cup)	112	26
Pear (1)	98	25
Pineapple (1 cup)	77	19
Prunes, dried (10)	201	53
Raisins (2/3 cup)	300	79
Raspberries (1 cup)	61	14
Strawberries (1 cup)	45	11
Watermelon (1 cup)	50	12
Vegetables		
Three-bean salad (1/2 cup)	90	20
Carrots (1 medium)	31	8
Corn (1/2 cup)	89	21
Lima beans (1 cup)	217	40

(continued)

High-Carbohydrate Foods *(continued)*

Food group	Calories	Carbohydrates (grams)
Vegetables (continued)		
Peas, green (1/2 cup)	63	12
Potato (1 large)	220	50
Sweet potato (1 large)	118	28
Bread and cereals		
Bagel (1)	165	31
Biscuit (1)	103	13
Breadsticks (2 sticks)	77	15
Cereal, ready-to-eat (1 cup)	110	24
Cream of rice (3/4 cup, ckd)	95	21
Cream of wheat (3/4 cup, ckd)	96	20
Cornbread (1 square)	178	28
English muffin	154	30
Fig bar (1)	50	10
Flavored oatmeal, Quacker instant (1 packet)	110	25
Flour tortilla (6 1/2-inch diameter)	88	15
Granola bar (low-fat, 1)	109	16
Graham crackers (2 squares)	60	11
Hamburger bun (1)	123	22
Hotdog bun (1)	123	22
Noodles, spaghetti (1 cup, ckd)	197	40
Oatmeal (1 cup, ckd)	145	25
Oatmeal raisin cookie	62	9
Pancake (4-inch diameter)	84	11
Pizza (cheese, 1 slice)	290	39
Popcorn, plain (1 cup, popped)	26	6
Pretzels (1 oz)	106	21
Rice (1 cup, ckd)	226	50
Rice, brown (1 cup, ckd)	226	45
Saltines (5 crackers)	60	10
Triscuit crackers (3 crackers)	60	10
Waffles (2, 3.5″ x 5.5″)	230	30
White bread (1 slice)	61	12
Whole-wheat bread (1 slice)	55	11

Source: *Gatorade Sports Science Exchange,* 11(4):71.

Eating on the Run

Stocking Your Pantry

If you're like most athletes, you have the time to eat healthy meals and snacks. What you don't have time for is pedaling or hoofing it over to the nearest grocery store because you're missing some key ingredient or, worse, you look in the fridge and realize you forgot to go food shopping again. To avoid the minimalist look from overtaking your kitchen, keep a stash of these nutritious staples on hand in your pantry, refrigerator, and freezer. It makes grabbing healthy snacks and whipping up simple meals easy.

Breads, Pasta, Rice and Other Grains

Quick-cooking brown or white rice (cooking time: 10 minutes)

Pasta (cooking time: 10 minutes; fresh pasta: 3 to 5 minutes)

Other prepackaged quick-cooking pastas or grains: couscous (cooking time: 5 minutes), quinoa (cooking time: 10 to 15 minutes), cracked wheat bulgur, pasta and beans, wheat pilaf, tabouli (cooking time: 15 minutes)

Instant stuffing mixes (cooking time: 5 minutes)

Corn and flour tortillas

Whole-grain breads, bagels, rolls, pita bread, English muffins (store in the freezer)

Low-fat crackers (4 grams of fat or less per ounce)

Quick-cooking oatmeal, Farina, Wheatena (cooking time: 5 minutes)

Ready-to-eat cereals, breakfast bars, granola bars

Toaster waffles

Fruits and Vegetables

Potatoes or sweet potatoes (store in a cool, dark area; bake in the microwave)

Instant mashed potato mixes (cooking time: 5 minutes)

Frozen or canned vegetables (rinse canned varieties to reduce sodium content)

Bags of prewashed salad greens

Bags of mini-carrots

Prechopped vegetables or fruit from grocery store salad bars

Canned fruit

Oranges, apples, bananas (store in fridge to slow ripening), dates

Dried fruit such as raisins, pineapple, apples, prunes

Frozen juice concentrates and individual-serving juice boxes

Milk and Milk Products

Low-fat milk (regular or soy)

Low-fat yogurt

Low-fat cheese (for example, part-skim ricotta and mozzarella, Parmesan)

Meat and Meat Alternates

Boneless, skinless chicken breasts (store in the freezer)

Lean ground meat (ground round, sirloin, turkey breast)

Cubed meat for kebabs or stir-fries

Lean deli meats such as turkey, ham, or roast beef

Cans of tuna (packed in water), chicken

Canned chili

Canned beans such as kidney, pinto, black, chickpeas, low-fat refried beans

Frozen veggie or gardenburgers

Tofu

Eggs or egg substitutes (can be stored in the freezer)

Peanut or other nut butters

Others

Condiments such as low-fat salad dressing or mayonnaise, soft tub margarine, olive oil, mustard, ketchup, cocktail sauce, soy sauce, vinegar, jelly or jam

Seasonings such as onion and garlic powders, dried herbs

Spaghetti sauce

Canned soup

Instant "just add boiling water" cups of polenta, lentils, beans

Sports bars

Assorted nuts, sunflower seeds

Pretzels

Cookies

Note: Perishables, such as milk and yogurt, fresh fruit and vegetables, fresh pasta, and deli meats, need to be replaced weekly. Other staples can be stored for longer periods of time, especially if unopened.

Dining Out

Dining away from home doesn't mean giving up on a well-balanced, healthy diet. Keep the Food Guide Pyramid in mind and try to fill out the groups as you would at home. Choose the restaurant or eatery carefully, and you'll have plenty of options. It takes some creativity, but even convenience-store cuisine can offer acceptable fare. Although some endurance athletes can afford to consume higher fat items, this list emphasizes higher carbohydrate, lower fat selections for those who eat out regularly.

Convenience Stores and Minimarts

Carton of nonfat or low-fat milk

Low-fat yogurt or frozen yogurt

Part-skim string cheese (mozzarella sticks)

Pudding cups

Ice cream sandwiches

Bean burrito

Jerky

Snack-size cereal, cereal bars, low-fat granola bars

Bagels

Bananas, oranges, apples, raisins

Fruit juice, tomato, or vegetable juice

Frozen juice bars

Sports drinks

Bottled water

Low-fat muffins, brownies, or cookies—animal cookies, fig bars, graham crackers, ginger snaps, vanilla wafers

Lower-fat crackers such as rye crisps, saltines, melba rounds, Triscuits, Wheat Thins

Energy bars

Trail mix (dried fruit and nuts) or assorted nuts

Pretzels, popcorn, rice cakes

Baked or low-fat chips with salsa

Supermarkets

Bread, bagel, roll, or pita and sandwich fixings: lean deli meats, low-fat cheese, humus

Ready-made deli sandwiches or subs

Soup and salad bar

Pizza with vegetarian toppings

Precooked chicken to go

Bento or rice bowl with stir-fry (if Chinese take-out is available)

Fresh fruit, dried fruit, fruit juice

Bottled water

Skim milk or low-fat milk

Low-fat muffins, cookies, brownies

Pretzels or popcorn

Tips: Choose plain or barbecued chicken (discard skin) over fried chicken wings, broth-based, bean, or lentil soups over creamy soups, bread or roll over a croissant, deli sandwiches without mayonnaise (add your own or use mustard or ketchup), and pretzels over chips. Go easy on cream cheese, salad dressing, chips, and pasta, potato and other salads made with mayonnaise or oil-based dressings (tuna, chicken, egg salad).

Fast Food

Pizza with vegetarian toppings

Broiled burgers or grilled chicken with lettuce and tomato on whole-wheat bun

Sandwich or sub made with lean roast beef, ham, turkey or chicken

Chicken fajitas or soft tacos

Bean burrito

Salad bar

Soup

Baked potato with low-fat toppings

Chili with crackers

Bagel or English muffin – lightly buttered or with jam

Waffle or pancakes with syrup

Ready-to-eat cereal (hot or cold)

Low-fat muffins or cookies

Nonfat or low-fat milk

Low-fat milkshake

Frozen yogurt or soft-serve ice cream

Fruit juice

Tips: Go easy on extra cheese or meat toppings on pizza, supersize burgers and fries, fried chicken and fish sandwiches, creamy soups, salad dressings, breakfast biscuits, sausage and bacon, tartar sauce, mayonnaise, special sauces, Danish pastries, and soft drinks.

Restaurant Dining

Mexican. Fill up on gazpacho or bean soup, red or black beans, refried beans (made without lard or fat), Spanish rice, marinated vegetables, grilled shrimp, fish, and chicken, soft plain tortillas, burritos (not deep fried), soft tacos, fajitas, enchiladas, tamales, pico de gallo, salsa and baked tortilla chips.

Go easy on crispy fried tortillas (nachos) and taco shells, quesadillas, chile relleno, tostados, chimichangas, sour cream, cheese, and guacamole and always ask how the refried beans are prepared. Order a la carte if you can and choose your sides wisely.

Chinese—Fill up on wonton or hot and sour soup, steamed rice and vegetables, steamed dumplings, stir-fries with chicken, beef, scallops, shrimp, or tofu with vegetables, chow mein dishes, Moo goo gai pan, chicken or beef chop suey, and fortune cookies.

Go easy on fried rice, fried wontons, egg rolls, fried chow-mein noodles, spare ribs, sweet and sour dishes, crispy beef, Kung pao chicken, lemon chicken, General Tso's chicken, and Peking duck.

Italian. Fill up on minestrone soup, bread sticks or plain bread, pasta with lower-fat sauce (marinara, red clam, white clam), meat sauce rather than meatballs, chicken cacciatore or primavera, spinach or mushroom tortellini, thick-crust plain or vegetable pizza, salads with dressings on the side, and Italian ice or sorbert.

Go easy on antipasto plates, butter, margarine, or olive oil served with bread, creamy salad dressings, extra cheese and meat toppings on pizza, Alfredo or pesto sauce, Italian sausage, fried calamari, parmigian dishes, manicotti, and lasagna.

Indian. Fill up on dahl (bean soup), naam, roti (breads), basmati rice, shish kebab, and curries.

Go easy on fried appetizers, samosas, and dishes that load up on cheese or sauces, such as Palak or Saag Paneer. Ask how sauces are made because many restaurants add cream besides the ghee (clarified butter) and coconut milk (Malai) normally used.

Classic American Fare. Fill up on broth-based soups, plain bread, salad with dressing on the side, steamed vegetables, baked or mashed potatoes, rice, stir-fries, barbecue chicken, pot roast, turkey with stuffing, hamburger or gardenburger, filet mignon or sirloin steak, grilled, broiled, baked fish or chicken, fruit, sherbet or frozen yogurt, low-fat milk shakes.

Go easy on salads already dressed (for example, Caesar salad), buffalo wings, stuffed potato skins, French fries, onion rings, fried items (chicken, steak, and shrimp), extra gravy, tartar sauce, creamy and buttery sauces, sour cream or butter on baked potatoes, pot pies, cheesy items (for example, grilled cheese, cheese steak sandwich, patty melt) and New York strip, T-bone, and porterhouse steaks. Watch out for excessively generous serving sizes—split with a friend or request a doggy bag.

Selected Resources

Sport Nutrition Information

American Dietetic Association (ADA) Consumer Nutrition Hotline, 800-366-1655, **www.eatright.org**.

Ask the Dietitian, **www.dietitian.com**.

EndurePlus Online (sports nutrition and endurance training information), **www.endureplus.com**.

Gatorade Sports Science Institute, 800-616-4774, **www.gssiweb.com**.

International Food Information Council, **http://ificinfo.health.org**.

SCAN (Sports, Cardiovascular and Wellness Nutritionists—to locate a registered dietitian specializing in sports nutrition), 719-475-7751, **www.nutrifit.org**.

SportsMed Web (sports medicine site for endurance athletes), **www.riceinfo.rice.edu/~jenky/**.

Tufts University Nutrition Navigator, **www.navigator.tufts.edu**.

United States Olympic Training Center, 719-578-4500, **www.olympic-usa.org**.

Sport Nutrition Products

Athletica, 888-256-3787, **www.athletica.com**.

InterNutria Sports, 888-459-2376, **www.internutriasports.com**.

Longevity Plus (Spizerinctum), 800-548-4447, **www.bikescor.com**.

PeakPerformance Health, Inc., 888-609-7824, **www.peakhealth.net**.

Prolithic Sports, 800-969-6199, **www.prolithic.com**.

Ultrafit Products, (414) 495-3474, **www.ultrafit-endurance.com**.

Hydration Systems and Gear

Camelbak Hydration Systems, 800-767-8775, **www.camelbak.com**.

Campmor (selected outdoor gear), 800-230-2151, **www.campmor.com**.

Moletracks, 800-813-3217, **www.moletracks.com**.

Mountain Safety Research (beverage bags, water filters), 800-877-9677, **www.msrcorp.com**.

Nalgene Outdoor Products (flexible water bag, bottles, etc.), 800-872-4552, **www.nalgene-outdoor.com**.

Nashbar Bike Gear (hydration systems, insulated bottles, etc.), 800-627-4227, **www.bikenashbar.com**.

Outdoor Research (water-bottle cover), 888-467-4327, **www.orgear.com**.

Ultimate Direction, 800-426-7229, **www.ultdir.com**.

Dehydrated Food

Adventure Foods, (828) 497-4113, **www.adventurefoods.com**.

AlpineAire Foods, 800-322-6325, **www.alpineairefoods.com**.

Backpacker's Pantry, American Outdoor Products, 800-641-0500, ext.4 **www.backpackerspantry.com/**.

Mountain House, Oregon Freeze Dry, Inc., 800-547-0244, **www.ofd.com**.

MSR Cuisine (organic, vegetarian), 800-877-9677, **www.msrcorp.com**.

Outback Oven Foods, American Outdoor Products (800) 641-0500, ext.4, **www.backpackerspantry.com**.

Eating Disorders

American Anorexia/Bulimia Association, 212-575-6200, **www.aabainc.org**.

Anorexia Nervosa and Related Eating Disorders, **www.anred.com**.

Eating Disorders Awareness & Prevention, Inc., Eating Disorders Information and Referral Line, 800-931-2237, **www.edap.org**.

Something Fishy Website on Eating Disorders, **www.somethingfishy.org**.

Cookbooks, Dining Out, and Recipes

Dining Lean: How to Eat Healthy in Your Favorite Restaurants, Joanne Lichten, Nutrifit Publishing, 1988.

Eating on the Run, Evelyn Tribole, MS, RD, Leisure Press, 1992.

Eating Out Food Counter, Annette Natow, PhD, RD, and Jo-Ann Heslin, MA, RD, Pocket Books (Simon and Schuster), 1998.

Lickety-Split Meals for Health Conscious People on the Go!, Zonya Foco, RD, ZHI Publishing, 1998.

The New York City Marathon Cookbook, Nancy Clark, MS, RD, Rutledge Hill Press, 1994.

No Time to Cook, American Institute for Cancer Research, 800-843-8114 (free pamphlet).

Quick & Healthy Recipes and Ideas for People Who Say They Don't Have Time to Cook Healthy Meals, Volumes I & II, Brenda Ponichtera, RD, ScaleDown Publishing, 1991 (volume 1), 1995 (volume 2).

Stealth Health: How to Sneak Nutrition Painlessly into Your Diet, Evelyn Tribole, Viking Press, 1998.

Meals For You, **www.mealsforyou.com**.

Supplement Information

Health Care Reality Check, **www.hcrc.org**.

National Collegiate Athletic Association Banned Drug Classes, **www.ncaa.org/sports_sciences/drugtesting/banned_list.html**.

Quackwatch, **www.quackwatch.com**.

Supplement Watch, **www.supplementwatch.com**.

United States Olympic Committee, **www.olympic-usa.org,** select Search and type Nutrition, select Inside the USOC: Nutrition: Dietary Supplements.

United States Olympic Committee Drug Education Department (Drug Reference Hotline), 800-233-0393.

Vegetarianism

The Vegetarian Food Guide and Nutrition Counter, Suzanne Havala, MS, RD, The Berkeley Publishing Group, 1997.

Vegetarian Nutrition & Health Letter, 888-558-8703, **www.llu.edu/llu/vegetarian**.

Vegetarian Resource Group, 410-366-8343, **www.vrg.org**.

The Vegetarian Sports Nutrition Guide, Lisa Dorfman, MS, RD, John Wiley & Sons, 1999.

Women's Health

Before Your Pregnancy, **www.b4yourpregnancy.com**.

Melpomene Institute for Women's Health Research, 612-642-1951, **www.melpomene.org**.

Weight Management

Power Systems (skinfold calipers), 800-321-6975.

Tanita Body Fat Monitor/Scale (for home use), 800-Tanita-8, **www.tanita.com**.

Adventure Sports/Racing

Adventure Racing Association, **www.adventureracing.org**.

Adventure World Magazine, 408-997-3581.

Beyond Adventure Sports, **www.beyondadventure.com**.

Ecochallenge, **www.ecochallenge.com**.

Cycling

Bicycling, 800-666-2806, **www.bicyclingmagazine.com**.

Bike Site, **www.bikesite.com**.

Cyber Cycling, **www.cycling.org**.

Cycling Performance Tips, **www.halcyon.com/gasman**.

Race Across America, **www.raceacrossamerica.org**.

Ultra-Marathon Cycling Association, 303-545-9566, **www.ultracycling.com**.

USA Cycling, 719-578-4581, **www.usacycling.org**.

Mountain Biking

International Mountain Bicycling Association, 303-545-9011, **www.outdoorlink.com/IMBA**.

MOUNTAIN Bike, 800-666-1817, **www.mountainbike.com**.

Outdoor Recreation

Backpacker, 800-666-3434, **www.backpacker.com**.

Climbing, 800-829-5895, **www.climbing.com**.

Great Outdoor Recreation Pages, **www.gorp.com**.

Mountain Zone (skiing, mountain biking, hiking, climbing, expeditions, adventure racing), **www.mountainzone.com**.

Outdoor Life Network, **www.greatoutdoors.com**.

Outside, 800-678-1131, **www.outsidemag.com**.

Running

All American Trail Running Association, 719-570-9795, **www.trailrunner.com**.

American Running Association, 800-776-ARFA, **www.americanrunning.org**.

Marathon and Beyond, 217-359-9345, **www.marathonandbeyond.com**.

Marathon des Sables (Toughest Footrace on Earth), **www.sandmarathon.com**.

The Running Network, **www.runningnetwork.com**.

Running Research News, (517) 371-4897, **www.rrnews.com**.

Road Runners Club of America, 703-836-0558, **www.rrca.com**.

Running Times, 800-816-4735, **www.runningtimes.com**.

Runner's World, 800-666-2828, **www.runnersworld.com**.

Ultramarathon World, **http://fox.nstn.ca/~dblaikie**.

Ultrarunning, 888-858-7203, **www.ultrarunning.com**.

Skiing

American Alpine Club, 303-384-0110, **www.americanalpineclub.com**.

American Birkebeiner, 800-872-2753, **www.birkie.com**.

Cross Country Ski World, **www.xcskiworld.com**.

Nordic ski racing, **www.skiracing.com**.

U.S. Ski and Snowboard Association, 435-649-9090, **www.usskiteam.com**.

Swimming

Swim Sport, **www.swimsport.com**.

United States Swimming, 719-578-4578, **www.usswim.org**.

Triathlon

Insidetriathlon, 800-494-1413, **www.insidetri.com**.

Triathlete, 800-441-1666, **www.triathletemag.com**.

Triathlon & Duathlon News, **www.duathlon.com**.

USA Triathlon, 719-597-9090, **www.usatriathlon.org**.

Bibliography

Anderson, O. 1998. Athletes use Coca-Cola as sports drink, but does running really go better with Coke? *Running Research News* 14(6): 1–5.

_____. 1997. Making your marathons jell with gels—and other topics. *Running Research News* 13(8): 1, 7–9.

_____. 1998. Why your creatine consumption is costing you too much. *Running Research News* 14(7): 1–4.

Antonio, J., C. Street, D. Kalman and C. Colker. 1999. Dietary supplements used by athletes. *AMAA Quarterly* 13: 6-8.

Applegate, L. 1998. Supplement speak. *Runner's World*, Feb., 30–31.

_____. 1997. Vegetable matter. *Runner's World*, April, 26–27.

Aravjo, D. 1997. Expecting questions about exercise and pregnancy? *The Physician and Sportsmedicine* 25: 85-93

Armsey, T.D. and G.A. Green. 1997. Nutrition supplements: Science vs hype. *The Physician and Sportsmedicine* 25: 77–92.

Armstrong, L.E et al. 1996. Heat and cold illnesses during distance running. American College of Sports Medicine position stand. Medicine and Science in Sports and Exercise 28: i–x.

Askew, E.W. 1989. Nutrition for a cold environment. *The Physician and Sportsmedicine* 17: 77–89.

Barr, S.I. 1998. Muscle sprouts-vegetarian eating. *Bicycling*, March, 46-47.

Barr, S.I. 1998. Stamp out cramps. *Bicycling*, April, 46-47.

Beals, K.A. and M.M. Manore. 1994. The prevalence and consequences of subclinical eating disorders in female athletes. *International Journal of Sport Nutrition* 4: 175–195.

Benson J.E., K.A. Englebert-Fenton, and P.A. Eisenman. 1996. Nutritional aspects of amenorrhea in the female athlete triad. *International Journal of Sport Nutrition* 6: 134–145.

Berning, B. and S. Nelson Steen. 1998. Nutrition for sport & exercise. Gaithersburg, MD: Aspen Publishers, Inc.

Burke, E.R. and J.R. Berning. 1996. Training nutrition. Carmel, IN: Cooper Publishing Group.

Burke, L.M., G.R. Collier, and M. Hargreaves. 1998. Glycemic index—a new tool in sport nutrition? *International Journal of Sport Nutrition* 8: 401–415.

Bursztyn, P.G. 1990. Physiology for sportspeople. Manchester, England: Manchester University Press.

Calcium: the queen of nutrients. 1999. Women's Health Advisor 3: 1-3.

Clapp, J., F. 1998. Exercising through your pregnancy. Champaign, IL: Human Kinetics.

Clark, N. 1994. The New York City Marathon cookbook. Nashville, TN: Rutledge Hill Press.

Clark, N. 1995. Water—the ultimate nutrient. *The Physician and Sportsmedicine* 23: 32g-32h.

Clinical Sports Nutrition. 1994, ed. L. Burke and V. Deakin. Sydney, Australia: McGraw-Hill Book Company.

Coleman, E.J. 1996. The biozone nutrition system: A dietary panacea? *International Journal of Sports Nutrition* 6: 69–71.

Coyle, E.F. 1995. Fat metabolism during exercise. *Sports Science Exchange* 8: 1–6.

Davis, J.M. 1996. Carbohydrates, branched-chain amino acids and endurance: The central fatigue hypothesis. *Sports Science Exchange* 9: 1–5.

Dietary fat and physical activity: 1996. Fueling the controversy. *Sports Science Exchange* 7(3): 1–4.

Doubt, T.J. 1991. Physiology of exercise in the cold. *Sports Medicine* 11: 367–381.

Downes, S. 1998. Running on empty? *Running Times* Oct., 53–56.

Engelhardt, M., G. Neumann, A. Berbalk and I. Reuter. 1998. Creatine supplementation in endurance sports. *Medicine and Science in Sports and Exercise* 30: 1123-1129.

Farquhar, B. and W.L. Kennedy. 1997. Anti-inflammatory drugs, kidney function, and exercise. *Sports Science Exchange* 11(4): 1–6.

The female athlete triad. 1997. *Sports Science Exchange* 8(1): 1–4.

Food allergies, How worried should you be? 1999. Tufts University Health and Nutrition Letter, April 6.

Girard Eberle, S. 1997. The vegetarian runner. *Marathon & Beyond* Sept./Oct., 69–77.

Harris, S.S. 1995. Helping active women avoid anemia. *The Physician and Sportsmedicine* 23(5): 35–48.

Hawley, J.A. 1998. Fat burning during exercise—can ergogenics change the balance? *The Physician and Sportsmedicine* 26(9): 56–68.

Ivy, J.L. 1998. Glycogen resynthesis after exercise: Effect of carbohydrate intake. *International Journal of Sports Medicine* 19: S142–S145.

Jeukendrup, A.E., W.H. Saris, and J.M. Wagenmakers. 1998. Fat metabolism during exercise: A review (part I). *International Journal of Sports Medicine* 19: 231–244.

_____. 1998. Fat metabolism during exercise: a review (part II). *International Journal of Sports Medicine* 19: 293–302.

Kayser, B. 1994. Nutrition and energetics of exercise at altitude. *Sports Medicine* 17: 309–323.

Kleiner, S.M. 1995. The role of meat in an athlete's diet: Its effect on key macro- and micronutrients. *Sports Science Exchange* 8(58): 1–6.

Lemon, P.W. 1995. Do athletes need more dietary protein and amino acids? *International Journal of Sport Nutrition* 5: S39–S61.

Levey, J.M. 2000. Runner's diarrhea: an overview. *AMAA Quarterly* 14: 6-7.

Levine, M.P. and M.D. Maine. 1997. A guide to the primary prevention of eating disorders. Eating Disorders Awareness & Prevention pamphlet.

Lindeman, A.K. 1994. Self-esteem: Its application to eating disorders and athletes. *International Journal of Sport Nutrition* 4: 237–252.

Loosli, A.R. and J.S. Rudd. 1998. Meatless diets in female athletes: A red flag. *The Physician and Sportsmedicine* 26: 45–48.

Maughan, R.J, J.B. Leiper, and S.M. Shirreffs. 1996. Rehydration and recovery after exercise. *Sports Science Exchange* 9(3): 1–6.

Maughan, R.J. 1997. Preparing athletes for competition in the heat: Developing an effective acclimatization strategy. *Sports Science Exchange* 10(2): 1–4.

Messina, V. and M. Messina. 1996. The vegetarian way. New York: Three Rivers Press.

Miller, D. 1998. The backcountry cupboard. *Backpacker* May, 30–37.

Murphy, T.J. 1999. You are what you drink. *Triathlete* 181: 36-45.

Murray, R. 1995. Fluid needs in hot and cold environments. *International Journal of Sport Nutrition* 5: S62–S73.

Nelson Steen, S. 1998. Eating on the road: Where are the carbohydrates? *Sports Science Exchange* 11 (4): 1-5.

Nielsen, P. and D. Nachtigall. 1998. Iron supplementation in athletes. *Sports Medicine* 26(4): 207–216.

Nieman, D.C. 1998. Immunity in athletes: current issues. Sports Science Exchange 11(2): 1–6.

Otis, C.L., B. Drinkwater, M. Johnson, A. Loucks, and J. Wilmore. 1997. American College of Sports Medicine position stand: The female athlete triad. *Medicine and Science in Sports and Exercise* 29(5): i–v.

O'Toole, L. and P.S. Douglas. 1995. Applied physiology of triathlon. *Sports Medicine* 19(4): 251–267.

Pfitzinger, P. 1999. Don't just hydrate . . . "hyperhydrate" in the heat with glycerol. *Running Times* June, 16.

Pfitzinger, P. 1999. Fat facts. *Running Times* September, 19.

Putukian, M. and C. Potera. 1997. Don't miss gastrointestinal disorders in athletes. *The Physician and Sportsmedicine* 25: 80-94.

Questioning 40/30/30—a guide to understanding nutrition advice. 1997. American Dietetic Association pamphlet.

Rosenbloom, C. 1996. The dietary supplement health and education act (DSHEA): what you should know. SCAN's PULSE 15(4): 7–8.

SCAN (Sports, Cardiovascular and Wellness Nutritionists) Professional Development Workshop on Disordered Eating. 1998. Dieting: The on ramp to the eating disorder highway. The American Dietetic Association.

SCAN (Sports and Cardiovascular Nutritionists). 1993. Sports nutrition—a guide for the professional working with active people, ed. D. Benardot. American Dietetics Association.

Screening for iron overload proposed for more people. 1999. Tufts University Health and Nutrition Letter, February 3.

Seiler, S. 1992. Partial zone defense. *Running Times* 12–141996.

Shephard, R.J. 1993. Metabolic adaptations to exercise in the cold. *Sports Medicine* 16(4) 266–289.

Sherman, W.M., and N. Leenders. 1995. Fat loading: The next magic bullet? *International Journal of Sports Nutrition* 5: S1–S12.

Singh A., P.A. Pelletier, and P.A. Deuster. 1994. Dietary requirements for ultra-endurance exercise. *Sports Medicine* 18(5): 301–308.

Sports foods for athletes: What works? *Sports Science Exchange* 9(2): 1–6.

Spriet, L.L. 1995. Caffeine and performance. *International Journal of Sport Nutrition* 5: S84–S99.

Stamford, B. 1993. Muscle cramps: Untying the knots. *The Physician and Sportsmedicine* 21(7): 115–116.

Sykora, C., C.M. Grilo, D.E. Wilfley, and K.D. Brownell. 1993. Eating, weight, and dieting disturbances in male and female lightweight and heavyweight rowers. *International Journal of Eating Disorders* 14: 203-211.

Tribole, E. 1992. Eating on the Run. Champaign, IL: Leisure Press.

Tribole, E. and E. Resch. 1995. Intuitive eating—a recovery book for the chronic dieter. New York: St. Martin's Press.

Wagner, D.R. 1999. Hyperhydrating with glycerol: Implications for athletic performance. *Journal of the American Dietetic Association* 99(2): 207–212.

Walberg Rankin, J. 1997. Glycemic index and exercise metabolism. *Sports Science Exchange* 10: 1-7.

Williams, M. 1998. Creatine supplementation and exercise performance. *Journal of the American College of Nutrition* 17: 216–234.

Williams, M.H. 1999. Pumping dietary iron. *ACSM's Health and Fitness Journal* 3: 15-22.

_____. 1998. The ergogenics edge. Champaign, IL: Human Kinetics.

Wilmore, J.H. and D.L. Costill. 1994. Physiology of sport and exercise. Champaign, IL: Human Kinetics.

Winter sports. 1998. *Sports Science Exchange* 9(4): 1–6.

Index

About the Author

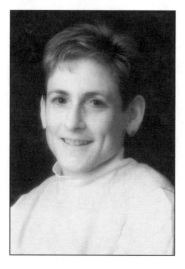

Suzanne Girard Eberle, MS, RD, is a registered dietician who practices what she teaches. As a multisport athlete, Girard Eberle has 25 years of competitive endeavors under her belt. She is a former All-America runner for Georgetown University and a national 5K track champion who has competed around the world in running competitions. Today, she runs over 50 miles per week and enjoys hiking, climbing, cycling, cross-country skiing, and participating in adventure races. She has climbed Mount Blanc, the highest mountain in the Alps, and Mount Kilimanjaro, the highest mountain in Africa.

As a sports nutrition expert, Girard Eberle regularly counsels athletes of all levels, beginners to world-class, on how to improve their performance by paying more attention to their nutrition habits. A contributing editor for *Running Times,* her nutrition articles have also appeared in *Women's Sports & Fitness, SELF, Footnotes,* and *Marathon & Beyond.* She created and teaches a sport nutrition class at Portland State University, as well as the Smart CHOICES weight management program for a local hospital.

Girard Eberle holds a master's degree in clinical nutrition from Boston University. She is a member of the American College of Sports Medicine, the American Dietetic Association, and its Sports, Cardiovascular and Wellness Nutritionists Practice Group. She lives in Portland, Oregon, with her husband John and retired racing greyhound Flip.